Genitourinary Imaging
A Core Review

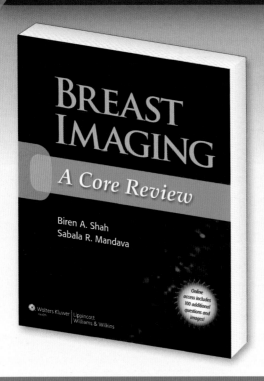
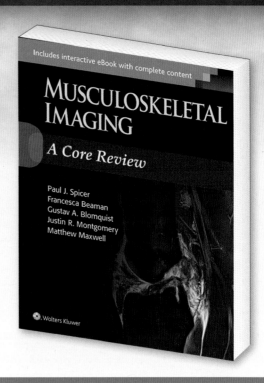
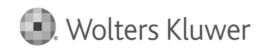

Genitourinary Imaging
A Core Review

Matthew S. Davenport, MD

Assistant Professor
Division of Abdominal Imaging
Department of Radiology
University of Michigan Health System
Ann Arbor, Michigan

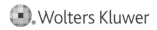. Wolters Kluwer

Philadelphia · Baltimore · New York · London
Buenos Aires · Hong Kong · Sydney · Tokyo

Acquisitions Editor: Ryan Shaw
Product Development Editor: Amy Dinkel
Production Project Manager: Priscilla Crater
Design Coordinator: Stephen Druding
Manufacturing Coordinator: Beth Welsh
Prepress Vendor: SPi Global

9 8 7 6 5 4 3 2 1

Printed in China

Library of Congress Cataloging-in-Publication Data
Davenport, Matthew S., author.
Genitourinary imaging : a core review / Matthew S. Davenport.
p. ; cm. — (Core review series)
Includes bibliographical references and index.
ISBN 978-1-4511-9407-4
I. Title. II. Series: Core review series.
[DNLM: 1. Female Urogenital Diseases—diagnosis—Examination Questions. 2. Male Urogenital Diseases—diagnosis—Examination Questions. 3. Diagnostic Imaging—Examination Questions. 4. Urogenital Neoplasms—diagnosis—Examination Questions. WJ 18.2]
RC874
616.6'0754076—dc23
2014024091

Care has been taken to confirm the accuracy of the information presented and to describe generally accepted practices. However, the author, editors, and publisher are not responsible for errors or omissions or for any consequences from application of the information in this book and make no warranty, expressed or implied, with respect to the currency, completeness, or accuracy of the contents of the publication. Application of this information in a particular situation remains the professional responsibility of the practitioner; the clinical treatments described and recommended may not be considered absolute and universal recommendations.

The author, editors, and publisher have exerted every effort to ensure that drug selection and dosage set forth in this text are in accordance with the current recommendations and practice at the time of publication. However, in view of ongoing research, changes in government regulations, and the constant flow of information relating to drug therapy and drug reactions, the reader is urged to check the package insert for each drug for any change in indications and dosage and for added warnings and precautions. This is particularly important when the recommended agent is a new or infrequently employed drug.

Some drugs and medical devices presented in this publication have Food and Drug Administration (FDA) clearance for limited use in restricted research settings. It is the responsibility of the health care provider to ascertain the FDA status of each drug or device planned for use in his or her clinical practice.

LWW.com

RRS1410

To the residents: May your questions have answers, and your answers, more questions.

SERIES FOREWORD

Genitourinary Radiology: A Core Review is the third book in the *Core Review Series*. This book covers the most important aspects of genitourinary radiology in a manner that I believe will serve as a guide for residents to be able to assess their knowledge and review the material in a format that is similar to the ABR core examination.

Dr. Davenport has succeeded in producing a book that exemplifies the philosophy and goals of the *Core Review Series*. He has done a meticulous job in covering key topics and providing quality images. The questions have been divided logically into chapters so as to make it easy for learners to work on particular topics as needed. There are mostly multiple choice questions with some extended matching questions. Each question has a corresponding answer with an explanation of not only why a particular option is correct but also why the other options are incorrect. There are also references provided for each question for those who want to delve more deeply into a specific subject. This format is also useful for radiologists preparing for Maintenance of Certification (MOC).

The intent of the *Core Review Series* is to provide the resident, fellow, or practicing physician a review of the important conceptual, factual, and practical aspects of a subject by providing approximately 300 multiple choice questions, in a format similar to the ABR core examination. The *Core Review Series* is not intended to be exhaustive but to provide material likely to be tested on the ABR core exam and that would be required in clinical practice.

As series editor of the *Core Review Series*, I have had the pleasure to work with many outstanding individuals across the country who contributed to the series. This series represents countless hours of work and involvement by many, and it would not have come together without their participation.

Dr. Matthew Davenport is to be commended for an outstanding job. I believe *Genitourinary Radiology: A Core Review* will serve as a valuable resource for residents during their board preparation and a valuable reference for fellows and practicing radiologists.

Biren A. Shah, MD, FACR
Series Editor

PREFACE

This book was crafted to serve as a valuable multidisciplinary tool for learners studying for the ABR core examination and for practicing radiologists preparing for Maintenance of Certification. It covers many aspects of genitourinary radiology, including image acquisition physics, contrast media administration, iatrogenic adverse events, image-based diagnosis, percutaneous biopsy and drainage catheter techniques, disease management, research study design, and medical ethics. Though it is not possible to cover the breadth of radiology in a single 300-question book, I have tried to hit the highlights and have provided references for each question to propel further independent study. Where possible, I have included and cited modern established guidelines for safe and effective practice.

Much thanks to Christi and Quinn, Patricia Quinn Davenport, Jim Ellis, Tom Chenevert, Elaine Caoili, Jonathan Rubin, Rich Cohan, Hero Hussain, Ellen Higgins, Anna Fox, Anastasia Hryhorczuk, Jonathan Dillman, Bill Masch, Sarah Abate, Bill Weadock, Joel Platt, N. Reed Dunnick, Jeff Nadig, Biren Shah, Ronald Buckwalter, and the Wolters Kluwer staff.

I would like to make specific mention of Jim Ellis, who tried his utmost to cleanse the errors from the entire text. What you don't see are his successes; what you do see are my failures. If only Jim were on hire for the other typos in my life.

Matthew S. Davenport, MD

CONTENTS

1 Contrast Media

1 A 60-year-old female presents with anaphylactic shock following an intravenous dose of nonionic low-osmolality iodinated contrast material. Which of the following is the correct dose of the pictured medication?

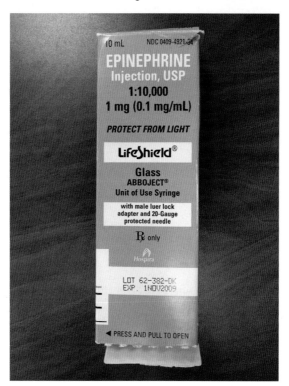

A. 0.1 mg intravenously
B. 1.0 mg intravenously
C. 0.1 mg intramuscularly
D. 1.0 mg intramuscularly
E. The pictured drug is contraindicated for the treatment of anaphylactic shock.

2   What is the principal effect of gadolinium-based contrast media on T1?

   A. Directly shortens T1
   B. Indirectly shortens T1
   C. Indirectly lengthens T1
   D. Directly lengthens T1

3   A 42-year-old female complains of increasing injection site pain 2 hours following the attempted administration of 125 mL of nonionic low-osmolality iodinated contrast material through a peripheral intravenous catheter in the antecubital fossa. The injection was halted after 100 mL was injected. Which factor most strongly indicates that a surgical consultation may be necessary?

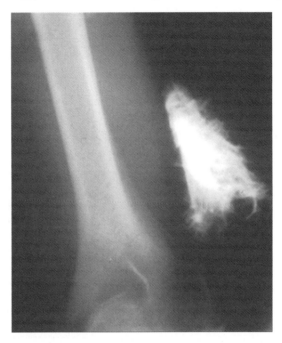

   A. The patient's symptoms (increasing pain)
   B. The patient's age (42 years)
   C. The attempted injection volume (125 mL)
   D. The actual injection volume (100 mL)
   E. The injection site (antecubital fossa)

4   A 68-year-old male with prostate cancer and an estimated glomerular filtration rate (eGFR) of 31 mL/min/1.73 m^2 presents for magnetic resonance imaging (MRI) of the pelvis. The patient is concerned about nephrogenic systemic fibrosis (NSF). Among the following contrast media, which has been associated with the least number of unconfounded cases of NSF?

   A. Gadodiamide (Omniscan)
   B. Gadopentetate dimeglumine (Magnevist)
   C. Gadoversetamide (OptiMARK)
   D. Gadoteridol (ProHance)

5   What is the most important factor used to discriminate vasovagal reaction from anaphylactic shock?

   A. Blood pressure
   B. Blood oxygen saturation
   C. Heart rate
   D. Body temperature

6 A 55-year-old male with hypertension complains of light-headedness and nausea 1 minute following the intravenous administration of 120 mL of nonionic low-osmolality iodinated contrast material. While the patient's vital signs (shown below) are being measured, he loses consciousness. Despite laying the patient supine, raising his legs, and administering an intravenous fluid bolus, he remains unconscious with a palpable pulse at an unchanged rate. What is the best next step?

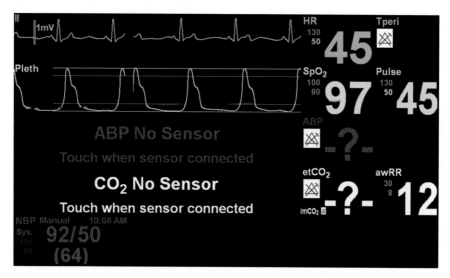

A. Administer epinephrine 0.1 mg intravenously.

D. Administer diphenhydramine 50 mg intravenously.

C. Administer atropine 0.6 mg intravenously.

D. Administer methylprednisolone 125 mg intravenously.

7 A 62-year-old male with severe hypertension, peripheral vascular disease, and stage IIIb chronic kidney disease (eGFR is 35 mL/min/1.73 m^2) presents for a CT angiogram of the renal arteries. What is the most effective way to improve or maintain vascular attenuation while simultaneously reducing the iodinated contrast material dose?

A. Decrease mA

B. Decrease kVp

C. Increase mA

D. Increase kVp

8 A 66-year-old male with type 2 diabetes mellitus, coronary artery disease, hypertension, arrhythmia, and an estimated glomerular filtration rate of 40 mL/min/1.73 m^2 presents for a triple-phase contrast-enhanced CT of the abdomen for abnormal liver function tests. He is taking the following medications: glipizide 5 mg PO daily; metoprolol 50 mg PO twice daily; metformin 500 mg PO daily; and amiodarone 400 mg PO daily. Which of the following is the best next step?

A. Proceed with the test. No special precautions are needed.

B. Reschedule the test, and tell the patient to hold his metformin 24 hours prior.

C. Proceed with the test, and tell the patient to hold his metformin afterward.

D. Reschedule the test and discuss holding the amiodarone with the patient's cardiologist.

E. Proceed with the test, and tell the patient to hold his amiodarone afterward.

9 A 51-year-old female imaged with contrast-enhanced CT for evaluation of right lower quadrant pain develops an estimated 125 mL extravasation into her right forearm. What is the approximate likelihood that she will develop a compartment syndrome?

   A. <2%
   B. 5%
   C. 20%
   D. 50%

10 What is the primary mechanism of parenterally administered ultrasmall superparamagnetic iron oxide particle (USPIO) nodal imaging with MRI?

   A. Shortens T1
   B. Chemical shift artifact
   C. Lengthens T2
   D. Susceptibility artifact

11 Which imaging finding is most suggestive of malignancy within a 5-mm short-axis perirectal lymph node before and after intravenous ultrasmall superparamagnetic iron oxide particle (USPIO) administration on T2*-weighted imaging?

   A. Diffuse signal void after USPIO administration
   B. Homogeneously hyperintense to muscle after USPIO administration
   C. Homogeneously hyperintense to muscle before USPIO administration
   D. Heterogeneously hypointense to muscle before USPIO administration

12 Human plasma osmolality is approximately 285 to 295 mOsm/kg. What is the approximate osmolality of most low-osmolality iodinated contrast media?

   A. 300 mOsm/kg
   B. 600 mOsm/kg
   C. 900 mOsm/kg
   D. 1,200 mOsm/kg

13 In contrast to most low-osmolality iodinated contrast media, what is the approximate osmolality of most high-osmolality iodinated contrast media?

   A. 300 mOsm/kg
   B. 600 mOsm/kg
   C. 900 mOsm/kg
   D. 1,200 mOsm/kg

14 Which of the following contrast media is considered to be iso-osmolar?

   A. Iodixanol 652 mg/mL (Visipaque 320)
   B. Iohexol 647 mg/mL (Omnipaque 300)
   C. Iopamidol 61% (Isovue 300)
   D. Ioversol 64% (Optiray 300)

15 A 38-year-old female with stage III cervical cancer and a prior allergic-like reaction to iodinated contrast material (reaction: bronchospasm) presents for a contrast-enhanced CT of the chest, abdomen, and pelvis. She has not been premedicated with corticosteroids. What is the shortest length of time of oral corticosteroid premedication that has been shown to be efficacious in the prevention of a future contrast reaction?

   A. 2 hours
   B. 4 hours
   C. 12 hours
   D. 20 hours

16 A 24-year-old female in her third trimester of pregnancy presents to an urgent care clinic with right lower quadrant pain. Pelvic ultrasound is negative, and an abdominal/pelvic MRI is not possible. A contrast-enhanced CT of the abdomen and pelvis is performed without oral contrast material following the intravenous administration of 100 mL of nonionic low-osmolality iodinated contrast material. What is the predicted effect of this contrast material bolus on neonatal thyroid function?

A. 90% chance of neonatal hypothyroidism
B. 50% chance of neonatal hypothyroidism
C. 20% chance of neonatal hypothyroidism
D. 5% chance of neonatal hypothyroidism
E. <1% chance of neonatal hypothyroidism

17 Some patients with chronic kidney disease are at risk of developing nephrogenic systemic fibrosis following the intravascular administration of gadolinium-based contrast media. What estimated glomerular filtration rate range is cited by the U.S. Food and Drug Administration as contraindicated for the highest-risk agents?

A. <60 mL/min/1.73 m^2
B. <45 mL/min/1.73 m^2
C. <30 mL/min/1.73 m^2
D. <15 mL/min/1.73 m^2

18 A 51-year-old female was imaged with contrast-enhanced CT for evaluation of right lower quadrant pain. One hundred and twenty-five milliliters of nonionic low-osmolality iodinated contrast material was administered intravenously. An incidental abnormality was detected in the right kidney. What is the best next step?

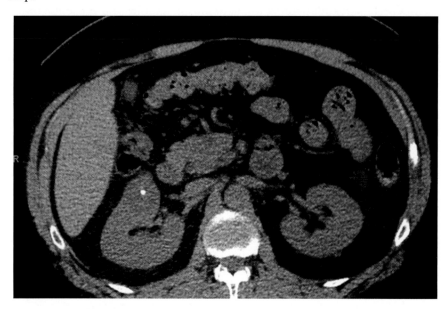

A. Perform a physical examination.
B. Recommend MRI.
C. Recommend 6-month follow-up.
D. Recommend urology consultation.

19 A 32-year-old lactating female with normal renal function who is 4 weeks postpartum presents with pleuritic chest pain. A contrast-enhanced CT pulmonary angiogram is performed with 100 mL of nonionic low-osmolality iodinated contrast material. The patient would like to know what to do regarding breast-feeding her infant after the test. What is the most appropriate advice?

A. The risk to the infant is small but has been confirmed in small series. The mother should be advised to pump and discard her milk for 3 days.

B. The risk to the infant is small but has been confirmed in small series. The mother should be advised to pump and discard her milk for 1 day.

C. The risk to the infant is likely negligible or nonexistent, but the mother may choose to pump and discard her milk for 3 days if she chooses.

D. The risk to the infant is likely negligible or nonexistent, but the mother may choose to pump and discard her milk for 1 day if she chooses.

20 A 22-year-old male was involved in a serious motor vehicle collision. A contrast-enhanced portal venous phase CT of the abdomen and pelvis performed 6 hours ago at an outside hospital confirmed hepatic, splenic, and renal lacerations. The clinical service would like to evaluate for ureteric injury and asks if another contrast material bolus is required. What is the approximate half-life of most intravenously administered nonionic low-osmolality iodinated contrast media in patients with normal renal function?

A. 30 minutes

B. 2 hours

C. 4 hours

D. 8 hours

21 An 82-year-old female with hypertension, peripheral vascular disease, a 2 pack-per-day smoking habit, and bilateral calf claudication presents for a CT angiogram with runoff to the lower extremities. Preprocedural estimated glomerular filtration rate is 28 mL/min/1.73 m². Six months ago, it was 27 mL/min/1.73 m². Which of the following measures has most consistently been shown to mitigate the risk of contrast-induced nephrotoxicity?

A. 600 mg *N*-acetylcysteine PO every 12 hours twice before and twice after the scan

B. 1,000 mL 0.45% NaCl IV bolus once before and once after the scan

C. 1,200 mg *N*-acetylcysteine PO every 12 hours twice before and twice after the scan

D. 1,000 mL 0.9% NaCl IV bolus once before and once after the scan

22 A 66-year-old male with a left subclavian pacemaker is being evaluated for possible spinal cord compression. A STAT myelogram CT is requested. Due to the urgency of the request, the myelogram will be performed in the gastrointestinal radiology suite. What is the most important thing to ensure with respect to the administered contrast material before proceeding with the test?

A. Only nonionic iodinated contrast media should be used.

B. Only iodinated contrast media with an osmolality of approximately 300 mOsm/kg should be used.

C. Only iodinated contrast media warmed to human body temperature should be used.

D. Only iodinated contrast media with meglumine salts should be used.

23 A 33-year-old female with a recent diagnosis of Graves disease and normal renal function presents for an I-131 therapy session 1 week after a contrast-enhanced CT of the chest was performed. Eighty milliliters of nonionic low-osmolality iodinated contrast material was administered. For how long should the practitioner wait before administering the I-131 treatment dose to be certain that the nonradioactive iodine from the contrast material bolus has first cleared from the patient's thyroid gland?

A. No additional waiting is necessary (total waiting time: 1 week).
B. One additional week (total waiting time: 2 weeks)
C. Three additional weeks (total waiting time: 4 weeks)
D. Seven additional weeks (total waiting time: 8 weeks)

24 A 50-year-old male with multiple food and drug allergies and a history of hypertension exhibits diffuse erythema and altered mental status following the intra-arterial administration of approximately 50 mL of iso-osmolality iodinated contrast material. Vital signs were obtained (shown below) while the patient was receiving supplemental oxygen (4 L by nasal cannula) and following a 1 L 0.9% NaCl intravenous fluid bolus. 1:1,000 epinephrine is available. What is the ideal site for injection?

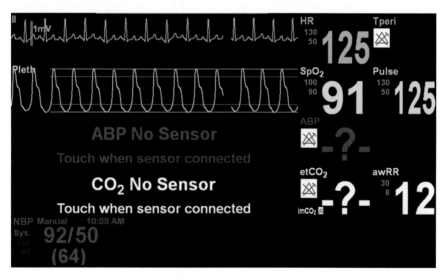

A. Myocardium
B. Peripheral vein
C. Subcutaneous tissue
D. Quadriceps
E. Epinephrine is not indicated.

25 A 60-year-old male with left lower quadrant pain and two prior allergic-like reactions to nonionic low-osmolality iodinated contrast material (both prior reactions: hives) presents for a contrast-enhanced CT of the abdomen and pelvis. He has received a standard oral corticosteroid regimen and states that all doses were taken as scheduled. The patient reports that following his last contrast-enhanced CT, he experienced hives despite receiving the same regimen. What is the likelihood that this patient will experience a severe contrast reaction following this contrast-enhanced study?

A. <1%
B. 10%
C. 25%
D. 50%
E. 100%

26 A 39-year-old female with Raynaud syndrome and systemic lupus erythematosus presents with 2 months of progressive digital claudication in her right hand. Digital subtraction angiography with provocative testing is planned. Which of the following contrast media would be predicted to cause the least amount of discomfort during this procedure?

A. Iopamidol 61% (Isovue 300)
B. Ioversol 64% (Optiray 300)
C. Iodixanol 652 mg/mL (Visipaque 320)
D. Iohexol 647 mg/mL (Omnipaque 300)

27 What contrast material is depicted by the following chemical structure?

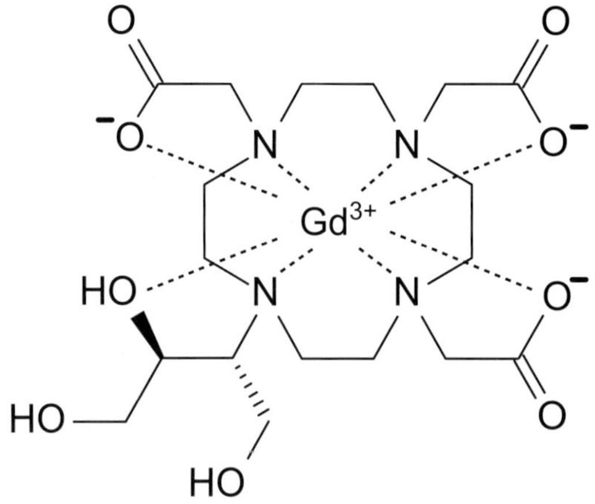

A. Gadofosveset trisodium (Ablavar)
B. Gadopentetate dimeglumine (Magnevist)
C. Gadoversetamide (OptiMARK)
D. Gadobenate dimeglumine (MultiHance)
E. Gadobutrol (Gadavist)

28 A 30-year-old male with multiple endocrine neoplasia (MEN) type 2b and early-onset hypertension presents for an adrenal protocol CT of the abdomen. The patient had a prophylactic thyroidectomy many years ago and has no allergies or other medical conditions. Based on this information, what is the risk of administering 125 mL of nonionic low-osmolality iodinated contrast material to this patient?

A. No increased risk above the general population
B. Higher likelihood of severe allergic-like reaction
C. Higher likelihood of hypertensive crisis
D. Higher likelihood of thyroid storm

29 A 28-year-old female with seasonal allergies and asthma complains of throat tightness and hoarseness following the intravenous administration of 125 mL of iodinated contrast material. She is producing an audible high-pitched noise during inspiration. Which of the following is the optimal dose of 1:1,000 epinephrine?

A. 0.1 mg
B. 0.3 mg
C. 0.7 mg
D. 1.0 mg
E. Epinephrine is not indicated.

30   A 75-year-old male with peripheral vascular disease and hypertension presents with acute anemia and hematochezia. His estimated glomerular filtration rate is 25 mL/min/1.73 m². A tagged red blood cell scan was conducted (shown below). If angiography is performed, which of the following contrast media contributes the least nephrotoxic risk?

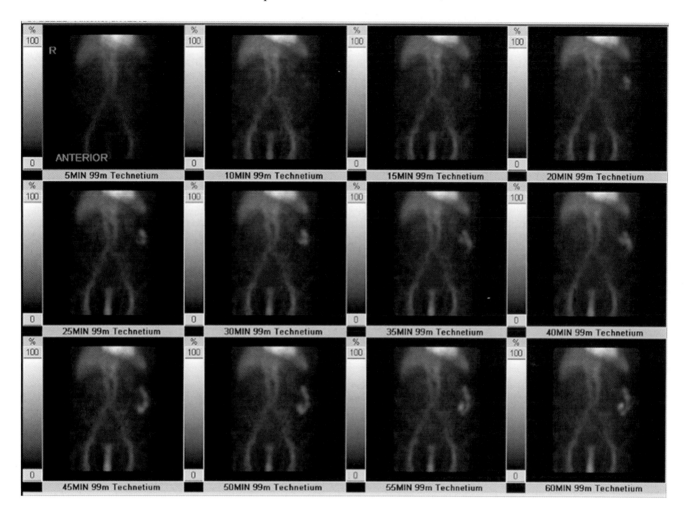

A. Iopamidol 61.2% (Isovue 300)
B. Iodixanol 652 mg/mL (Visipaque 320)
C. Gadopentetate dimeglumine (Magnevist)
D. Carbon dioxide
E. Iothalamate meglumine 60% (Conray 280)

ANSWERS AND EXPLANATIONS

1   Answer A.   The pictured medication is 1:10,000 epinephrine. This concentration is used for intravenous administration. It is 10-fold less concentrated than doses used for intramuscular administration (1:1,000). The recommended dose of IV epinephrine (1:10,000) is 0.1 mg, which equals 1 mL of a 1:10,000 solution. A 1.0-mg dose (10 mL) is the dose used for the treatment of cardiopulmonary arrest (e.g., pulseless electrical activity) and should not be used for the treatment of anaphylaxis. Overdose of intravenous epinephrine has been associated with cardiovascular toxicity, including myocardial infarction and stroke.

Reference: American College of Radiology Committee on Drugs and Contrast Media. *Manual on contrast media*, 9th ed. Reston, VA: American College of Radiology, 2013.

2   Answer B.   Gadolinium ions have seven unpaired electrons. Fields produced by these unpaired electrons oscillate near the Larmor frequency, generating tiny magnetic moments. These tiny magnetic fields interact with hydrogen protons of water and fat to promote electron–nuclear–dipole interactions. This process speeds up spin transfers, promotes relaxation from high-energy states to low-energy states, and indirectly shortens T1. Shortening T1 increases T1-weighted signal intensity. Lengthening T1 decreases T1-weighted signal intensity. The signal intensity generated from gadolinium-based contrast media is indirect— one does not observe the contrast material itself, but rather the effect it is having on the local proton environment.

Reference: McRobbie DW, Moore EA, Graves MJ, et al. *MRI: From proton to picture.* Cambridge, UK: Cambridge University Press, 2007.

3   Answer A.   This scenario describes a contrast material extravasation event. Most extravasations are minor with no lasting effects, but rarely an extravasation can result in compartment syndrome. This serious complication causes tissue necrosis from increased compartment pressures. The patient's symptoms are the best indicator of whether a surgical consultation is necessary. Minor and/or improving symptoms are typically benign, while severe, unrelenting, and/or progressive symptoms should be taken seriously. Predictors of greater risk for an extravasation event occurring include elderly patients, patients who are unable to effectively communicate, pediatric patients, injections through metal intravenous catheters, intravenous catheters with an extended indwelling time, large-volume injections (>50 mL), patients with difficult intravenous access, and injections into small veins (e.g., dorsum of the hand). Predictors of greater risk for moderate or severe postextravasation injury include progressive swelling or pain, altered tissue perfusion or sensation in the affected extremity, and skin ulceration and blistering.

References: American College of Radiology Committee on Drugs and Contrast Media. *Manual on contrast media*, 9th ed. Reston, VA: American College of Radiology, 2013.
Wang CL, Cohan RH, Ellis JH, et al. Frequency, management, and outcome of extravasation of nonionic iodinated contrast material in 69,657 intravenous injections. *Radiology* 2007;243:80–87.

4   Answer D.   Nephrogenic systemic fibrosis (NSF) is a rare, life-threatening disease that develops in patients with acute kidney injury and severe chronic kidney disease (particularly stage IV and stage V chronic kidney disease) who receive gadolinium-based contrast material. It is believed to result from the disassociation of gadolinium ions from their chelates, with subsequent deposition of free gadolinium into tissue leading to fibroblastic proliferation. Patients with NSF develop painful joint contractures, a "woody" appearance of the skin, end-organ damage and, in some cases, death. Three gadolinium-based contrast media have been associated with the greatest number of unconfounded cases ("unconfounded" refers to development of NSF following exposure to only one agent). These include gadodiamide (Omniscan), gadopentetate dimeglumine (Magnevist), and gadoversetamide (OptiMARK). Gadoteridol (ProHance) is a macrocyclic gadolinium-based contrast agent. Macrocyclic agents likely have a lower risk of NSF because their chemical structure permits a stronger bond between the gadolinium ion and its chelate, preventing disassociation and resultant tissue deposition.

References: American College of Radiology Committee on Drugs and Contrast Media. *Manual on contrast media*, 9th ed. Reston, VA: American College of Radiology, 2013.

U.S. Food and Drug Administration. *FDA drug safety communication: New warnings for using gadolinium-based contrast agents in patients with kidney dysfunction.* December 2010 update. Accessed September 2013.

5 **Answer C.**   Anaphylactic shock and vasovagal reactions can present with hypotension. In both, the oxygen saturation and body temperature may initially be relatively normal. The key factor discriminating the two is the patient's heart rate. Anaphylactic shock is accompanied by tachycardia (>100 bpm), which is a physiologic response to peripheral vasodilation, while vasovagal reactions are accompanied by bradycardia (<60 bpm), which is due to parasympathetic output by the vagus nerve.

Reference: American College of Radiology Committee on Drugs and Contrast Media. *Manual on contrast media*, 9th ed. Reston, VA: American College of Radiology, 2013.

6 **Answer C.**   The scenario (bradycardia [45 bpm] and hypotension [92/50]) describes a vasovagal reaction, which typically presents as bradycardia, hypotension, mental status changes and, occasionally, loss of consciousness. The presence of bradycardia (<60 bpm) distinguishes a vasovagal reaction from anaphylactic shock. Anaphylactic shock usually presents with tachycardia (>100 bpm). The management of a vasovagal reaction that is unresponsive to conservative measures (i.e., laying the patient supine, raising the patient's legs, administering isotonic intravenous fluids) is 0.6 to 1.0 mg intravenous atropine.

Diphenhydramine (Answer B) and methylprednisolone (Answer D) are medications used in the treatment of an allergic-like reaction. Epinephrine (Answer A) is the treatment of choice for anaphylactic shock and other severe allergic-like reactions. Vasovagal reactions are physiologic reactions (non–allergic-like) and therefore should not be treated like an allergic-like reaction.

Reference: American College of Radiology Committee on Drugs and Contrast Media. *Manual on contrast media*, 9th ed. Reston, VA: American College of Radiology, 2013.

7 **Answer B.**   kVp indicates the peak energy contained within the polychromatic x-ray beam. Lowering kVp will have the desired effect of increasing the attenuation of iodine by moving the average energy of the beam closer to the k-edge of iodine (33.2 keV). This effectively increases the attenuating effect of iodine while increasing image noise and is best suited to high-contrast examinations such as CT angiography that are less negatively affected by the cost of increased noise. Increasing kVp will have the opposite effect, increasing the aggregate energy of the x-ray beam farther away from the k-edge of iodine and decreasing the attenuating effects of iodinated contrast material. mA reflects the current applied to the x-ray tube and affects the number of x-rays released by the tube. Changing mA does not change attenuation.

References: Heyer CM, Mohr PS, Lemburg SP, et al. Image quality and radiation exposure at pulmonary CT angiography with 100- or 120-kVp protocol: prospective randomized study. *Radiology* 2007;245:577–583.

Yeh BM, Shepherd JA, Wang ZJ, et al. Dual energy and low kVp CT in the abdomen. *AJR Am J Roentgenol* 2009;193:47–54.

8 **Answer C.** Patients taking metformin-containing products are at rare risk of life-threatening lactic acidosis if they develop acute kidney injury. Because of the possible risk of contrast-induced nephrotoxicity in patients with moderate to severe chronic renal impairment, patients receiving metformin-containing drugs should stop taking their metformin-containing medication at the time of the contrast-enhanced study and not restart it until at least 48 hours later. If there is no evidence of acute kidney injury after 48 hours, the drug can be restarted.

Both amiodarone and iodinated contrast media contain iodine, but there is no significant interaction between these agents. It is important to remember that allergic-like reactions to iodinated contrast media are not due to the presence of iodine. Iodine is a physiologic element in humans. Iodine-containing products such as amiodarone and topical iodine have no cross-reactivity with iodinated contrast material.

References: American College of Radiology Committee on Drugs and Contrast Media. *Manual on contrast media*, 9th ed. Reston, VA: American College of Radiology, 2013.
Lakshmanadoss U, Lindsley J, Glick D, et al. Incidence of amiodarone hypersensitivity in patients with a previous allergy to iodine or iodinated contrast agents. *Pharmacotherapy* 2012;32:618–622.

9 **Answer A.** It is extremely uncommon for an extravasation event to result in compartment syndrome, even when the extravasated volume is large (e.g., >100 mL). The literature suggests that this rate is <2%. In a large series of 475 extravasation events (Wang, 2007), compartment syndrome resulted from 0 of 61 extravasation events associated with an extravasation volume of 100 to 150 mL and 1 of 54 extravasation events associated with an extravasation volume of 50 to 99 mL. The rate is likely even lower for smaller-volume extravasation events <50 mL (0 of 321 in the same series).

References: American College of Radiology Committee on Drugs and Contrast Media. *Manual on contrast media*, 9th ed. Reston, VA: American College of Radiology, 2013.
Wang CL, Cohan RH, Ellis JH, et al. Frequency, management, and outcome of extravasation of nonionic iodinated contrast material in 69,657 intravenous injections. *Radiology* 2007;243:80–87.

10 **Answer D.** Ultrasmall superparamagnetic iron oxide particles (USPIO) are scavenged by circulating macrophages and deposited in normal lymphatic tissue where the iron distorts the local magnetic environment and generates metallic susceptibility effects. This creates "negative contrast" in which normal lymph nodes (which contain macrophages) are devoid of signal, and neoplastic lymph nodes (which lack macrophages) remain visible. Neoplastic lymph nodes are replaced entirely or in part by tumor cells, preventing the circulating macrophages from delivering the iron ions into the affected portion(s) of the lymph nodes.

T1 shortening (Answer A) is the primary mechanism of signal creation for gadolinium-containing contrast media on T1-weighted imaging. Although USPIO shorten T1, it is not the primary mechanism: T2 shortening and T2* effects dominate.

T2 prolongation (Answer C) creates increased signal intensity on T2-weighted images (e.g., water has a long T2) and is not a feature of USPIO; iron ions decrease T2.

Chemical shift artifact (Answer B) is an unrelated type of artifact that occurs because of the differential resonance frequency of fat and water protons (~3.5 ppm or ~220 Hz at 1.5 Tesla). It manifests in two ways. Chemical shift artifact of the first kind causes displacement of fat protons in the frequency-encoding direction, creating a dark band where signal is lost and a bright band where signal is added. Chemical shift artifact of the second kind causes signal loss in voxels containing both fat and water protons when the spins of the fat and water protons are 180 degrees out of phase.

References: Lahaye MJ, Engelen SME, Kessels AGH, et al. USPIO-enhanced MR imaging for nodal staging in patients with primary rectal cancer: predictive criteria. *Radiology* 2008;246:804–811.

Leyendecker JR, Brown JJ, Merkle EM. *Practical guide to abdominal MRI*, 2nd ed. Philadelphia PA: Lippincott Williams & Wilkins, 2010.

11 **Answer B.** Abnormal lymph nodes on ultrasmall superparamagnetic iron oxide particle (USPIO)-enhanced T2*-weighted MRI will exhibit absent uptake of iron particles, resulting in preserved T2-weighted signal intensity (hyperintense to muscle). Lymph nodes infiltrated entirely by neoplasm do not contain normal macrophages and therefore will not contain scavenged iron. Normal lymph nodes have iron-scavenging macrophages and will appear as homogeneously hypointense signal voids.

Morphologic criteria on unenhanced T2-weighted images (e.g., irregular margins, heterogeneous signal intensity) have a weaker positive predictive value than does the USPIO enhancement pattern. Remember that USPIO enhancement is "negative enhancement." USPIO uptake causes loss of signal intensity (signal void) and is a predictor of benignancy. Lack of USPIO uptake permits the lymph node to retain its usual signal intensity and is a predictor of malignancy. This is opposite from the pattern seen with traditional gadolinium-containing contrast media and directly relates to the mechanism causing "enhancement" in each case.

References: Bellin MF, Roy C, Kinkel K, et al. Lymph node metastases: safety and effectiveness of MR imaging with ultrasmall superparamagnetic iron oxide particles—initial clinical experience. *Radiology* 1998;207:799–808.

Koh DM, George C, Temple L, et al. Diagnostic accuracy of nodal enhancement pattern of rectal cancer at MRI enhanced with ultrasmall superparamagnetic iron oxide: findings in pathologically matched mesorectal lymph nodes. *AJR Am J Roentgenol* 2010;194: W505–W513.

12 **Answer B.** The following table demonstrates the approximate osmolality of iodinated contrast media relative to human plasma when the iodinated media has around 300 mgI/mL.

Substance	Approximate Osmolality
Human plasma	285–295 mOsm/kg
Iso-osmolality iodinated contrast media	~300 mOsm/kg
Low-osmolality iodinated contrast media	~600 mOsm/kg
High-osmolality iodinated contrast media	~1,200 mOsm/kg

Human plasma has an osmolality of approximately 290 mOsm/kg. Therefore, so-called "low-osmolality" iodinated contrast media actually have approximately double the osmolality of human plasma. They are termed "low osmolality" for historical reasons. Older contrast media ("high-osmolality" iodinated contrast media) have an osmolality that is roughly quadruple that of human plasma (~1,200 vs. ~290 mOsm/kg).

Reference: American College of Radiology Committee on Drugs and Contrast Media. *Manual on contrast media*, 9th ed. Reston, VA: American College of Radiology, 2013.

13 **Answer D.** The following table demonstrates the approximate osmolality of iodinated contrast media relative to human plasma when the iodinated media has around 300 mgI/mL.

Substance	Approximate Osmolality
Human plasma	285–295 mOsm/kg
Iso-osmolality iodinated contrast media	~300 mOsm/kg
Low-osmolality iodinated contrast media	~600 mOsm/kg
High-osmolality iodinated contrast media	~1,200 mOsm/kg

High-osmolality iodinated contrast media have substantially more side effects than low- and iso-osmolality iodinated contrast media when administered intravascularly. Therefore, high-osmolality iodinated contrast media are no longer used for routine intravascular administration; they are now instead most often used for intracavitary studies like cystograms and enemas. Osmolality and ionicity are related but not interchangeable concepts. Ionic contrast media often disassociate in solution, effectively doubling the number of particles and therefore increasing the osmolality (osmolality is an expression of the number of particles of solute per kilogram of water). Although high-osmolality iodinated contrast media are commonly ionic, and low- and iso-osmolality iodinated contrast media are commonly nonionic, this is not a fixed rule (e.g., ioxaglate meglumine sodium [Hexabrix] is ionic but has a "low" osmolality of ~600 mOsm/kg).

Reference: American College of Radiology Committee on Drugs and Contrast Media. *Manual on contrast media*, 9th ed. Reston, VA: American College of Radiology, 2013.

14 **Answer A.** The following table demonstrates the relative osmolality of the contrast media from the question. The weight–volume ratio listed after each generic name (i.e., mg/mL, or expressed as a percentage) indicates the weight of contrast material molecules in each milliliter of solution. The number listed after each trade name indicates the milligrams of iodine per milliliter of solution.

Substance	Osmolality (mOsm/kg)	Class
Iodixanol 652 mg/mL (Visipaque 320)	290	Iso-osmolality
Iohexol 647 mg/mL (Omnipaque 300)	672	Low osmolality
Iopamidol 61% (Isovue 300)	616	Low osmolality
Ioversol 64% (Optiray 300)	651	Low osmolality

Of the listed iodinated contrast media, only iodixanol (Visipaque) is "iso-osmolality." It is not important for you to remember the individual osmolality of each of the various contrast media, but you should be generally familiar with which contrast media belong to which class. Low-osmolality iodinated contrast media have been repeatedly shown to cause fewer side effects than high-osmolality iodinated contrast media, but iso-osmolality contrast media (e.g., iodixanol) do not have the same clear relationship with respect to low-osmolality contrast media. Although originally thought to cause a lesser incidence of contrast-induced nephrotoxicity, subsequent publications have cast that in doubt, and routine use of iodixanol for the prevention of contrast material–related complications other than discomfort from peripheral angiography is of questionable benefit.

Reference: American College of Radiology Committee on Drugs and Contrast Media. *Manual on contrast media*, 9th ed. Reston, VA: American College of Radiology, 2013.

15 **Answer C.** The shortest oral corticosteroid premedication regimen shown to be efficacious in the prevention of contrast reactions to iodinated contrast media is 12 hours. There are two widely used protocols, referred to as the "Lasser prep" (12-hour regimen using two doses of 32-mg oral methylprednisolone 12 and 2 hours prior to contrast material administration) and the "Greenberger prep" (13-hour regimen using three doses of 50-mg oral prednisone 13, 7, and 1 hours prior to contrast material administration combined with 50-mg oral diphenhydramine 1 hour prior to contrast material administration). The "Lasser prep" has the strongest evidence to support it, but both regimens see widespread clinical use. Shorter oral dosing 2 hours prior to contrast material administration has been shown to be not effective. Oral regimens between 2 and 12 hours prior to contrast material administration have not been rigorously tested.

References: Greenberger PA, Patterson R, Radin RC. Two pretreatment regimens for high-risk patients receiving radiographic contrast media. *J Allergy Clin Immunol* 1984;74:540–543.
Lasser EC, Berry CC, Mishkin MM, et al. Pretreatment with corticosteroids to prevent adverse reactions to nonionic contrast media. *AJR Am J Roentgenol* 1994;162:523–526.
Lasser EC, Berry CC, Talner LB, et al. Pretreatment with corticosteroids to alleviate reactions to intravenous contrast material. *N Engl J Med* 1987;317:845–849.
O'Malley RB, Cohan RH, Ellis JH, et al. A survey on the use of premedication prior to iodinated and gadolinium-based contrast material administration. *J Am Coll Radiol* 2011;345–354.

16 **Answer E.** There has been an historic concern that maternal exposure to intravascular iodinated contrast material will result in neonatal hypothyroidism. Iodinated contrast media cross the placenta and enter the fetal circulation, exposing the fetus to high doses of iodine. However, studies on low-osmolality iodinated contrast media find the risk of neonatal hypothyroidism to be negligible (<1% incidence). For example, in one study of 344 maternal exposures to a single dose of low-osmolality iodinated contrast material (Bourjeily, 2010), only a single neonate experienced transient thyroid-stimulating hormone (TSH) elevation, and that contrast material administration was confounded by other drug exposures.

References: Atwell TD, Lteif AN, Brown DL, et al. Neonatal thyroid function after administration of IV iodinated contrast agent to 21 pregnant patients. *AJR Am J Roentgenol* 2008;191:268–271.
Bourjeily G, Chalhoub M, Phornphutkul C, et al. Neonatal thyroid function: effect of a single exposure to iodinated contrast medium in utero. *Radiology* 2010;256:744–750.
Rajaram S, Exley CE, Fairlie F, et al. Effect of antenatal iodinated contrast agent on neonatal thyroid function. *Br J Radiol* 2012;85:e238–242.

17 **Answer C.** The U.S. Food and Drug Administration (FDA) has contraindicated gadodiamide (Omniscan), gadopentetate dimeglumine (Magnevist), and gadoversetamide (OptiMARK) for patients with acute kidney injury and/or an estimated glomerular filtration rate (eGFR) <30 mL/min/1.73 m^2 due to the risk of nephrogenic systemic fibrosis. These three "highest-risk" agents were specifically singled-out by the FDA because they are associated with the greatest number of unconfounded cases of NSF (unconfounded means that NSF developed after exposure to only a single agent). However, many gadolinium-containing contrast media other than these three have been associated with unconfounded cases of NSF; the incidence is simply much less. Therefore, the FDA recommends caution prior to the administration of all gadolinium-containing contrast media in patients with acute kidney injury and/or an eGFR <30 mL/min/1.73 m².

References: American College of Radiology Committee on Drugs and Contrast Media. *Manual on contrast media*, 9th ed. Reston, VA: American College of Radiology, 2013.

U.S. Food and Drug Administration. *FDA drug safety communication: New warnings for using gadolinium-based contrast agents in patients with kidney dysfunction.* December 2010 update. Accessed September 2013.

18 Answer A. The CT image shows no enhancement despite the administration of intravenous contrast material. This indicates one of several possibilities: (1) contrast material extravasation (as in this case), (2) intravenous catheter malfunction (no or minimal contrast material traversed the catheter), (3) scan timing error (unlikely given that there is no visible contrast material), (4) protocol error (contrast material ordered but not given), or (5) incorrect patient (the images are from a different patient who used a different protocol).

When contrast material is given but is not evident on the scan, an extravasation should be suspected and the patient should be examined for evidence of this. Symptoms of an extravasation include injection site redness, swelling, and pain.

Because there are no contrast-enhanced images, the right renal mass cannot be characterized on this study, making 6-month follow-up (Answer C) and urology consultation (Answer D) not the best choices. MRI could be considered (Answer B), although it would likely be easier to place a new intravenous catheter in the contralateral extremity and repeat the current scan. However, in any case, the possible acute extravasation event takes priority over characterizing the renal mass.

Reference: American College of Radiology Committee on Drugs and Contrast Media. *Manual on contrast media*, 9th ed. Reston, VA: American College of Radiology, 2013.

19 Answer D. Due to its low lipid solubility, <1% of administered low-osmolality iodinated contrast material is excreted into breast milk, and <1% of that would be subsequently absorbed by the infant's gastrointestinal tract. Therefore, the systemic dose to the infant is <1/10,000ths the maternal dose. The American College of Radiology's *Manual on Contrast Media* (9th ed.) states that the risk to the infant is likely extremely small and no special precautions are required. However, if the mother wishes to avoid any secondary exposure to her infant, she can choose to pump and discard her milk for 24 hours. The half-life of most low-osmolality iodinated contrast media is close to 2 hours in individuals with normal renal function, which means that the concentration within the mother will be nonexistent after approximately 20 hours (10 half-lives). Therefore, if the mother pumps and discards her milk for 1 day, that should be a sufficient length of time to avoid any secondary exposure.

References: American College of Radiology Committee on Drugs and Contrast Media. *Manual on contrast media*, 9th ed. Reston, VA: American College of Radiology, 2013.

Webb JAW, Thomsen HS, Morcos S, et al. The use of iodinated and gadolinium contrast media during pregnancy and lactation. *Eur Radiol* 2005;15:1234–1240.

20 Answer B. The half-life of most low-osmolality iodinated contrast media is approximately 2 hours in individuals with normal renal function. Therefore, if the patient is re-presenting for excretory-phase imaging only 6 hours after the original contrast material bolus, a second dose is probably not needed (i.e., the patient could be reimaged without a second bolus and achieve the same effect). If the patient is re-presenting for excretory-phase imaging 20 hours after the original contrast material bolus (10 half-lives), the entire dose will have been already excreted, and a second dose will be needed. In patients with acute kidney injury and/or chronic kidney disease, the half-life can be substantially prolonged. Low-osmolality iodinated contrast media are excreted primarily by the kidneys.

Reference: American College of Radiology Committee on Drugs and Contrast Media. *Manual on contrast media*, 9th ed. Reston, VA: American College of Radiology, 2013.

21 Answer D.   The only adjunctive measure consistently shown to reduce the incidence of contrast-induced nephrotoxicity (CIN) is intravenous volume expansion. Volume expansion with isotonic intravenous fluids (e.g., 0.9% NaCl ["normal saline"]) has been shown superior to volume expansion with hypotonic intravenous fluids (e.g., 0.45% NaCl ["half-normal saline"]). Other measures, including but not limited to the use of iso-osmolality contrast media (e.g., iodixanol [Visipaque]) instead of low-osmolality contrast media, pre- and/or postprocedure *N*-acetylcysteine administration, and volume expansion with sodium bicarbonate, have had conflicting results and are not generally advocated.

References: American College of Radiology Committee on Drugs and Contrast Media. *Manual on contrast media*, 9th ed. Reston, VA: American College of Radiology, 2013.
Weisbord SD, Palevsky PM. Prevention of contrast-induced nephropathy with volume expansion. *Clin J Am Soc Nephrol* 2008;3:273–280.

22 Answer A.   It is critically important that only nonionic low-osmolality iodinated contrast media be used for intrathecal administration. Ionic iodinated contrast media can cause seizures and death if administered into the thecal space. Only a small subset of low-osmolality iodinated contrast media is approved for intrathecal use. These agents are specifically labeled for this indication and include iohexol (Omnipaque 180, Omnipaque 240, Omnipaque 300) and iopamidol (Isovue-M 200, Isovue-M 300). Ionic contrast media are often used for gastrointestinal (e.g., enemas) and genitourinary (e.g., cystograms) radiology studies. Therefore, it is generally good practice not to perform intrathecal and intracavitary studies in the same room to avoid an accidental misadministration.

The agents approved for intrathecal use have an approximate osmolality of 400 to 700 mOsm/kg. Contrast media for intrathecal use are often stored at room temperature, not human body temperature (Answer C). Contrast media containing meglumine salts are by definition ionic and should not be used for intrathecal opacification (Answer D).

References: American College of Radiology Committee on Drugs and Contrast Media. *Manual on contrast media*, 9th ed. Reston, VA: American College of Radiology, 2013.
McClennan BL. Contrast media alert. *Radiology* 1993;189:35.

23 Answer C.   The Society of Nuclear Medicine recommends a withdrawal period of 3 to 4 weeks (if normal renal function) following intravenous iodinated contrast material exposure prior to the administration of therapeutic I-131. If this withdrawal period is ignored, the thyroid gland will be saturated with nonradioactive iodine from the contrast material bolus that will compete with I-131, resulting in an undesired subtherapeutic dose to the gland. It is important to note that the 3- to 4-week waiting period is not directly related to the circulating half-life of contrast material, which for most commonly used iodinated contrast media is approximately 2 hours. This is because iodine trapped by the thyroid gland first must undergo organification before it can again enter the systemic circulation.

Reference: Society of Nuclear Medicine treatment guideline for therapy of thyroid disease with Iodine-131 (sodium iodide), version 2.0. 1-8. Accessed April 2014. http://interactive.snm.org/docs/Therapy%20of%20Thyroid%20Disease%20with%20Iodine-131%20v2.0.pdf

24   **Answer D.**   The scenario describes the life-threatening condition of anaphylactic shock (hypotension, tachycardia). The treatment is epinephrine. 1:1,000 epinephrine is the concentration used for intramuscular and subcutaneous dosing, with subcutaneous doses discouraged for hypotensive patients due to poorer absorption and slower drug delivery. The optimal site for the intramuscular administration of 1:1,000 epinephrine is in the anterolateral thigh (quadriceps), which has been shown to have superior drug delivery compared to the shoulder (deltoid). 1:1,000 epinephrine should not be administered intravascularly because it can cause severe cardiovascular toxicity (e.g., myocardial infarction, stroke).

References: American College of Radiology Committee on Drugs and Contrast Media. *Manual on contrast media*, 9th ed. Reston, VA: American College of Radiology, 2013.
Chowdhury BA, Meyer RJ. Intramuscular versus subcutaneous injection. *J Allergy Clin Immunol* 2001;108:871–873.
Simons FER, Roberts JR, Gu X, et al. Epinephrine absorption in children with a history of anaphylaxis. *J Allergy Clin Immunol* 1998;101:33–37.

25   **Answer A.**   The risk of this patient developing a severe breakthrough contrast reaction (i.e., a severe allergic-like reaction that develops in spite of corticosteroid premedication) is <1%. In patients who have had a prior breakthrough reaction of any severity, the majority (88% [174/197]) will not experience a repeat breakthrough reaction on a future contrast-enhanced study using similar contrast media. When a breakthrough reaction does occur, breakthrough reactions are usually similar in severity or less severe than the original contrast reaction (92% [118/128]). In patients with a mild index reaction, severe breakthrough reactions are rare (0% [0/103]).

Reference: Davenport MS, Cohan RH, Caoili EM, et al. Repeat contrast medium reactions in premedicated patients: frequency and severity. *Radiology* 2009;253:372–379.

26   **Answer C.**   Iodixanol, an iso-osmolality contrast material, has been shown to cause less discomfort and lesser sensations of warmth during peripheral angiography compared to low-osmolality iodinated contrast media. For this reason, it is often preferred for catheter-directed angiograms targeting small arteries. Iodixanol is a dimer, and its characteristic chemical composition is shown below.

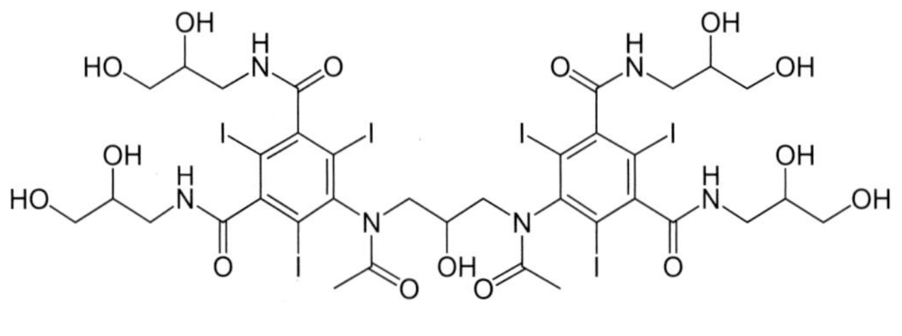

References: McCullough PA, Capasso P. Patient discomfort associated with the use of intra-arterial iodinated contrast media: a meta-analysis of comparative randomized controlled trials. *BMC Med Imaging* 2011;11:12.
Pugh ND, Sissons GR, Ruttley MS, et al. Iodixanol in femoral arteriography (phase III): a comparative double-blind parallel trial between iodixanol and iopromide. *Clin Radiol* 1993;47:96–99.
Rosenblum JD, Siegel EL, Leef J, et al. Iodixanol and ioxaglate in adult aortography and peripheral angiography: a phase III clinical trial. *Acad Radiol* 1996;3:S514–S518.

27 Answer E. The depicted molecule has a macrocyclic structure. Specifically, the gadolinium ion is surrounded by a "cage" of molecular bonds. Gadolinium ions in macrocyclic contrast media have much stronger bonds with their chelates compared to many linear gadolinium-based contrast media.

Gadolinium stability is of primary interest in the prevention of nephrogenic systemic fibrosis (NSF), which is believed to result from disassociation of gadolinium from its chelate and subsequent deposition of free gadolinium in tissue. Among the contrast media listed as possible answers, only gadobutrol is a macrocyclic contrast agent. Other macrocyclic contrast media include gadoteridol (ProHance) and gadoterate meglumine (Dotarem).

Although it is not important to know the specific chemical structure of each of the contrast media, it is important to know their general molecular classification because it has relevance for clinical practice. The other two primary classifications of gadolinium-based contrast media include linear nonionic (e.g., gadoversetamide [OptiMARK] and gadodiamide [Omniscan], both of which are considered "high risk" for NSF and both of which have the least chemical stability of the available gadolinium-based contrast media) and linear ionic (e.g., essentially all remaining gadolinium-based agents other than those already listed).

References: Morcos SK. Nephrogenic systemic fibrosis following the administration of extracellular gadolinium based contrast agents: is the stability of the contrast agent molecule an important factor in the pathogenesis of this condition? *Br J Radiol* 2007;80:73–76.
Rofsky NM, Sherry AD, Lenkinski RE. Nephrogenic systemic fibrosis: a chemical perspective. *Radiology* 2008;247:608–612.

28 Answer A. Patients with MEN 2B syndrome are at risk for medullary thyroid cancer and pheochromocytoma. Prophylactic thyroidectomy is often performed to prevent the development of medullary thyroid cancer. In a patient with MEN 2B syndrome and early-onset hypertension, pheochromocytoma should be strongly suspected. There has been historic concern that administration of iodinated contrast media to a patient with pheochromocytoma might induce a hypertensive crisis if the patient is not provided preprocedural alpha-adrenergic blockade. However, data have shown that the risk of this occurring in patients administered intravascular nonionic low-osmolality iodinated contrast material is negligible, and no special precautions are needed in this patient population.

References: Baid SK, Lai EW, Wesley RA, et al. Brief communication: radiographic contrast infusion and catecholamine release in patients with pheochromocytoma. *Ann Intern Med* 2009;150:27–32.
Bessell-Browne R, O'Malley ME. CT of pheochromocytoma and paraganglioma: risk of adverse events with i.v. administration of nonionic contrast material. *AJR Am J Roentgenol* 2007;188:970–974.
Mukherjee JJ, Peppercorn PD, Reznek RH, et al. Pheochromocytoma: effect of nonionic contrast medium in CT on circulating catecholamine levels. *Radiology* 1997;202:227–231.

29 Answer B. The scenario describes the life-threatening condition of laryngeal edema. Stridor, which is an audible high-pitched noise during inspiration, is an indicator of upper airway constriction (i.e., laryngeal swelling). This is distinguished from wheezing, which is an audible high-pitched noise during end expiration, and is an indicator of lower airway constriction (i.e., bronchospasm). The treatment for laryngeal edema is epinephrine, and the dose is 0.3 mg (0.3 mL of 1:1,000 epinephrine). If the epinephrine is given intravenously, the dose would be 0.1 mg (1 mL of 1:10,000 epinephrine).

The first-line pharmaceutical for the treatment of wheezing (lower airway constriction) is an inhaled β_2-adrenergic agonist (e.g., albuterol). If bronchospasm progresses and is unresponsive to inhaled β_2-adrenergic agonist therapy, epinephrine should be administered.

Reference: American College of Radiology Committee on Drugs and Contrast Media. *Manual on contrast media*, 9th ed. Reston, VA: American College of Radiology, 2013.

30 **Answer D.**   Carbon dioxide is a low-viscosity gas that can be used as a negative contrast agent for angiographic procedures. It carries no significant nephrotoxic risk and is an option for patients with acute kidney injury or severe chronic kidney disease. However, because it is a gas, it has different properties than liquid-based contrast media. For example, the low viscosity of carbon dioxide may increase the sensitivity for active extravasation, but its tendency to travel along nondependent surfaces can limit assessment of the dependent vascular lumen. Additionally, if the carbon dioxide reservoir is contaminated with air, arterial injections can cause gas emboli resulting in downstream ischemia. Similarly, excessive venous-side injection of carbon dioxide, even without contamination, can displace the blood within the right heart, prevent pulmonary artery outflow, and cause cardiac arrest. It is not a feasible contrast agent for CT or MRI.

References: Hawkins IF, Cho KJ, Caridi JG. Carbon dioxide in angiography to reduce the risk of contrast-induced nephropathy. *Radiol Clin North Am* 2009;47:813–825.
Nadolski GJ, Stavropoulos SW. Contrast alternatives for iodinated contrast allergy and renal dysfunction: options and limitations. *J Vasc Surg* 2013;57:593–598.

2 Kidneys (Native and Transplant)

1 A 63-year-old male with oliguria and systemic inflammatory response syndrome presents for a CT of the abdomen and pelvis. What is the most likely explanation for the imaging findings?

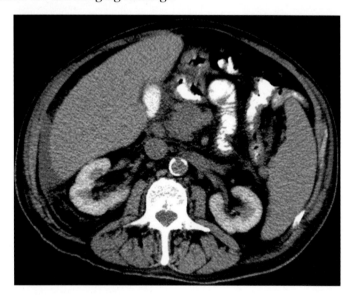

   A. Contrast-induced nephrotoxicity
   B. Acute tubular necrosis
   C. Pyelonephritis
   D. Recent exposure to gadolinium-based contrast material

2 A 61-year-old female with an incidentally discovered renal mass undergoes an abdominal MRI. Which finding on T1-weighted dual-echo gradient-recalled echo (GRE) imaging at 1.5 Tesla is most indicative of a benign histology?

   A. Homogeneous signal loss at a TE of 2.2 msec
   B. Homogeneous signal loss at a TE of 4.4 msec
   C. India ink artifact at the interface between the mass and the perinephric fat
   D. India ink artifact at the interface between the mass and the kidney

3   A 52-year-old male with autosomal dominant polycystic kidney disease presents with 12 hours of anuria and abdominal pain postoperative day 1 status post renal transplantation. Which of the following is the most likely explanation for the spectral waveform?

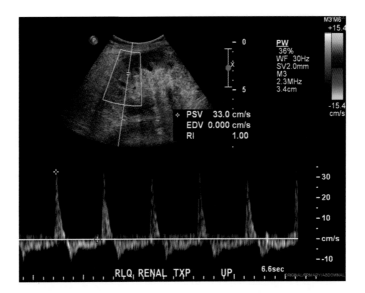

A. Renal artery stenosis
B. Renal arteriovenous fistula
C. Renal vein thrombosis
D. Normal superimposed waveforms

4   A 50-year-old male with hematuria and a renal transplant presents for Doppler imaging. What is the most likely explanation for the finding in the lower pole?

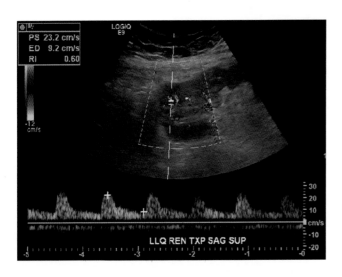 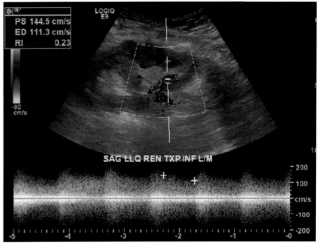

A. Polyarteritis nodosa
B. Iatrogenic injury
C. Congenital malformation
D. Renal artery thrombosis
E. Acute tubular necrosis

5 A 49-year-old male with an incidentally discovered renal mass undergoes a multiphasic renal mass protocol CT. This demonstrates a solitary exophytic 5.5-cm hypervascular heterogeneous solid right renal mass that lacks macroscopic fat and has a central scar. Which of the following is most correct?

A. The mass is a renal cell carcinoma.
B. The mass is an oncocytoma.
C. The mass is an angiomyolipoma.
D. The mass is a lymphoma.
E. The mass is a urothelial carcinoma.
F. The mass is indeterminate.

6 A 34-year-old female with numerous small solid echogenic renal masses undergoes a set of screening examinations. Which of the following studies is most likely to have been obtained in this patient?

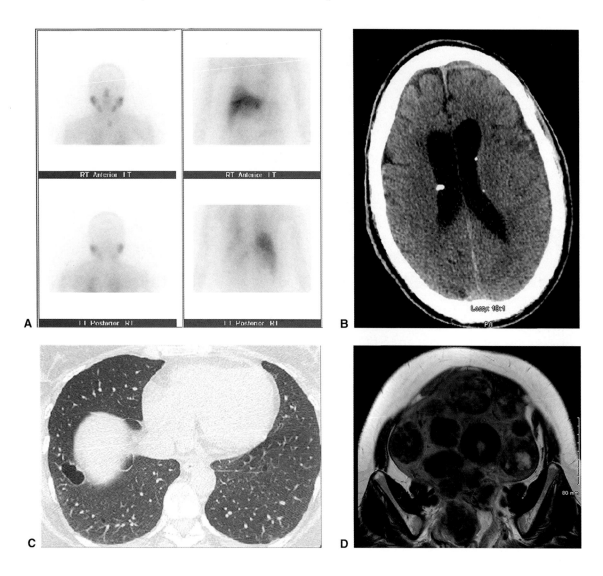

A.
B.
C.
D.

7 A 42-year-old male with diabetes mellitus type I complicated by end-stage renal disease undergoes a renal transplant. A percutaneous renal biopsy is performed 6 months later due to an elevated serum creatinine, and a subsequent renal ultrasound demonstrates an intrarenal arteriovenous fistula. What spectral Doppler waveform is characteristic of this entity?

A. High velocity, high resistance
B. High velocity, low resistance
C. Low velocity, high resistance
D. Low velocity, low resistance

8 A 67-year-old male with a solid right renal mass undergoes percutaneous biopsy confirming clear cell renal cell carcinoma. Which artifact best explains the finding within the mass on T1-weighted dual-echo gradient-recalled echo (GRE) imaging at 1.5 Tesla?

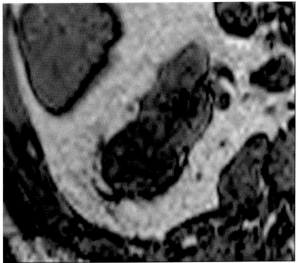 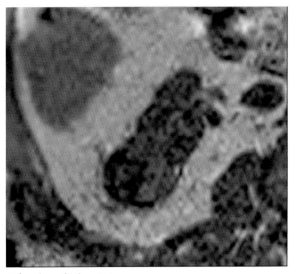

Echo time (TE) = 2.2 msec   *Echo time (TE) = 4.4 msec*

A. Chemical shift artifact of the first kind
B. Chemical shift artifact of the second kind
C. Chemical shift artifact of the third kind
D. Chemical shift artifact of the fourth kind

9 A 60 year-old male with malaise and weight loss presents for contrast-enhanced CT, which demonstrates multiple bilateral non–contour-deforming low-attenuation renal masses (30 to 50 Hounsfield units). They are confirmed to be solid on MRI. Which of the following is the most likely diagnosis?

A. Tuberous sclerosis
B. Birt-Hogg-Dubé syndrome
C. Renal cell carcinoma
D. Urothelial carcinoma
E. Renal sarcoma
F. Lymphoma
G. von Hippel-Lindau syndrome

10 A 37-year-old female is found to have an incidental cystic renal mass. The highest attenuation component measures 180 Hounsfield units on postcontrast imaging (below) and 30 Hounsfield units on unenhanced imaging (not shown). What is the most appropriate Bosniak classification?

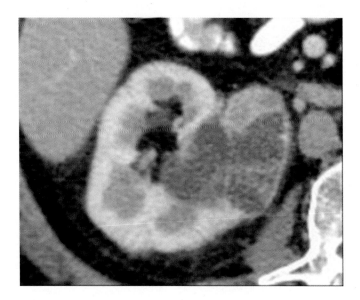

A. Bosniak I
B. Bosniak II
C. Bosniak IIF
D. Bosniak III
E. Bosniak IV

11 A 30-year-old female with chronic urolithiasis and multiple prior CT studies (one of which, performed 3 years ago, is shown below) presents with flank pain and hematuria. A renal stone CT is ordered. What is the best way to ensure that the radiation dose be as low as reasonably achievable (ALARA)?

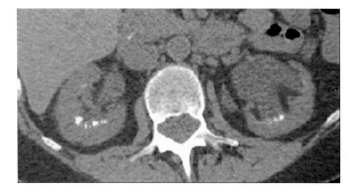

A. Reduce the beam energy from 120 kVp to 80 kVp.
B. Reduce the tube current from 400 mA to 200 mA.
C. Enable tube current modulation.
D. Increase the pitch from 1.0 to 1.25.
E. Perform a renal ultrasound instead of a CT.
F. Enable adaptive statistical iterative reconstruction.
G. Apply breast and thyroid shielding.

12 A 59-year-old female with hypertension treated with two oral medications has the following incidental finding. What is the best next step?

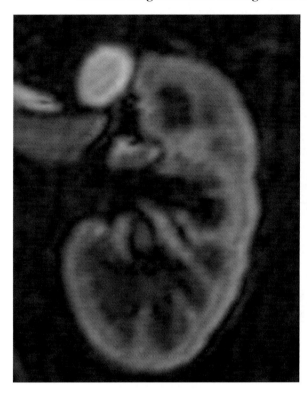 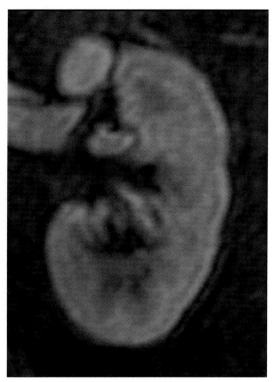

    A. Partial nephrectomy
    B. Percutaneous biopsy
    C. Further imaging
    D. Ignore. The finding is a normal variant.

13 A 43-year-old female undergoes a multiphasic renal mass protocol CT of the abdomen demonstrating a 1.4-cm right renal mass. The attenuation measurements are 32 Hounsfield units on unenhanced images and 50 Hounsfield units on postcontrast images. An MRI is then obtained and is shown below. Given the MR findings, what is the best explanation for the measured attenuation difference on the unenhanced and postcontrast CT images?

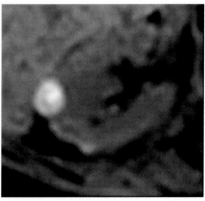 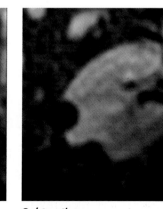

T1-weighted precontrast   *T1-weighted postcontrast*   *Subtraction*

    A. Solid enhancing tissue
    B. Application of tube current modulation
    C. Erroneous beam hardening correction
    D. Respiratory motion artifact

14   A 40-year-old female with recalcitrant hypertension undergoes CT angiography of the renal arteries. Which of the following would be treated best with balloon angioplasty alone?

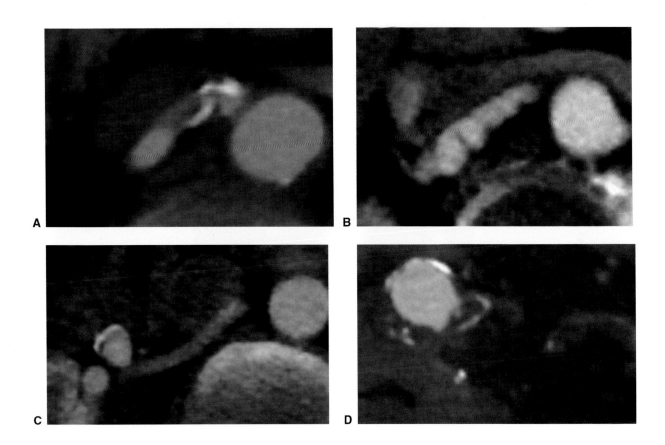

A.
B.
C.
D.

15   A 59-year-old male with urosepsis and hypotension presents with 6 hours of absent urine output. A renal Doppler study is performed. Which of the following spectral Doppler waveforms is most characteristic of acute tubular necrosis?

A. Resistive index = 1.0 and minimal diastolic flow
B. Resistive index = 0.7 and intact diastolic flow
C. Resistive index = 0.4 and blunted systolic upstroke
D. Resistive index = 0.2 and elevated arterial velocity

16 A 62-year-old male with hematuria is found to have a large left renal mass. Which risk factor has the strongest association with the imaging findings?

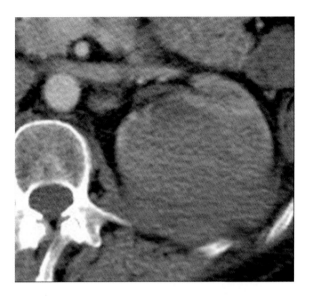

A. Solid organ transplant
B. Obesity
C. Hypertension
D. von Hippel-Lindau syndrome

17 In which retroperitoneal space is the fluid collection predominantly located?

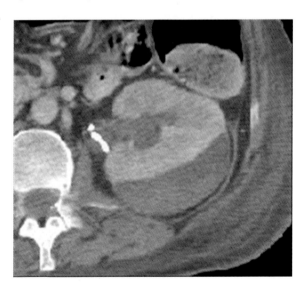

A. Anterior pararenal space
B. Posterior pararenal space
C. Perirenal space
D. Subcapsular space

18 A 45-year-old male was involved in a motor vehicle collision, and his left kidney was lacerated. Two weeks later, a contrast-enhanced CT was performed for persistent abdominal pain. What late-term complication is most strongly associated with the depicted abnormality?

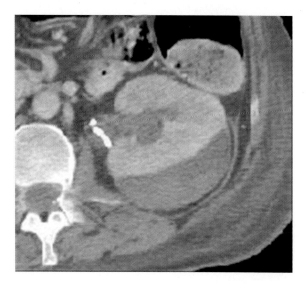

A. Nephrolithiasis
B. Hypertension
C. Pyelonephritis
D. Fistula formation

19 A 55-year-old female undergoes an unenhanced CT of the abdomen demonstrating a renal mass that measures 62 Hounsfield units. There are no comparison studies. What is the best next step?

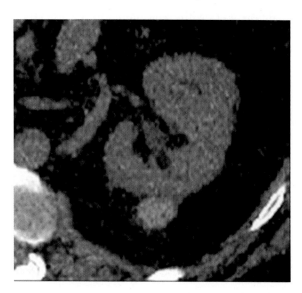

A. Observation
B. More imaging
C. Renal mass biopsy
D. Partial nephrectomy

20   A 2-year-old girl with abdominal swelling and pain undergoes a CT of the abdomen and pelvis. Which of the following organisms most likely colonizes this patient's urinary tract?

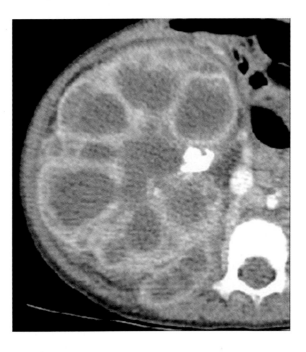

A. *Schistosoma haematobium*
B. *Proteus mirabilis*
C. *Mycobacterium tuberculosis*
D. *Staphylococcus aureus*
E. *Echinococcus multilocularis*

21   A 52-year-old male presents with flank pain and dysuria, and a CT is performed 120 seconds after intravenous contrast material administration. Which of the following best describes the imaging finding in the left kidney?

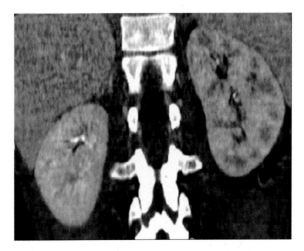

A. Striated nephrogram
B. Delayed nephrogram
C. Absent nephrogram
D. Dense nephrogram

22 A 62-year-old male smoker with chronic obstructive pulmonary disease, coronary artery disease, hypertension, and peripheral vascular disease undergoes a CT angiogram of the abdomen and pelvis that demonstrates a 1.8-cm indeterminate homogeneous low-attenuation left renal mass (35 Hounsfield units). A renal mass protocol MRI is performed. What is the most likely explanation for the imaging findings?

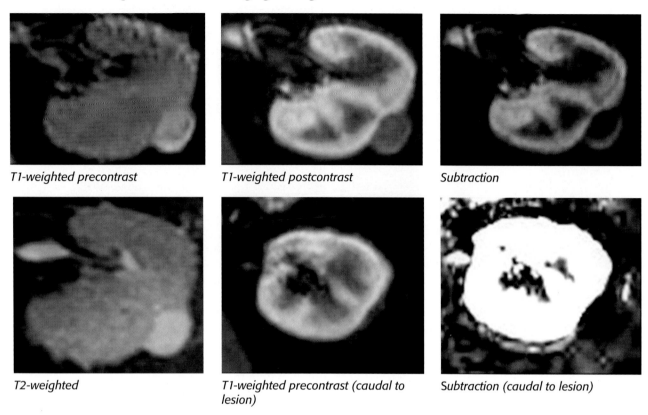

T1-weighted precontrast   *T1-weighted postcontrast*   *Subtraction*

T2-weighted   *T1-weighted precontrast (caudal to lesion)*   *Subtraction (caudal to lesion)*

A. Chemical shift artifact
B. Misregistration artifact
C. Mural calcifications
D. Mural soft tissue

23 A 76-year-old patient with back pain undergoes a digital subtraction angiogram of the left kidney. What is the best next step?

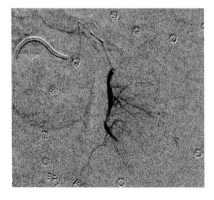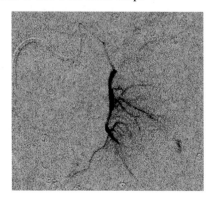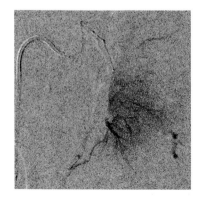

A. Covered stent
B. Balloon angioplasty
C. Embolization
D. Observation
E. Surgery

24 A 52-year-old male with biopsy-confirmed pancreatic adenocarcinoma undergoes a pancreaticoduodenectomy. During the postoperative course, a complication is suspected, and a contrast-enhanced CT of the abdomen is performed (shown below). Which of the following is the most specific imaging sign of acute renal infarction?

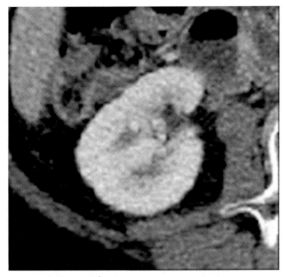
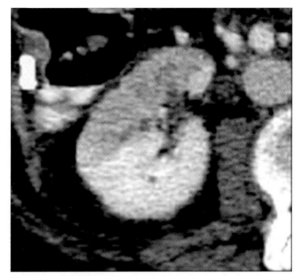

Preoperative study

Postoperative study (2 weeks later)

A. Alternating bands of hyper- and hypoattenuation extending to the capsule

B. Sharply demarcated cortical defect with an underlying calyceal diverticulum

C. Global delayed nephrogram with collecting system dilation and urothelial enhancement

D. Wedge-shaped focal delayed nephrogram with a thin enhancing capsular rim

25 A 51-year-old male with diabetes mellitus type II presents with right flank pain and dysuria. He has not seen a physician in many years. What is the best next step?

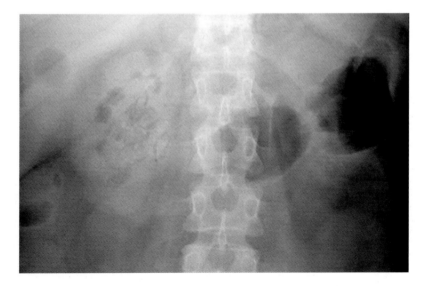

A. Operative debridement

B. Simple nephrectomy

C. Extracorporeal shock wave lithotripsy

D. Intravenous antibiotics

26 A 52-year-old female presents with acute right flank pain. A contrast-enhanced CT is performed. Which of the following risk factors is most likely to be present in this patient?

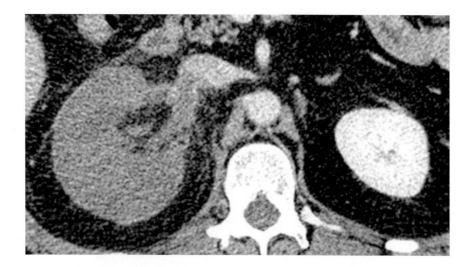

A. Relapsing urinary tract infection
B. Bladder cancer
C. Liver transplant recipient
D. Polycythemia vera
E. Recurrent nephrolithiasis

27 A 1-month-old infant presents with abnormal kidneys. Which of the following structures is likely to be also involved by this disease?

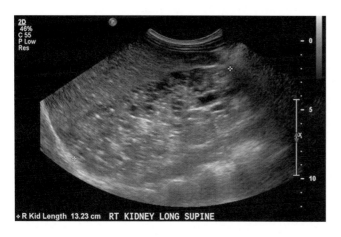
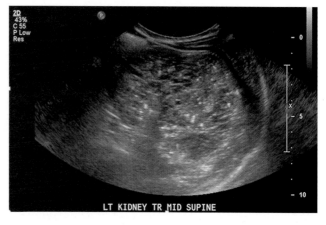

A. Spleen
B. Liver
C. Adrenal glands
D. Pancreas
E. Spinal cord

28 A 62-year-old male with diabetes mellitus type II, benign prostatic hypertrophy, and urinary retention presents with a 2-cm ill-defined left renal mass that is new since a comparison CT 6 months ago. Following a 2-week course of antibiotics, the imaging is repeated, demonstrating persistence of the finding. The mass enhances 30 Hounsfield units. What is the best next step?

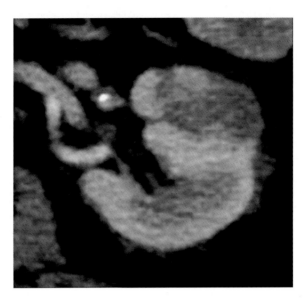

A. Thermal ablation
B. Partial nephrectomy
C. Percutaneous biopsy
D. MRI

29 A 54-year-old male with no significant past medical history presents with fever, leukocytosis, tachycardia, hypotension, and dysuria. What is the definitive management for this condition?

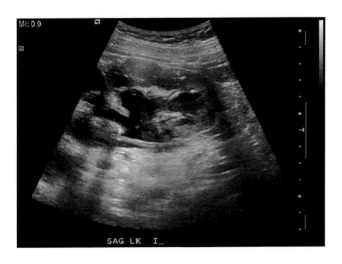
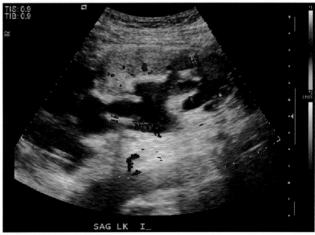

A. Antibiotics
B. Percutaneous nephrostomy
C. Nephrectomy
D. Observation

30　A 60-year-old male presents for a contrast-enhanced CT of the abdomen, and an abnormality is noted in the kidneys. Which of the following is most strongly associated with this finding?

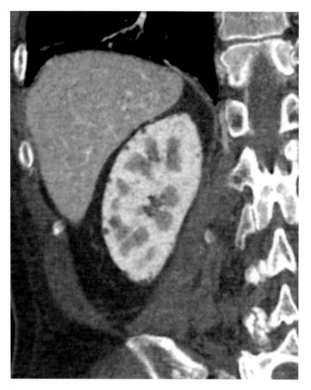 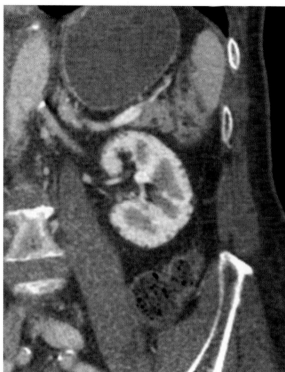

A. Hepatorenal syndrome
B. Mood disturbances
C. Untreated hypertension
D. Antihypoglycemic medications

ANSWERS AND EXPLANATIONS

1 **Answer B.** The images demonstrate contrast material in the kidneys (corticomedullary phase), gallbladder (vicarious excretion), and bowel (oral contrast material), but no contrast material within the vasculature or other upper abdominal viscera. This suggests recent exposure to intravascular contrast material that is being abnormally retained within the kidneys (i.e., bilateral delayed nephrograms). The most common antecedent history in this context is a recent contrast-enhanced CT or coronary angiogram in the setting of hypotension. The generic differential diagnosis for a delayed nephrogram can be oversimplified as follows:

- "Blood in": renal artery stenosis/thrombosis/laceration
- "Blood out": renal vein thrombosis
- "Urine in": acute tubular necrosis, pyelonephritis, glomerulonephritis
- "Urine out": collecting system obstruction

In this case, the delayed nephrogram is diffuse and bilateral. Therefore, acute tubular necrosis is the best answer. Contrast-induced nephrotoxicity (Answer A) could cause this appearance, but it is not the best answer because it is an uncommon and specific cause of acute kidney injury. Although pyelonephritis can be bilateral (Answer C), it would more likely present with striated nephrograms. In this case, the pattern of enhancement is globally delayed, not striated. Although extracellular gadolinium-based contrast material can resemble dilute iodinated contrast material on CT (Answer D), it in general follows the same dynamic enhancement pattern. In this case, the enhancement pattern is abnormal; therefore, gadolinium-based contrast material exposure is not the best answer.

References: Dyer RB, Munitz HA, Bechtold R, et al. The abnormal nephrogram. *Radiographics* 1986;6:1039–1063.
Saunders HS, Dyer RB, Shifrin RY, et al. The CT nephrogram: implications for evaluation of urinary tract disease. *Radiographics* 1995;15:1069–1085.
Wolin EA, Hartman DS, Olson JR. Nephrographic and pyelographic analysis of CT urography: differential diagnosis. *AJR Am J Roentgenol* 2013;200:1197–1203.

2 **Answer D.** T1-weighted dual-echo gradient-recalled echo (GRE) imaging can be used to help characterize renal masses. At 1.5 Tesla, fat and water protons are in opposite phase (180 degrees opposed) at echo time (TE) 2.2 msec, and in phase (dipole pointing in the same direction) at TE 4.4 msec. Therefore, at TE 2.2 msec, there will be signal loss in voxels that share fat and water protons, while at TE 4.4 msec the signal will be additive (NB: the echo times where fat and water protons are in and out of phase varies with the field strength of the magnet).

At TE 2.2 msec (1.5 Tesla) in masses that contain "intracellular lipid" (i.e., "microscopic fat"), there will be signal loss in voxels that contain both fat and water protons. The signal loss will be sheet-like in appearance, not linear. Both benign (e.g., angiomyolipoma) and malignant (e.g., clear cell renal cell carcinoma) renal masses can exhibit "intracellular lipid." Therefore, "intracellular lipid" cannot be used in isolation to discriminate benign from malignant renal masses (i.e., Answers A and B are not correct).

In masses that contain "macroscopic fat," the portions of the mass that contain solely fat protons will cause no signal loss at TE 2.2 msec (1.5 Tesla), but rather linear signal loss along the periphery where this "macroscopic fat" abuts soft tissue containing water protons (e.g., normal renal parenchyma or nonfatty elements within the mass). Again, this is due to the presence of fat and water protons sharing the same voxel. Peripheral signal loss at the interface of "macroscopic fat" with water protons from adjacent soft tissue is known as India ink artifact because it creates a solid dark line. However, at a fundamental level, India ink artifact and "intracellular lipid" are caused by the same process; their different names refer to their differing appearance on imaging.

No India ink artifact is created at the boundary of fat and fat (e.g., fat within a mass and fat in the perinephric space [Answer C is not correct]) because both fat and water protons sharing the same voxel is required for phase cancellation. Renal masses containing macroscopic fat, regardless of quantity, almost always represent angiomyolipoma (Answer D is correct). The exceptions are rare (e.g., osseous metaplasia within a renal cell carcinoma) and, when present, often demonstrate calcifications and/or invasion of adjacent structures.

References: Bosniak MA, Megibow AJ, Hulnick DH, et al. CT diagnosis of renal angiomyolipomas: the importance of detecting small amounts of fat. *AJR Am J Roentgenol* 1988;151:497–501.

Hindman N, Ngo L, Genega EM, et al. Angiomyolipoma with minimal fat: can it be differentiated from clear cell renal cell carcinoma by using standard MR techniques? *Radiology* 2012;265:468–477.

Hood MN, Ho VB, Smirniotopoulos JG, et al. Chemical shift: the artifact and clinical tool revisited. *Radiographics* 1999;19:357–371.

Israel GM, Hindman N, Hecht E, et al. The use of opposed-phase chemical shift MRI in the diagnosis of renal angiomyolipomas. *AJR Am J Roentgenol* 2005;184:1868–1872.

3 **Answer C.** The images demonstrate holodiastolic reversal of flow within the intrarenal arcuate arteries. This indicates that higher-velocity systolic flow can enter the kidney, but lower-velocity diastolic flow must return retrograde out of the kidney via the arteries (as opposed to the veins). Note the absence of flow below the baseline during systole. This is an important feature to differentiate this clinically significant waveform from superimposition of simultaneously acquired arterial and venous waveforms (which is common and not inherently pathologic, Answer D).

Holodiastolic reversal of flow within the intrarenal arcuate arteries of a renal transplant can be seen in the setting of renal vein thrombosis, acute tubular necrosis, or acute rejection. In all cases, presence of this waveform portends a poor prognosis for the graft. Holodiastolic reversal of flow combined with absent venous flow is highly suggestive of renal vein thrombosis, which has a high rate of graft failure and can lead to transplant nephrectomy. Some grafts can be salvaged with urgent thrombectomy and/or urgent thrombolysis. The role of catheter-directed thrombolysis and percutaneous thrombectomy for the management of this condition is evolving.

References: Fathi T, Samhan M, Gawish F, et al. Renal allograft venous thrombosis is salvageable. *Renal Transplant* 2007; 39:1120–1121.

Kaveggia LP, Perrella RR, Grant EG, et al. Duplex Doppler sonography in renal allografts: the significance of reversed flow in diastole. *AJR Am J Roentgenol* 1990;155:295–298.

Kim HS, Fine DM, Atta MG. Catheter-directed thrombectomy and thrombolysis for acute renal vein thrombosis. *J Vasc Interv Radiol* 2006;17:815–822.

4 **Answer B.** The images demonstrate a tangle of vessels within the lower pole of the renal transplant. Spectral analysis is consistent with a high-velocity low-resistance waveform characteristic of an arteriovenous fistula. In this setting, blood travels from the high-velocity arteries directly into the low-resistance veins without an intervening capillary bed. The lack of significant flow impedance results in a low-resistance pattern. Renal arteriovenous fistulae are most commonly caused by renal biopsy, in which the biopsy needle creates an aberrant communication between an intrarenal artery and an intrarenal vein. Renal arteriovenous fistulae are not often congenital (Answer C).

Polyarteritis nodosa (Answer A) is a vasculitis characterized by numerous small intrarenal aneurysms. Renal artery thrombosis (Answer D) and acute tubular necrosis (Answer E) are both high-resistance conditions in which arterial flow has a difficult time passing through to the vein(s); that is the opposite of what is shown here.

Reference: Brown ED, Chen MYM, Wolfman NT, et al. Complications of renal transplantation: evaluation with US and radionuclide imaging. *Radiographics* 2000;20:607–622.

5 **Answer F.** Although the mass is most likely to represent renal cell carcinoma on a statistical probability basis, there are no reliable imaging features that allow foolproof noninvasive differentiation of solid enhancing renal masses that lack macroscopic fat. The large hypervascular mass described in this question could represent malignant renal cell carcinoma (most likely), benign oncocytoma, or a rare alternative etiology. The presence of a central scar, the morphology, and the enhancement pattern are not reliable features. Therefore, enhancing solid renal masses that lack macroscopic fat require histologic sampling (percutaneous or surgical) for definitive diagnosis. Urothelial carcinoma and lymphoma are unlikely given the exophytic nature of the mass, and angiomyolipoma is unlikely because minimal fat angiomyolipoma (angiomyolipoma lacking evident macroscopic fat) is usually small (<4 cm).

References: Israel GM, Bosniak MA. How I do it: evaluating renal masses. *Radiology* 2005;236:441–450.
Silverman SG, Gan YU, Mortele KJ, et al. Renal masses in the adult patient: the role of percutaneous biopsy. *Radiology* 2006;240:6–22.

6 **Answer B.** Multiple small bilateral echogenic renal masses in a young patient are most likely to represent angiomyolipomas (AML) in the setting of tuberous sclerosis. Tuberous sclerosis is associated with renal angiomyolipomas (both typical AML [benign] and epithelioid variant AML [aggressive]), renal cysts, renal cell carcinoma, calcifying subependymal nodules (shown in Answer B), subependymal giant cell astrocytoma (SEGA), cortical tubers, cardiac rhabdomyomas, cutaneous angiofibromas, and pulmonary lymphangioleiomyomatosis (LAM).

The other images demonstrate pheochromocytoma on MIBG in the setting of von Hippel-Lindau syndrome (Answer A), occasional thin-walled pulmonary cysts of varying sizes in the setting of Birt-Hogg-Dubé syndrome (Answer C; pulmonary LAM cysts are usually more numerous and similar in size), and uterine fibroids in the setting of HLRCC (Answer D; hereditary leiomyomatosis and renal cell cancer syndrome, characterized by uterine leiomyomas [fibroids], cutaneous leiomyomas, and renal cell carcinoma [typically type II papillary—an aggressive variant of papillary renal cell carcinoma]). Although von Hippel-Lindau syndrome (Answer A) can cause bilateral renal lesions, these are typically a combination of renal cysts and renal cell carcinomas; bilateral echogenic renal masses without cysts would be atypical.

Both angiomyolipoma and renal cell carcinoma can appear echogenic on ultrasound. Therefore, presence of an echogenic renal mass usually prompts further imaging (CT or MRI) to determine whether the mass has evidence of macroscopic fat. Some reports indicate that a small homogeneous echogenic mass with posterior acoustic shadowing is always consistent with angiomyolipoma, but most echogenic renal masses do not have all these features.

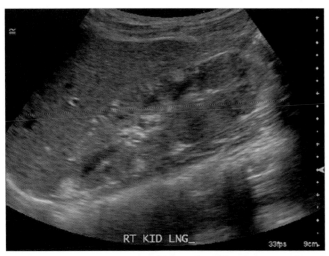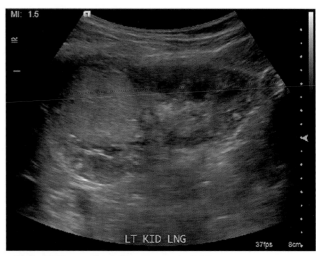

7-year-old female with tuberous sclerosis, multiple AMLs, and a left upper pole RCC

Reference: Choyke PL, Glenn GM, McClellan MW, et al. Hereditary renal cancers. *Radiology* 2003;226:33–46.

7 **Answer B.** The typical spectral Doppler waveform of a renal arteriovenous fistula is high velocity and low resistance. This is because high velocity arterial flow directly enters the vein(s) without an intervening capillary bed, allowing it to immediately exit without resistance. The measured resistive index in this setting is typically <0.5.

Reference: Brown ED, Chen MYM, Wolfman NT, et al. Complications of renal transplantation: evaluation with US and radionuclide imaging. *Radiographics* 2000;20:607–622.

8 **Answer B.** Dual-echo gradient-recalled echo (GRE) imaging exploits the difference in resonance frequency between fat and water protons (~3.5 ppm, or ~220 Hz at 1.5 Tesla and ~440 Hz at 3.0 Tesla). The first image was acquired at an echo time where the phase of fat and water protons are 180 degrees opposed (2.2 msec at 1.5 Tesla), causing diffuse signal loss in regions of "intracellular lipid" (present in this case). The second image was acquired at an echo time where the phase of fat and water protons are directly aligned, or in-phase (4.4 msec at 1.5 Tesla), causing their signals to be additive. The second, in-phase image serves as the comparator for the opposed-phase image.

Signal loss secondary to such phase cancellation artifact is known as chemical shift artifact of the second kind (Answer B). Chemical shift artifact of the first kind occurs for the same fundamental reason as does chemical shift artifact of the second kind (differing resonance frequency between fat and water protons), but has a different appearance, manifesting solely in the frequency-encoding direction along fat–water interfaces. Because spatial location along the frequency-encoding direction is determined by the resonance frequency of water protons, the different resonance frequency of fat protons causes these protons to be shifted erroneously on the image (the MRI device assumes them to be water protons and maps them incorrectly). In the space where the fat protons are actually present will be a dark band (absent signal from displaced fat protons), simultaneously creating a white band at the space into which the shifted protons are erroneously mapped onto preexisting water protons. Chemical shift artifacts of the third (Answer C) and fourth (Answer D) kind are not entities in medical imaging.

References: Hood MN, Ho VB, Smirniotopoulos JG, et al. Chemical shift: the artifact and clinical tool revisited. *Radiographics* 1999;19:357–371.
Merkle EM, Dale BM. Abdominal MRI at 3.0 T: the basics revisited. *AJR Am J Roentgenol* 2006;186:1524–1532.

9   **Answer F.**   Bilateral hypovascular endophytic non–contour-deforming solid renal masses are most likely to represent renal lymphoma. The differential diagnosis includes metastatic disease, a hereditary papillary renal cell carcinoma syndrome, renal infection, and IgG4-related disease. The other provided options are less likely.

Tuberous sclerosis (Answer A) is also associated with solid bilateral low-attenuation renal masses, but the majority of these will be angiomyolipomas containing macroscopic fat (<–10 Hounsfield units). Birt-Hogg-Dubé syndrome (Answer B) is associated with chromophobe renal cell carcinoma and oncocytoma, but it is much rarer than lymphoma, and if multiple bilateral masses are present, it would be unlikely for them all to be entirely endophytic. Sporadic renal cell carcinoma (Answer C), sporadic urothelial carcinoma (Answer D), and sporadic renal sarcoma (Answer E) are typically solitary masses. von Hippel-Lindau syndrome (Answer G) is associated with renal cysts and renal cell carcinoma, but like Birt-Hogg-Dubé syndrome (Answer B), the cysts and masses in von Hippel-Lindau syndrome, when numerous, are unlikely to be all endophytic.

References: Choyke PL, Glenn GM, McClellan MW, et al. Hereditary renal cancers. *Radiology* 2003;226:33–46.

Dyer R, DiSantis DJ, McClennan BL. Simplified imaging approach for evaluation of the solid renal mass in adults. *Radiology* 2008;247:331–343.

Sheth S, Ali S, Fishman E. Imaging of renal lymphoma: patterns of disease with pathologic correlation. *Radiographics* 2006;26:1151–1168.

10   **Answer E.**   This mass has a solid enhancing nodule, consistent with a Bosniak IV cystic neoplasm. The Bosniak classification system is widely accepted as a method for stratifying malignant risk within cystic renal lesions. The imaging features that define each Bosniak category are detailed in the table.

Category	Characteristics	Malignant Risk	Measurable Enhancement?
Bosniak I	Simple cyst. Thin imperceptible wall. Resembles simple water. No septations.	0%	No
Bosniak II	"Few" hairline septations. Fine calcifications, or minimal thicker calcification. "Hyperdense" cysts <3 cm.	~0%	No
Bosniak IIF	"Multiple" hairline septations and/or a thin perceptible wall. Thick or nodular calcifications. Endophytic "hyperdense" cysts ≥3 cm.	10%–20%	No
Bosniak III	Thickened septations and/or a thickened wall (irregular and/or smooth). No enhancing nodules.	55%–60%	Possibly
Bosniak IV	Enhancing nodule(s).	95%	Yes

References: Harisinghani MG, Maher MM, Gervais DA, et al. Incidence of malignancy in complex cystic renal masses (Bosniak category III): should imaging-guided biopsy precede surgery? *AJR Am J Roentgenol* 2003;180:755–758.

Israel GM, Bosniak MA. How I do it: evaluating renal masses. *Radiology* 2005;236:441–450.

Smith AD, Remer EM, Cox KL, et al. Bosniak category IIF and III cystic renal lesions: outcomes and associations. *Radiology* 2012; 262:152–160.

11 **Answer E.** All of the listed options have been used alone or in combination with other methods to reduce the radiation dose to the patient. Only Answer E avoids the use of ionizing radiation. In patients with relapsing urolithiasis and recurrent identical symptoms, ultrasound can be performed instead of CT. It may take many hours for the collecting system to dilate in the setting of obstruction (particularly if the patient is not "hydrated" before the study), and so a "negative" sonogram is less helpful than is a "positive" sonogram showing new or progressive collecting system dilation. However, starting with the least ionizing study first while applying ALARA principles (As Low As is Reasonably Achievable) can decrease radiation exposure to this overimaged patient population.

Reference: American College of Radiology. ACR Appropriateness Criteria. Acute onset flank pain—suspicion of stone disease. Last review date: 2011. Date of origin: 1995. http://www.acr.org/~/media/ACR/Documents/AppCriteria/Diagnostic/AcuteOnsetFlankPainSuspicionStoneDisease.pdf. Accessed September 2013.

12 **Answer C.** Hypervascular masses that follow the blood pool are suspicious for vascular anomalies. In this case, the "mass" is actually an aneurysm. Notice that it is isointense to the inflowing renal artery on both arterial and venous phases. Further imaging (Answer C; e.g., other MR pulse sequences, Doppler ultrasound) can confirm that this is an aneurysm and permit proper management.

Partial nephrectomy (Answer A) is not an appropriate treatment for a renal artery aneurysm, although simple nephrectomy can be considered in cases of aneurysm rupture or end-stage ischemic nephropathy. Percutaneous biopsy (Answer B) of an aneurysm is dangerous and can lead to life-threatening hemorrhage. Renal artery aneurysms are not normal variants (Answer D), although observation can be pursued when the aneurysm is small and the patient is asymptomatic. Specific size thresholds indicating therapy are controversial. In general, renal artery aneurysms >1.0 cm in patients with severe hypertension, most renal artery aneurysms 1.5 to 2.0 cm in all patients regardless of symptoms, and all renal artery aneurysms >2.0 cm in all patients regardless of symptoms should be considered for treatment. Hypertension and female sex are supporting indications for definitive management.

Reference: Henke PK, Cardneau JD, Welling TH, et al. Renal artery aneurysms: a 35-year clinical experience with 252 aneurysms in 168 patients. *Ann Surg* 2001;234:454–463.

13 **Answer C.** The measured attenuation change on CT was likely due to pseudoenhancement, which is commonly attributed to faulty correction for beam hardening artifact prevalent with multidetector CT. Pseudoenhancement effects are greatest in small (<20 mm) renal cysts with an endophytic growth pattern (i.e., intrarenal) that are adjacent to brightly enhancing renal parenchyma. This is a major reason why definitive enhancement on multidetector CT is ≥20 Hounsfield units, while "enhancement" of 11 to 19 Hounsfield units is considered equivocal.

The MR images demonstrate intracystic hemorrhagic or proteinaceous content (hyperintensity to water on unenhanced T1-weighted imaging), and absent internal enhancement (confirmed on subtraction imaging). MRI is an excellent tool for small renal masses that exhibit equivocal enhancement on CT because it is not susceptible to pseudoenhancement effects. Cysts <5 mm are often "too small to characterize" by CT, but can be characterized easily with subtraction MRI if the patient is able to reliably hold his or her breath (to avoid subtraction misregistration artifact).

References: Israel GM, Bosniak MA. How I do it: evaluating renal masses. *Radiology* 2005;236:441–450.
Maki DD, Birnbaum BA, Chakraborty DP, et al. Renal cyst pseudoenhancement: beam-hardening effects on CT numbers. *Radiology* 1999;213:468–472.

14 **Answer B.**   The four images depict ostial renal artery stenosis secondary to atherosclerotic disease (Answer A), fibromuscular dysplasia (Answer B), a distal renal artery aneurysm (Answer C), and long-segment renal artery occlusion (Answer D). Of these, the option treated most often with balloon angioplasty alone is fibromuscular dysplasia. Stent placement is generally only indicated for renal artery fibromuscular dysplasia if angioplasty alone fails or for the treatment of iatrogenic renal artery dissection occurring during angioplasty. In contradistinction, stent placement is typical for ostial stenosis secondary to atherosclerotic disease (Answer A). Angioplasty is not indicated for the treatment of renal artery aneurysms (Answer C) or long-segment renal artery occlusions (Answer D).

References: Olin JW. Recognizing and managing fibromuscular dysplasia. *Cleve Clin J Med* 2007;74:273–274.

Olin JW, Sealove BA. Diagnosis, management, and future developments of fibromuscular dysplasia. *J Vasc Surg* 2011;53:826–836.

15 **Answer A.**   Acute tubular necrosis (ATN) typically manifests as a high-resistance spectral waveform with minimal, absent, or reversed diastolic flow. ATN is caused by hypotension, which leads to global compromise of the kidney, diffuse ischemia, and vasoconstriction. A normal renal resistive index is 0.5 to 0.7 in the general population (Answer B) and 0.5 to 0.8 in the elderly. An elevated resistive index (0.8 to 1.0) is nonspecific and indicates acute or chronic renal, renovascular, or obstructive pathology. A low resistive index (0.1 to 0.4) indicates renal artery stenosis when low velocity (Answer C, with or without a blunted systolic upstroke; almost exclusively in transplant renal artery stenosis) or an arteriovenous fistula when high velocity (Answer D). In general, the resistive index is not a specific or sensitive marker for renal disease.

References: Platt JF, Ellis JH, Rubin JM, et al. Intrarenal arterial Doppler sonography in patients with nonobstructive renal disease: correlation of resistive index with biopsy findings. *AJR Am J Roentgenol* 1990;154:1223–1227.

Platt JF, Rubin JM, Ellis JH. Acute renal failure: possible role of duplex Doppler US in distinction between acute prerenal failure and acute tubular necrosis. *Radiology* 1991;179:419–423.

Tublin ME, Bude RO, Platt JF. Review: the resistive index in Doppler sonography: where do we stand? *AJR Am J Roentgenol* 2003;180:885–892.

16 **Answer A.**   The image demonstrates a large homogeneous left renal mass that largely preserves the reniform shape of the kidney. There is extension of the mass into the perirenal fat. The infiltrative nature of the mass favors lymphoma and urothelial carcinoma over renal cell carcinoma. The homogeneous appearance favors lymphoma over urothelial carcinoma.

Common manifestations of renal lymphoma include (1) bilateral endophytic hypovascular hypoechoic renal masses, (2) infiltrative perirenal or hilar masses with or without direct renal invasion, and (3) bilateral nephromegaly. Of the listed risk factors, a history of solid organ transplant is most strongly associated with lymphoma (posttransplant lymphoproliferative disease [PTLD]). Obesity (Answer B), hypertension (Answer C), and von Hippel-Lindau syndrome (Answer D) are all risk factors for renal cell carcinoma, which is not as likely as lymphoma based on the appearance. Renal cell carcinoma is typically a cortically based, contour-deforming mass.

References: Hartman DS, Davidson AJ, Davis CJ, et al. Infiltrative renal lesions: CT-sonographic-pathologic correlation. *AJR Am J Roentgenol* 1988;150:1061–1064.

Sheth S, Ali S, Fishman E. Imaging of renal lymphoma: patterns of disease with pathologic correlation. *Radiographics* 2006;26:1151–1168.

17 **Answer D.** The fluid collection deforms the renal parenchyma and therefore is within the subcapsular space. Subcapsular collections are located between the renal parenchyma and the renal capsule, causing direct mass effect on the adjacent renal parenchyma. Fluid collections within the perirenal space are not constrained by the renal capsule and can diffuse without deforming the kidney.

The following image obtained in a 55-year-old male with acute pancreatitis depicts four major retroperitoneal spaces referent to the left kidney. The posterior pararenal fascia divides the perirenal space and posterior pararenal space. The anterior pararenal fascia divides the perirenal space and anterior pararenal space. The renal capsule divides the perirenal space and subcapsular space.

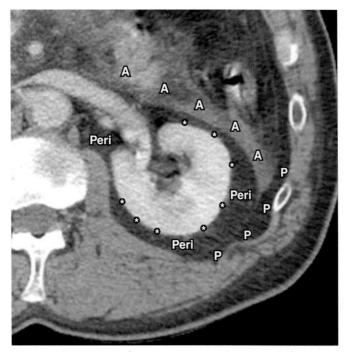

A = anterior pararenal space; P = posterior pararenal space;
*Peri = perirenal space; * = subcapsular space (potential space)*

Reference: Korobkin M, Silverman PM, Quint LE, et al. CT of the extraperitoneal space: normal anatomy and fluid collections. *AJR Am J Roentgenol* 1992;159:933–942.

18 **Answer B.** Chronic pressure on the renal parenchyma secondary to a subcapsular collection can result in "Page kidney," which is characterized by renin-mediated systemic arterial hypertension invoked by ischemia of the affected segment that is resistant to medical therapy. It can develop within weeks of the initial insult, and is managed with either drainage of the collection (percutaneous or operative) or nephrectomy.

Reference: Page IH. The production of persistent arterial hypertension by cellophane perinephritis. *JAMA* 1939;113:2046–2048.

19 **Answer B.** The differential diagnosis for a renal mass that measures 20 to 70 Hounsfield units on unenhanced CT includes a hemorrhagic/proteinaceous cyst or a solid renal mass. The two entities cannot be distinguished without further imaging. If there are no contraindications, either renal mass protocol CT or MRI (with pre- and postcontrast imaging) is the best next step. Ultrasound is an option, but sometimes it can be difficult to confirm sonographically that a hemorrhagic/ proteinaceous cyst is not solid (i.e., it may appear hypoechoic instead of anechoic).

Observation (Answer A) is not the best choice because the mass has not yet been characterized, and renal cell carcinoma is possible. Percutaneous (Answer C) and operative (Answer D) options are not appropriate because the mass could be a benign cyst. Percutaneous biopsy of a hemorrhagic cyst often will be nondiagnostic, and subjects the patient to a potentially unneeded invasive procedure (the diagnosis of a cyst should be made noninvasively).

Reference: Israel GM, Bosniak MA. How I do it: evaluating renal masses. *Radiology* 2005;236:441–450.

20 Answer B.   This is an example of xanthogranulomatous pyelonephritis (XGP), which classically presents on imaging with obstructing central urolithiasis, nephromegaly, and a "bear paw" sign within the renal parenchyma (rounded or oval-shaped noncommunicating low-attenuation mass-like abnormalities throughout the kidney representing infected purulent necrosis and lipid-laden foamy macrophages). XGP is an aggressive process that does not respect tissue planes, causes abscesses, and forms sinus tracts and fistulae. The urinary tracts of patients with XGP are often colonized with *Proteus mirabilis* (Answer B) and/or *Escherichia coli*. Management is surgical.

Schistosoma haematobium (Answer A) ascends the urinary tract from the urethra following direct inoculation and is associated with hemorrhagic cystitis, bladder wall calcifications, squamous cell carcinoma of the bladder, upper tract inflammation and stricture formation, and occasionally pyelonephritis. *Mycobacterium tuberculosis* (Answer C) descends the urinary tract from the kidneys following hematogenous seeding and is associated with pyelonephritis, amorphous renal parenchymal calcifications, "putty kidney" (atrophic calcified kidney), "cold" abscesses (false-negative results using traditional Gram stain and culture techniques), and urinary tract stricture formation. *Staphylococcus aureus* (Answer D) seeds the kidneys hematogenously and can cause multifocal pyelonephritis and abscess formation, particularly in patients with endocarditis (e.g., IV drug abuse); *Staphylococcus aureus* infection is not strongly associated with calculus disease and *Echinococcus multilocularis* (Answer E) is not typically a urinary tract pathogen.

References: Dyer RB, Chen MY, Zagoria RJ. Classic signs in uroradiology. *Radiographics* 2004;24:S247–S280.
Korkes F, Favoretto RL, Bróglio M, et al. Xanthogranulomatous pyelonephritis: clinical experience with 41 cases. *Urology* 2008;71:178–180.
Oyediran ABOO. Renal disease due to schistosomiasis of the lower urinary tract. *Kidney Int* 1979;16:15–22.
Pasternak MS, Rubin RH. Urinary tract tuberculosis. In: Schrier RW, eds. *Diseases of the kidney and urinary tract*. 7th ed. Philadelphia, PA: Lippincott Williams & Wilkins, 2001;910–929.

21 Answer B.   The left kidney exhibits a delayed nephrogram (Answer B). Specifically, the left kidney is in the corticomedullary phase and the right kidney is in the nephrographic/early pyelographic phase. In general, when one kidney (or a portion of a kidney) is in a different phase than the other kidney (or the rest of the ipsilateral kidney), the earlier-phase parenchyma is the abnormal parenchyma (i.e., delayed).

A striated nephrogram (Answer A) differs from corticomedullary phase imaging by the presence of alternating low-attenuation bands extending through the cortex. In the image from the question, the low-attenuation regions are medullary pyramids.

An "absent nephrogram" (Answer C) indicates that the kidney is not visible on projection imaging (e.g., IVP); examples include acute global infarction, congenital absence, severe chronic atrophy, and collecting system obstruction.

A "dense nephrogram" (Answer D) is the specific appearance of a global delayed nephrogram in the nephrographic phase, often visualized bilaterally hours or days after intravascular contrast-material exposure in the setting of acute tubular necrosis. Global hypotension of any cause (including an acute contrast reaction) can cause a bilateral "dense nephrogram."

The normal pattern of contrast-material uptake and excretion is shown below.

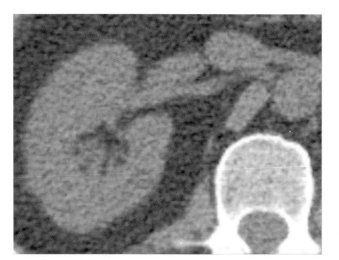

Unenhanced phase

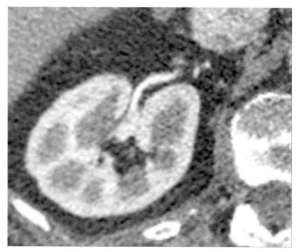

Corticomedullary phase

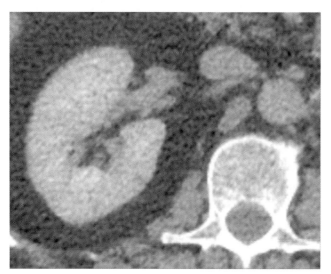

Nephrographic phase

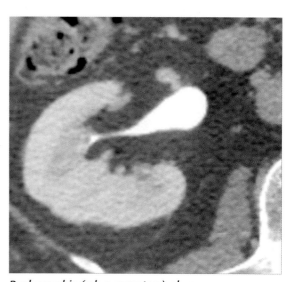

Pyelographic (a.k.a. excretory) phase

References: Dyer RB, Munitz HA, Bechtold R, et al. The abnormal nephrogram. *Radiographics* 1986;6:1039–1063.

Saunders HS, Dyer RB, Shifrin RY, et al. The CT nephrogram: implications for evaluation of urinary tract disease. *Radiographics* 1995;15:1069–1085.

Wolin EA, Hartman DS, Olson JR. Nephrographic and pyelographic analysis of CT urography: differential diagnosis. *AJR Am J Roentgenol* 2013;200:1197–1203.

22 **Answer B.** The images demonstrate subtraction misregistration artifact within a hemorrhagic cyst. Notice that the apparent curvilinear mural enhancement on the subtraction image corresponds to the most hyperintense component within the cyst on the unenhanced T1-weighted image. On the subtraction image caudal to the cyst, there is a signal void that is the same shape and in the same posterolateral axial location as the cyst.

Misregistration artifact is a common confounder that can impair characterization of a renal mass on MRI. Clues suggesting that perceived "enhancement" on subtraction imaging may be spurious include (1) motion artifact on the unenhanced image(s), postcontrast image(s), or both, (2) displacement of signal on the subtraction image outside the margins of the abnormality on the nonsubtracted image(s), (3) normal signal intensity within the region of apparent enhancement on other pulse sequences, (4) greater-than-expected apparent enhancement on subtraction images compared to the observed internal relative signal intensity on nonsubtracted postcontrast image(s), and (5) recognition that the apparent enhancement is along the margin of the abnormality. If the crescentic mural-based signal abnormality on the subtraction image in this case represented true enhancement, the abnormality would be characterized as a Bosniak III cystic mass (55% to 60% malignant risk) instead of a Bosniak II hemorrhagic/proteinaceous cyst (~0% malignant risk). Therefore, recognition of this artifact is important.

References: Nikken JJ, Krestin GP. MRI of the kidney—state of the art. *Eur Radiol* 2007;17:2780–2793.

Pedrosa I, Sun MR, Spencer M, et al. MR imaging of renal masses: correlation with findings at surgery and pathologic analysis. *Radiographics* 2008;28:985–1003.

23 **Answer C.** The images demonstrate active extravasation of contrast material from the lateral inferior left kidney. The appropriate next step is selective embolization (Answer C). Stent placement (Answer A), angioplasty (Answer B), and observation (Answer D) are not indicated. Surgery (Answer E) is not needed to treat this finding because the interventional radiologist has clear access to the bleeding vessel (as indicated by the images).

References: Chuang VP, Reuter SR, Schmidt RW. Control of experimental traumatic renal hemorrhage by embolization with autologous blood clot. *Radiology* 1975;117:55–58.

Mavili E, Dönmez H, Ozcan N, et al. Transarterial embolization for renal arterial bleeding. *Diagn Interv Radiol* 2009;15:143–147.

24 **Answer D.** Renal infarction, mediated by arterial (most common) or venous compromise, often presents as sharply defined wedge-shaped regions of delayed contrast material transit in the kidney (i.e., focal delayed nephrogram[s]). The appearance will vary depending on the location of the insult (proximal renal artery and distal renal vein compromise will result in global infarction, while peripheral arterial and/or venous compromise will result in regional infarction). The differential diagnosis for peripherally based wedge-shaped foci of delayed excretion (i.e., "striated nephrogram") includes pyelonephritis, vasculitis, embolic disease, and other causes of renal infarction (both arterial and venous).

Presence of a "cortical rim sign" (a thin rim of enhancing cortical tissue overlying the infarcted area) indicates that ischemia is the most likely etiology (Answer D). It takes between 8 hours and several days for the "cortical rim sign" to develop, and it is not pathognomonic for ischemia: it also can be seen with severe acute tubular necrosis (which is usually global and bilateral).

References: Frank PH, Nuttall J, Brander WL, et al. The cortical rim sign of renal infarction. *Brit J Radiol* 1974;47:875–878.

Glazer GM, Francis IR, Brady TM, et al. Computed tomography of renal infarction: clinical and experimental observations. *AJR Am J Roentgenol* 1983;140:721–727.

Kamel IR, Berkowitz JF. Assessment of the cortical rim sign in posttraumatic renal infarction. *J Comput Assist Tomogr* 1996;20:803–806.

Wolin EA, Hartman DS, Olson JR. Nephrographic and pyelographic analysis of CT urography: differential diagnosis. *AJR Am J Roentgenol* 2013;200:1197–1203.

25 Answer D.   The patient presents with a risk factor for urinary tract infection (diabetes mellitus type II), and imaging demonstrating stones and gas within the right collecting system. This is consistent with infectious emphysematous pyelitis. Recent instrumentation, a common benign cause of gas in the collecting system, is ruled out by history. The appropriate first step is intravenous antibiotics (Answer D). If the collecting system is obstructed, the best next step following parenteral antibiotics would be percutaneous nephrostomy.

Emphysematous pyelitis (gas within the collecting system) must be distinguished from emphysematous pyelonephritis (gas within the renal parenchyma) because the management is different (antibiotics [emphysematous pyelitis] vs. drainage/debridement/nephrectomy [emphysematous pyelonephritis]). Both conditions are more common in patients with diabetes mellitus. Shock wave lithotripsy (Answer C) is not appropriate in the acute setting.

References: Pontin AR, Barnes RD. Current management of emphysematous pyelonephritis. *Nat Rev Urol* 2009;6:272–279.

Roy C, Pfleger DD, Tuchmann CM, et al. Emphysematous pyelitis: findings in five patients. *Radiology* 2001;218:647–650.

26 Answer D.   The image demonstrates renal vein thrombosis with extensive venous infarction of the right kidney and a cortical rim sign. Renal vein thrombosis is more common in patients with hypercoagulable states, including malignancy, factor V Leiden, polycythemia vera (Answer D), and others. Bland renal vein thrombus is differentiated from neoplastic renal vein thrombus (e.g., renal cell carcinoma) by the absence of (bland) or presence of (neoplastic) enhancement or vasculature within the thrombotic material. The cortical rim sign can be seen in the setting of arterial and venous infarction (regional or global depending on the site[s] of thrombosis), as well as rarely acute tubular necrosis (global and bilateral).

References: Kim HS, Fine DM, Atta MG. Catheter-directed thrombectomy and thrombolysis for acute renal vein thrombosis. *J Vasc Interv Radiol* 2006;17:815–822.

Zigman A, Yazbeck S, Emil S, et al. Renal vein thrombosis: a 10-year review. *J Pediatr Surg* 2000;35:1540–1542.

27 Answer B.   This is an example of autosomal recessive polycystic kidney disease (ARPCKD), which is strongly associated with hepatic and periportal fibrosis (Answer B) that can result in biliary obstruction and portal hypertension. The kidneys in this patient are enlarged and contain numerous small cysts. Because of their small size, some of the cysts are hyperechoic (instead of anechoic) with parallel echogenic lines trailing from the far walls. This is due to reverberation artifact. Reverberation artifact is caused by repeated reflections of intracystic sound energy between the near and far walls of the cyst, creating aberrant "copies" of the cyst wall in the tissue beyond. This is due to a faulty assumption by the transducer that each echo it receives only encountered a single reflection. Because the distance of the reflector from the transducer is mapped based on a calculation contingent on the fixed speed of sound, echoes that are reflected more than once are artificially mapped deeper in tissue than they actually are. Multiple reflections create multiple lines deep to the cyst depending on the number of reflections each echo encounters (more reflections for a given echo equates to a greater mapped distance from the transducer).

References: Feldman MK, Katyal S, Blackwood MS. US artifacts. *Radiographics* 2009;29:1179–1189.

Lonergan GJ, Rice RR, Suarez ES. Autosomal recessive polycystic kidney disease: radiologic-pathologic correlation. *Radiographics* 2000;20:837–855.

28 Answer C.   The clinical scenario raises a number of differential diagnostic considerations: (1) incompletely treated pyelonephritis, (2) developing abscess or phlegmon, and (3) renal neoplasm. Given that antibiotic therapy has not clarified this, percutaneous biopsy (Answer C) is the best next step. Suspected infection is an accepted indication for percutaneous renal mass biopsy. Other accepted indications include (1) solid renal mass in the setting of a known extrarenal malignancy, (2) unresectable solid renal mass, and (3) solid renal mass in the setting of multiple medical comorbidities.

Percutaneous renal mass biopsy is growing in popularity as a way to stratify patient risk and to distinguish benign from malignant solid renal masses that lack macroscopic fat on imaging. Because infection is a strong possibility, thermal ablation (Answer A) and partial nephrectomy (Answer B) without histologic confirmation are not the best choices. MRI (Answer D) is unlikely to add additional value because the mass has already been confirmed to be solid (it enhanced 30 Hounsfield units; enhancement ≥20 Hounsfield units is diagnostic of solid enhancement).

References: Halverson SJ, Kunju LP, Bhalla R, et al. Accuracy of determining small renal mass management with risk stratified biopsies: confirmation by final pathology. *J Urol* 2013;189:441–446.

Silverman SG, Gan YU, Mortele KJ, et al. Renal masses in the adult patient: the role of percutaneous biopsy. *Radiology* 2006;240:6–22.

29 Answer B.   Percutaneous nephrostomy is the definitive treatment for patients with pyonephrosis. Pyonephrosis is characterized by urinary tract obstruction with superimposed infection. It can rapidly lead to sepsis and renal loss if not treated aggressively. The images demonstrate a dilated collecting system with echogenic filling defects. Filling defects alone are nonspecific (e.g., pus, blood, debris, cancer), so the history and ancillary laboratory findings are important to narrow the differential diagnosis.

Antibiotics (Answer A) should be given prior to percutaneous nephrostomy catheter placement, and play a major role in the treatment of pyonephrosis, but will not relieve the obstruction; therefore, antibiotics are not the definitive management for this condition. Nephrectomy (Answer C) is unnecessarily morbid as a first-line treatment. Retrograde ureteral stenting is not generally preferred in the setting of a clinically unstable patient, but some data have shown that the complication rates of retrograde stent placement and antegrade nephrostomy catheter placement are actually similar in this setting.

References: Ramsey S, Robertson A, Ablett MJ, et al. Evidence-based drainage of infected hydronephrosis secondary to ureteric calculi. *J Endourol* 2010;24:185–189.

Regalado SP. Emergency percutaneous nephrostomy. *Semin Intervent Radiol* 2006; 23:287–294.

30 Answer B.   The images demonstrate innumerable tiny (1 to 2 mm) cortically based renal cysts in a pattern characteristic of lithium nephropathy. Chronic lithium use causes a tubulointerstitial nephritis that can result in progressive renal impairment, nephrogenic diabetes insipidus, and end-stage renal disease. Key differentiators between this condition and other cystic diseases of the kidneys are (1) history of lithium use, (2) the size (1 to 2 mm) and location (cortical) of the cysts, (3) an absent history of dialysis, and (4) kidney size (normal to mildly decreased).

References: Farres MT, Ronco P, Saadoun D, et al. Chronic lithium nephropathy: MR imaging for diagnosis. *Radiology* 2003;229:570–574.

Presne C, Fakhouri F, Noël LH, et al. Lithium-induced nephropathy: rate of progression and prognostic factors. *Kidney Int* 2003;64:585–592.

Adrenal Glands

QUESTIONS

1   A 49-year-old male with a history of significant dehydration requiring intermittent hospitalization since 3 months of age presents with the following imaging findings on a venous-phase CT of the abdomen. What is the best next step?

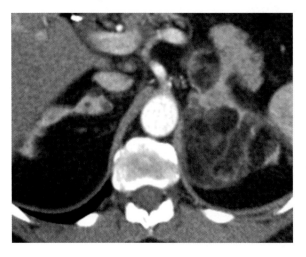 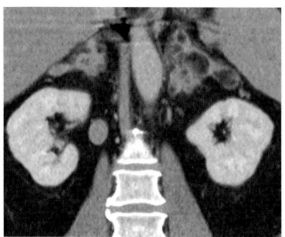

    A. Adrenal protocol CT
    B. PET
    C. Surgical referral
    D. Medical management

2   Attenuation measurements are the cornerstone of adrenal nodule characterization with CT. Which of the following adjustments will have the greatest effect on measured CT attenuation 1 minute after the administration of intravenous iopamidol 300 in a scan obtained and reconstructed with the following parameters: 120 kVp, 200 fixed mA, 5-mm collimation, and filtered back projection?

    A. Enabling statistical iterative reconstruction
    B. Increasing the mA from 200 to 400
    C. Decreasing the kVp from 120 to 80
    D. Exchanging iopamidol 300 for iohexol 300

3 A 50-year-old male with history of clear cell renal cell carcinoma status post–left nephrectomy presents for characterization of a right adrenal nodule detected on follow-up imaging. Images represent dual-echo gradient-recalled echo T1-weighted imaging with the following echo times at 1.5 Tesla: 2.2 msec (image on LEFT) and 4.4 msec (image on RIGHT). Signal intensity measurements within the adrenal mass are as follows: 144 (image on LEFT) and 175 (image on RIGHT) (18% signal loss). If there are no comparison studies, what is the best next step?

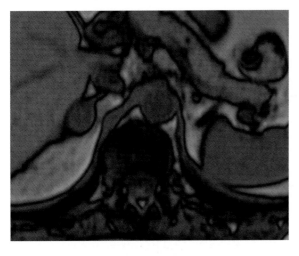 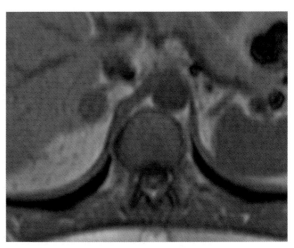

A. Tissue sampling
B. Follow-up in 12 months
C. Ignore (benign finding)
D. Adrenal protocol CT

4 A 63-year-old female with a history of gastric cancer presents for characterization of a 3.3-cm adrenal mass. There are no comparison images. Regions of interest drawn in the center of the mass on triphasic adrenal protocol CT are as follows: (a) unenhanced: 16 Hounsfield units; (b) 1-minute delay: 55 Hounsfield units; and (c) 15-minute delay: 28 Hounsfield units. What is the calculated absolute percent washout?

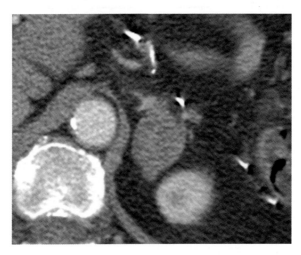

A. 29%
B. 49%
C. 69%
D. 89%

5 A 54-year-old female with node-positive invasive lobular breast cancer has a 2.1-cm homogeneous right adrenal mass. Adrenal protocol CT is performed utilizing 1-minute and 15-minute delays. Relative washout is calculated to be 50%. Which of the following is the most likely diagnosis?

A. Pheochromocytoma
B. Metastasis
C. Adenoma
D. Adrenocortical carcinoma

6 A 60-year-old male with hypertension and right lower quadrant pain undergoes a CT of the abdomen and pelvis to rule out appendicitis. An incidental 1.5-cm homogeneous right adrenal mass is identified. He has no other relevant medical history. What is the estimated risk that this adrenal nodule is malignant?

A. 1 in 5
B. 1 in 50
C. 1 in 500
D. <1 in 1,000

7 A 65-year-old male ICU patient with a complicated medical history presents with new findings in the adrenal glands. The unenhanced CT image on the left was obtained 2 weeks after the unenhanced CT image on the right. What is the best next step?

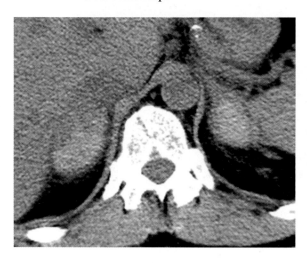 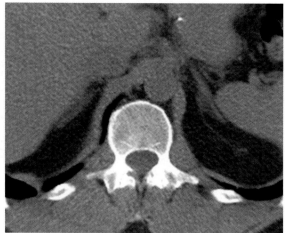

A. Adrenal protocol CT
B. Percutaneous biopsy
C. Medical management
D. Follow-up in 6 to 12 months

8 A 40-year-old female with postprandial pain and no other past medical history undergoes a right upper quadrant ultrasound. The gallbladder and biliary tree are normal, but an incidental 2.0-cm mass is identified in the right suprarenal fossa. An abdominal MRI follows confirming that the mass arises from the right adrenal gland. India ink artifact is observed within the mass encircling a 1.2-cm internal nodule. What is the most likely diagnosis?

A. Pheochromocytoma
B. Myelolipoma
C. Collision tumor
D. Adrenocortical carcinoma

9   A 23-year-old female with MEN-IIb syndrome and hypertension presents for an
I^{123}-MIBG scan. In which of the following organs is uptake on an I^{123}-MIBG scan
always abnormal?

A. Myocardium
B. Salivary glands
C. Adrenal glands
D. Bones
E. Colon

10   A 25-year-old male with a hereditary paraganglioma–pheochromocytoma
syndrome undergoes an I^{123}-MIBG study. What is the best diagnosis?

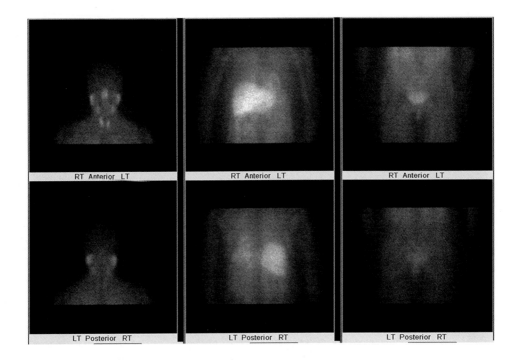

A. Myocarditis
B. Hepatic metastatic disease
C. Normal study
D. Nodal metastatic disease (neck)

11   T1-weighted dual-echo gradient-recalled echo imaging is used for the detection
of intracellular lipid and macroscopic fat. With this sequence, when fat and
water protons are out of phase, fat protons are shifted a certain distance along
the frequency-encoding axis depending on the receiver bandwidth and field
strength. What is the approximate calculated fat/water chemical shift at 1.5
Tesla? Use the following formula:

Shift = (fat / water resonant frequency separation [in ppm]) × (field strength [T])
$$\times 42 \text{ MHz} / \text{T}$$

A. 85 Hz
B. 220 Hz
C. 440 Hz
D. 550 Hz

12   A 56-year-old male with no history of malignancy and suspected primary hyperaldosteronism undergoes an adrenal protocol CT demonstrating a 1.5-cm left adrenal nodule with 70% absolute washout. The right adrenal gland is normal. What is the best next step?

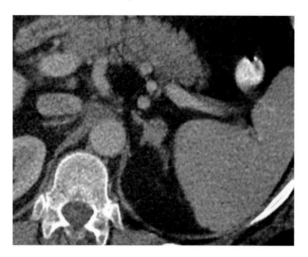

A. Adrenal protocol MRI
B. Left adrenalectomy
C. Percutaneous biopsy
D. Adrenal vein sampling

13   A 59-year-old female with suspected primary hyperaldosteronism and a 1.3-cm unilateral left adrenal nodule undergoes adrenal vein sampling. Which description best characterizes the adrenal venous anatomy?

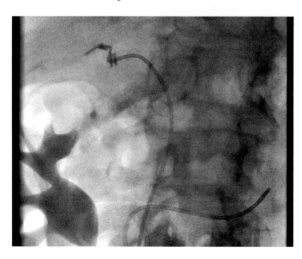 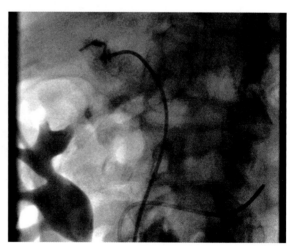

A. Right: A single vein drains into the IVC; Left: A single vein drains into the left renal vein.
B. Right: Three veins drain into the IVC; Left: Three veins drain into the left renal vein.
C. Right: A single vein drains into the right renal vein; Left: A single vein drains into the IVC.
D. Right: Three veins drain into the right renal vein; Left: Three veins drain into the IVC.

14 A 55-year-old male with non–small cell lung cancer and a 1.5-cm homogeneous right adrenal nodule presents for triphasic adrenal protocol CT. Which of the following image–time combinations has been shown to be most effective for adrenal nodule characterization?

    A. Unenhanced, 1 minute postcontrast, 20 minutes postcontrast
    B. Unenhanced, 1 minute postcontrast, 15 minutes postcontrast
    C. Unenhanced, 1 minute postcontrast, 10 minutes postcontrast
    D. Unenhanced, 1 minute postcontrast, 5 minutes postcontrast

15 A 62-year-old female with invasive ductal carcinoma of the breast and an indeterminate 1.5-cm left adrenal nodule undergoes a staging PET study. Which of the following adrenal nodule characteristics has the highest negative predictive value for metastasis?

    A. Standardized uptake value (SUV) maximum >5
    B. Standardized uptake value (SUV) maximum <5
    C. Qualitative uptake greater than background liver
    D. Qualitative uptake less than background liver

16 A 38-year-old female with early-onset diabetes mellitus presents with a dark rash covering her neck and armpits. CT imaging is performed and demonstrates a 4.9-cm left adrenal mass. An image representative of the entire mass is shown below. The patient has no history of malignancy. What is the best next step?

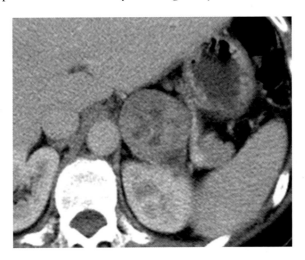

    A. Adrenal protocol CT
    B. Adrenal protocol MRI
    C. Percutaneous biopsy
    D. Open surgical resection

17 One of the fundamental sequences of adrenal protocol MR is T1-weighted dual-echo gradient-recalled echo imaging for the detection of intracellular lipid and macroscopic fat. Which of the following correctly describes a difference between gradient echo imaging and spin echo imaging?

    A. Gradient echo imaging usually has a longer TR.
    B. Gradient echo imaging usually has a larger flip angle.
    C. Gradient echo imaging has a refocusing RF pulse, and spin echo imaging does not.
    D. Gradient echo imaging is more affected by residual transverse magnetization.

18 A 70-year-old female with lung cancer and an indeterminate 2.2-cm left adrenal mass presents for percutaneous biopsy. Which of the following positional maneuvers will most effectively reduce the risk of pneumothorax during the biopsy while minimizing risk to other structures?

A. Decubitus, ipsilateral side down
B. Decubitus, contralateral side down
C. Prone
D. Supine

19 A 32-year-old male (body mass index: 22 kg/m²) with intermittent diaphoresis, palpitations, and early-onset hypertension (190/110) presents for adrenal protocol CT. What is the serious adverse event risk of administering intravenous low-osmolality iodinated contrast material to a patient with pheochromocytoma who is not receiving alpha- and beta-blockade?

A. 80% chance of a serious adverse event
B. 30% chance of a serious adverse event
C. 5% chance of a serious adverse event
D. <1% chance of a serious adverse event

20 A 62-year-old male with clinical-stage T1cN0Mx Gleason 5 + 4 = 9 prostate cancer and no signs of adrenal hyperactivity presents for MR characterization of a 2.4-cm right adrenal nodule. Images represent dual-echo gradient-recalled echo T1-weighted imaging with the following echo times at 1.5 Tesla: 2.2 msec (image on left) and 4.4 msec (image on right). What is the best next step?

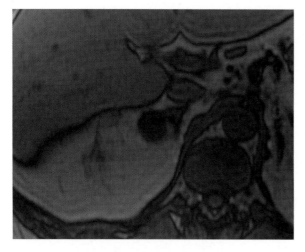 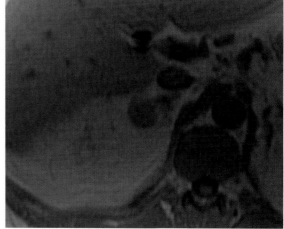

A. Ignore (benign finding)
B. Adrenal protocol CT
C. Percutaneous biopsy
D. Right adrenalectomy

21 Homogeneous loss of signal intensity within an adrenal nodule <4 cm on opposed-phase T1-weighted dual-echo gradient-recalled echo imaging is compatible with an adrenal adenoma in most cases. What organ is best used as an internal reference standard to determine the degree of signal loss within an adrenal nodule?

A. Liver
B. Pancreas
C. Kidney
D. Spleen

22 A 60-year-old female with right lower quadrant abdominal pain undergoes a CT of the abdomen and pelvis demonstrating perforated appendicitis and an incidental finding in the left adrenal gland. The following image is representative of the entire gland. Which of the following is most strongly associated with this abnormality?

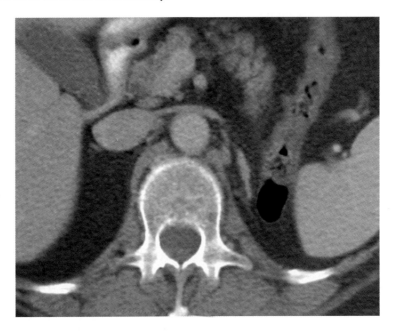

A. Hemangioblastoma
B. Renal agenesis
C. Pheochromocytoma
D. Polysplenia

23 A 58-year-old male with mild hypertension (140/90) managed with one medication and no history of malignancy undergoes an abdominal MRI that shows a 3.2-cm enhancing mass in the right adrenal gland. No intracellular lipid or macroscopic fat is identified. The left adrenal gland is normal, and the patient is asymptomatic. What is the best next step?

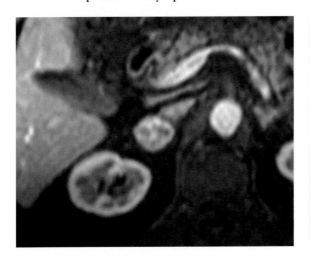
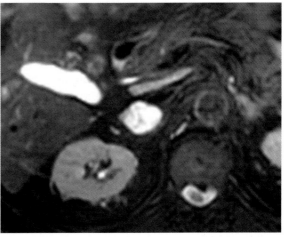

A. Right adrenalectomy
B. Alpha- and beta-adrenergic blockade
C. Percutaneous biopsy
D. Laboratory evaluation

24 A 45-year-old male with a right adrenal myelolipoma undergoes MR imaging. The following T2-weighted images were acquired without (left) and with (right) a conventional inversion recovery technique. Along what vector do the protons align in conventional inversion recovery imaging immediately following the preparation radiofrequency pulse (applied before the excitation pulse)?

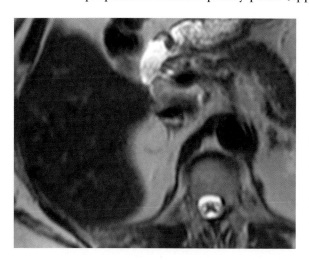
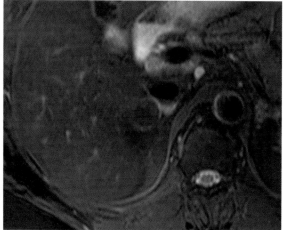

A. 0 degrees (with main magnetic field)
B. 90 degrees (perpendicular to main magnetic field)
C. 180 degrees (opposed to main magnetic field)
D. 270 degrees (perpendicular to main magnetic field)

25 A 51-year-old male with no comparison imaging and a recently diagnosed obstructing sigmoid colon cancer presents for staging CT of the chest, abdomen, and pelvis. Imaging demonstrates the known colon mass, enlarged regional lymph nodes, and a 2.2-cm left suprarenal abnormality. What is the best next step?

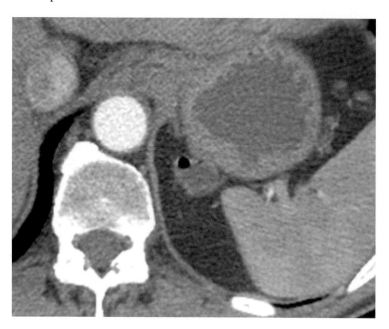

A. Adrenal protocol CT
B. Biopsy
C. Aspiration
D. Ignore (benign finding)

26 A 28-year-old male with suspected pheochromocytoma is scheduled to undergo an I^{131}-MIBG scan to confirm the diagnosis and evaluate for distant disease. Which organ is at greatest risk of radiation-induced carcinogenesis if no precautionary measures are taken?

A. Adrenal glands
B. Spleen
C. Myocardium
D. Thyroid

27 A 4-year-old girl with recurrent abdominal pain and unexplained fevers presents with a right suprarenal mass. What is the most likely diagnosis?

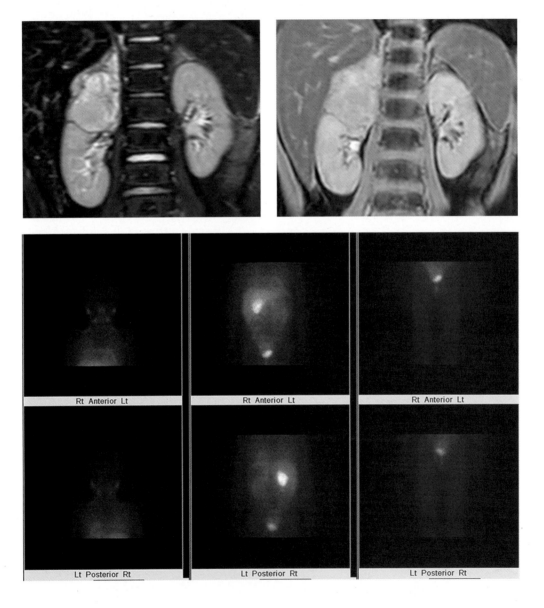

A. Sarcoma
B. Neuroblastoma
C. Adrenocortical carcinoma
D. Pheochromocytoma

28 Where is the organ of Zuckerkandl?

A. Near the carotid bifurcation
B. Near the aortic bifurcation
C. Within the middle ear
D. Along the urinary bladder wall

29 Pheochromocytoma is associated with several tumor-forming genetic syndromes. Which of the following is an example of that?

A. Multiple endocrine neoplasia (MEN) type I
B. Beckwith-Wiedemann syndrome
C. Neurofibromatosis type I
D. Hereditary leiomyomatosis renal cell cancer (HLRCC) syndrome

30 A 75-year-old male with altered mental status undergoes an abdominopelvic CT examination that demonstrates an abnormal left adrenal gland. The right adrenal gland is normal. Which of the following best explains this imaging finding?

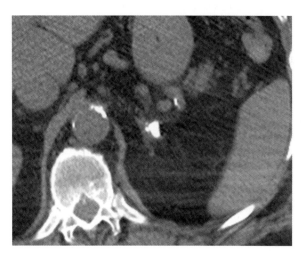

A. Pheochromocytoma
B. Metastasis
C. Remote hemorrhage
D. Adrenocortical carcinoma

ANSWERS AND EXPLANATIONS

1 **Answer D.** Large, bulky, bilateral macroscopic fat-containing adrenal masses is indicative of adrenal myelolipomas in the setting of congenital adrenal hyperplasia (CAH). These patients require medical management for their endocrine abnormalities. The most common cause of CAH is 21-hydroxylase deficiency, which results in salt wasting, female virilization, and hyperandrogenism. Most patients with 21-hydroxylase deficiency are detected during newborn screening. Adrenal protocol CT is not indicated for adrenal masses that contain macroscopic fat because it will add no additional information. PET and/or operative referral are not indicated because the masses are not malignant.

References: German-Mena E, Zibari GB, Levine SN. Adrenal myelolipomas in patients with congenital adrenal hyperplasia: review of the literature and a case report. *Endocr Pract* 2011;17:441–447.

Nermoen I, Rorvik J, Holmedal SH, et al. High frequency of adrenal myelolipomas and testicular adrenal rest tumours in adult Norwegian patients with classical congenital adrenal hyperplasia because of 21-hyroxylase deficiency. *Clin Endocrinol* 2011;75:753–759.

2 **Answer C.** Changing kVp has a direct effect on CT number measurements. Higher kVp imaging, particularly with multidetector CT, is susceptible to artificial increases in measured attenuation due to "pseudoenhancement" effects. Lower kVp imaging is closer to the k-edge of iodine, resulting in increased attenuation at lower kVp within iodine-containing (i.e., enhanced) structures. This fact is often exploited for high-contrast examinations like CT angiography. Lower kVp imaging is associated with greater image noise, less radiation dose, and greater measured iodine attenuation than higher kVp imaging. Changing mA, enabling statistical iterative reconstruction, and/or switching between contrast agents with similar iodine concentrations will have a negligible effect on CT number measurements.

References: Kaza RK, Platt JF, Goodsitt MM, et al. Emerging techniques for dose optimization in abdominal CT. *Radiographics* 2014;34:4–17.

Wang ZJ, Coakley FV, Fu Y, et al. Renal cyst pseudoenhancement at multidetector CT: what are the effects of number of detectors and peak tube voltage? *Radiology* 2008;248:910–916.

3 **Answer A.** The calculated signal intensity index ([IP − OP]/IP) of the right adrenal mass is 18% ([175 − 144]/175). Although the signal intensity index threshold varies with field strength (1.5 vs. 3.0 Tesla), sequence type (2D vs. 3D), and other parameters, homogeneous masses with a signal intensity index ≥16.5% are often thought to meet criteria for a lipid-rich adenoma. However, there are some exceptions (as in this case). Metastases known to contain "intracellular lipid" such as clear cell renal cell carcinoma and hepatocellular carcinoma can mimic adenomas on chemical shift imaging. Therefore, tissue sampling is the next best step (Answer A). This mass, though homogeneous and meeting the signal intensity index threshold, was proven to be a clear cell renal cell carcinoma metastasis. Another caveat to the use of the signal intensity index is for large masses (e.g., ≥4 cm) because adrenocortical carcinoma can also demonstrate signal loss on opposed-phase imaging. Chemical shift imaging is most helpful when the primary tumor is known not to contain intracellular lipid and the mass is <4 cm in size.

References: Blake MA, Cronin CG, Boland GW. Adrenal imaging. *AJR Am J Roentgenol* 2010;194:1450–1460.

Marin D, Dale BM, Bashir MR, et al. Effectiveness of a three-dimensional dual gradient echo two-point Dixon technique for the characterization of adrenal lesions at 3 Tesla. *Eur Radiol* 2012;22:259–268.

Shinozaki K, Yoshimitsu K, Honda H, et al. Metastatic adrenal tumor from clear-cell renal cell carcinoma: a pitfall of chemical shift MR imaging. *Abdom Imaging* 2001;26:439–442.

Sydow BD, Rosen MA, Siegelman ES. Intracellular lipid within metastatic hepatocellular carcinoma of the adrenal gland: a potential diagnostic pitfall of chemical shift imaging of the adrenal gland. *AJR Am J Roentgenol* 2006;187:W550–W551.

4 **Answer C.** The calculated absolute percent washout is 69%, and the calculated relative percent washout is 49%. Both are compatible with a lipid-poor adrenal adenoma, and both argue for a benign etiology (i.e., not a metastasis).

The formula for absolute washout is

$$100 \times \left(1\,\text{min HU} - 15\,\text{min HU}\right) / \left(1\,\text{min HU} - \text{pre HU}\right)$$

The formula for relative washout is

$$100 \times \left(1\,\text{min HU} - 15\,\text{min HU}\right) / \left(1\,\text{min HU}\right)$$

Where "pre-HU" is the measured attenuation on unenhanced CT, "1-min HU" is the measured attenuation on contrast-enhanced CT performed 1 minute after contrast material administration, and "15-min HU" is the measured attenuation on contrast-enhanced CT performed 15 minutes after contrast material administration.

Washout calculations are only applicable for homogeneous adrenal masses; they should not be used for heterogeneous, centrally necrotic, or calcified masses. It is important to recognize that adrenal washout calculations were derived from a select population of patients, namely, differentiating generic metastatic disease from adenomas. Washout calculations are less helpful in other settings, such as differentiating adenoma from primary adrenal neoplasms (e.g., pheochromocytoma) or differentiating adenoma from certain types of hypervascular metastases (e.g., hepatocellular carcinoma, renal cell carcinoma).

References: Caoili EM, Korobkin M, Francis IR, et al. Adrenal masses: characterization with combined unenhanced and delayed enhanced CT. *Radiology* 2002;222:629–633.

Choi YA, Kim CK, Park BK, et al. Evaluation of adrenal metastases from renal cell carcinoma and hepatocellular carcinoma: use of delayed contrast-enhanced CT. *Radiology* 2013;266:514–520.

Korobkin M, Brodeur JF, Francis IR, et al. CT time-attenuation washout curves of adrenal adenomas and nonadenomas. *AJR Am J Roentgenol* 1998;170:747–752.

Patel J, Davenport MS, Cohan RH, et al. Can established CT attenuation and washout criteria for adrenal adenoma accurately exclude pheochromocytoma? *AJR Am J Roentgenol* 2013;201:122–127.

5 **Answer C.** Relative washout calculations are designed for situations in which the unenhanced images were not acquired, but a patient has a homogeneous adrenal mass that needs to be characterized. Often, this occurs in cases where the adrenal mass is unsuspected. Relative washout calculations are based on attenuation measurements from the 1-minute and 15-minute delayed images, as follows:

$$\text{Relative washout}: 100 \times \left(1\,\text{min HU} - 15\,\text{min HU}\right) / \left(1\,\text{min HU}\right)$$

Obtaining a relative washout >40% in a homogeneous adrenal mass <4 cm in size indicates that adenoma is the most likely diagnosis. Although some masses can mimic this (e.g., pheochromocytoma, hepatocellular carcinoma metastasis, renal cell carcinoma metastasis), in a patient without risk factors for such masses, adenoma is the best choice and no further workup is generally required.

References: Caoili EM, Korobkin M, Francis IR, et al. Adrenal masses: characterization with combined unenhanced and delayed enhanced CT. *Radiology* 2002;222:629–633.

Choi YA, Kim CK, Park BK, et al. Evaluation of adrenal metastases from renal cell carcinoma and hepatocellular carcinoma: use of delayed contrast-enhanced CT. *Radiology* 2013;266:514–520.

Korobkin M, Brodeur JF, Francis IR, et al. CT time-attenuation washout curves of adrenal adenomas and nonadenomas. *AJR Am J Roentgenol* 1998;170:747–752.

Patel J, Davenport MS, Cohan RH, et al. Can established CT attenuation and washout criteria for adrenal adenoma accurately exclude pheochromocytoma? *AJR Am J Roentgenol* 2013;201:122–127.

6 **Answer D.** In a series by Song et al. (2008) of 1,049 adrenal masses in 973 consecutive patients without a history of malignancy or adrenal hyperfunction, the authors found zero malignant lesions. Incidental adrenal nodules <4 cm are incredibly unlikely to represent malignancy, and therefore adrenal protocol CT is not the best first step in the management of these patients. False positives are much more likely than true positives and would too often result in inappropriate management. Current guidelines state that patients with incidental adrenal nodule(s) should be referred instead for biochemical testing to determine whether the nodule(s) are hyperfunctioning.

References: American Medical Association of Clinical Endocrinologists and American Association of Endocrine Surgeons: Medical Guidelines for the Management of Adrenal Incidentalomas. AACE/AAES Guidelines, 2009.

Cawood TJ, Hunt PJ, O'Shea D, et al. Recommended evaluation of adrenal incidentalomas is costly, has high false-positive rates and confers a risk of fatal cancer that is similar to the risk of the adrenal lesion becoming malignant: time for a rethink? *Eur J Endocrinol* 2009;513–527.

Song JH, Chaudhry FS, Mayo-Smith WW. The incidental adrenal mass on CT: prevalence of adrenal disease in 1,049 consecutive adrenal masses in patients with no known malignancy. *AJR Am J Roentgenol* 2008;190:1163–1168.

7 **Answer C.** The image on the left depicts acute-onset bilateral adrenal masses that are high attenuation on unenhanced CT consistent with bilateral adrenal hemorrhage. Adrenal hemorrhage can lead to acute adrenal insufficiency (e.g., hypotension, hypoglycemia) and typically occurs in one of the following settings: (1) trauma (e.g., iatrogenic or otherwise); (2) sepsis (e.g., Waterhouse-Friderichsen syndrome); (3) hypercoagulable state (e.g., antiphospholipid antibody syndrome: due to thrombosis of the adrenal vein); (4) bleeding diathesis (e.g., heparin-induced thrombocytopenia); or (5) disseminated intravascular coagulation. Management of acute adrenal hemorrhage includes treatment of the underlying cause of hemorrhage and corticosteroid replacement. Failure to detect and address the hormone deficiencies resulting from adrenal insufficiency can lead to patient death. Adrenal hemorrhage should be suspected when acute-onset, high-attenuation adrenal masses (unilateral or bilateral) develop in the proper clinical setting (see above). Further imaging and/or biopsy are usually neither indicated nor helpful.

References: Jordan E, Poder L, Courtier J, et al. Imaging of nontraumatic adrenal hemorrhage. *AJR Am J Roentgenol* 2012;199:W91–W98.

Vella A, Nippoldt TB, Morris JC, III. Adrenal hemorrhage: a 25-year experience at the Mayo Clinic. *Mayo Clin Proc* 2001;76:161–168.

8 **Answer B.** The India ink artifact described in the question indicates that a large fraction of the mass is composed of macroscopic fat. Therefore, the most likely diagnosis is adrenal myelolipoma. Adrenal myelolipomas are benign, fat-containing masses that are generally hormonally inactive and require no further management. Rare adrenal masses that have been associated with macroscopic fat include (a) degenerated adenoma; (b) adrenal lipoma; (c) collision tumor within a myelolipoma (Answer C); (d) adrenocortical carcinoma (Answer D), when present the fat is usually <10% of the mass volume; and (e) pheochromocytoma (Answer A, a mimicker of many entities; presence of macroscopic fat would be very rare).

References: Blake MA, Kalra MK, Maher MM, et al. Pheochromocytoma: an imaging chameleon. *Radiographics* 2004;24:S87–S99.

Johnson PT, Horton KM, Fishman EK. Adrenal mass imaging with multidetector CT: pathologic conditions, pearls, and pitfalls. *Radiographics* 2009;29:1333–1351.

Musso S, Columbier D, Mazerolles C, et al. Imaging features of uncommon adrenal masses with histopathologic correlation. *Radiographics* 1999;19:569–581.

9 **Answer D.** I^{123}-MIBG uptake in the bones is always abnormal; when present, this indicates metastases from an adrenergic and/or catecholamine-expressing neoplasm (e.g., pheochromocytoma). The normal biodistribution of I^{123}-MIBG includes the liver, spleen, myocardium, salivary glands, and adrenal glands. Normal adrenal gland uptake should be mild and symmetric. Variable low-level uptake can be seen in the skeletal muscle, nasal mucosa, lungs, urinary tract, colon, gallbladder, and thyroid. Radioactive free iodine (i.e., iodine dissociated from the I^{123}-MIBG tracer) can be taken up into the normal thyroid gland, exposing it to unnecessary and potentially dangerous radiation; this action should be blocked with inert iodine (potassium iodide) tablets or perchlorate administered prior to the study.

References: Nakajo M, Shapiro B, Copp J, et al. The normal and abnormal distribution of the adrenomedullary imaging agent m-[I-131]iodobenzylguanidine (I-131 MIBG) in man: evaluation by scintigraphy. *J Nucl Med* 1983;24(8):672–682.

Olivier P, Colarinha P, Fettich J, et al. Guidelines for radioiodinated MIBG scintigraphy in children. Paediatric Committee of the European Association of Nuclear Medicine. *Eur J Nucl Med Mol Imaging* 2003;30(5):B45–B50.

10 **Answer C.**   The images demonstrate the normal biodistribution of I^{123}-MIBG. It is important to know the normal distribution of nuclear medicine tracers so that abnormal uptake can be differentiated from normal uptake. The normal biodistribution of I^{123}-MIBG includes the liver, spleen, myocardium, salivary glands, and adrenal glands. Normal adrenal gland uptake should be mild and symmetric. Variable low-level uptake can be seen in the skeletal muscle, nasal mucosa, lungs, urinary tract, colon, gallbladder, and thyroid.

References: Olivier P, Colarinha P, Fettich J, et al. Guideline for radioiodinated MIBG scintigraphy in children. Paediatric committee of the European Association of Nuclear Medicine. *Eur J Nucl Med Mol Imaging* 2003;30(5):B45–B50.

Nakajo M, Shapiro B, Copp J, et al. The normal and abnormal distribution of the adrenomedullary imaging agent m-[I-131]iodobenzylguanidine (I-131 MIBG) in man: evaluation by scintigraphy. *J Nucl Med* 1983;672–682.

11 **Answer B.**   Fat and water protons precess at different frequencies, and this principle is the foundation for chemical shift imaging. If the field strength is known, the fat/water chemical shift can be calculated by inserting the fat/water resonant frequency separation (3.5 ppm) and field strength into the following formula:

$$\text{Shift} = \left(\text{Fat / water resonant frequency separation}\left[\text{in ppm}\right]\right) \times \left(\text{field strength}\left[\text{T}\right]\right) \times 42 \text{ MHz / T}$$

At 1.5 Tesla, the fat/water chemical shift is approximately 220 Hz. This indicates that fat will be displaced approximately 220 Hz along the frequency-encoding axis in most pulse sequences. To convert this frequency into a distance, the matrix size (256 pixels) and receiver bandwidth (i.e., sampling frequency) must be known. For example, if the receiver bandwidth is 30 kHz, the shift at 1.5 Tesla is approximately 1.9 pixels.

$$30,000\,\text{Hz / 256 pixel matrix} = 117.2\,\text{Hz / pixel}$$
$$220\,\text{Hz} \times 1\,\text{pixel / } 117.2\,\text{Hz} = 1.9\,\text{pixels}$$

References: Bushong SC. *Magnetic resonance imaging: Physical and biological principles*, 3rd ed. St. Louis: Mosby Publishing, 2003.

McRobbie DW, Moore EA, Graves MJ, et al. *MRI: From picture to proton*, 2nd ed. New York: Cambridge University Press, 2007.

12 **Answer D.** The best next step is adrenal vein sampling. Biopsy and/or further imaging are not required. Patients over the age of 40 with suspected primary hyperaldosteronism and a unilateral adrenal nodule >1 cm should undergo adrenal vein sampling to determine whether the nodule visualized on CT is responsible or incidental. Because many patients over the age of 40 have nonfunctional adrenal nodules (i.e., an estimated 4% to 5% of patients over the age of 40 have an adrenal nodule of any type), the positive predictive value of an adrenal nodule in this population is low. In this setting, if CT alone is trusted and adrenal vein sampling is not used, as many as 40% to 50% of patients would be inappropriately managed (i.e., receive unneeded or wrong-site surgery, or fail to undergo needed surgery). This is a classic example of how positive predictive value varies depending on disease prevalence. In patients ≤40 years of age, the incidence of nonfunctional adrenal nodules is much less; therefore, in a patient ≤40 years of age with suspected primary hyperaldosteronism, presence of a unilateral adrenal nodule >1 cm is a sufficient indication for ipsilateral adrenalectomy without confirmation by adrenal vein sampling.

References: American Medical Association of Clinical Endocrinologists and American Association of Endocrine Surgeons: Medical Guidelines for the Management of Adrenal Incidentalomas. AACE/AAES Guidelines. 2009.

Bovio S, Cataldi A, Reimondo G, et al. Prevalence of adrenal incidentaloma in a contemporary computerized tomography series. *J Endocrinol Invest* 2006;29:298–302.

Nwariaku FE, Miller BS, Auchus R, et al. Primary hyperaldosteronism: effect of adrenal vein sampling on surgical outcome. *Arch Surg* 2006;141:497–503.

Tan YY, Ogilvie JB, Triponez F, et al. Selective use of adrenal venous sampling in the lateralization of aldosterone-producing adenomas. *World J Surg* 2006;30:879–887.

Young WF, Stanson AW, Thompson GB, et al. Role for adrenal venous sampling in primary aldosteronism. *Surgery* 2004;136:1227–1235.

13 **Answer A.** In most patients, a single right suprarenal vein drains into the IVC, and a single left suprarenal vein drains into the left renal vein. The images from the question demonstrate the normal position of adrenal vein sampling catheters within the suprarenal veins. Although the venous drainage is solitary, each adrenal gland typically is supplied by at least three small arteries (superior, middle, and inferior suprarenal arteries). Knowledge of adrenal venous anatomy is essential for performance of adrenal vein sampling. Because of the small size of the adrenal veins, the difficult angle of the right adrenal vein with the IVC, and the infrequent nature of these cases, adrenal vein sampling has a high failure rate when performed by inexperienced interventional radiologists.

References: American Medical Association of Clinical Endocrinologists and American Association of Endocrine Surgeons: Medical Guidelines for the Management of Adrenal Incidentalomas. AACE/AAES Guidelines, 2009.

Netter FH. *Atlas of human anatomy*, 5th ed. Philadelphia: Saunders Publishing, 2010.

White ML, Gauger PG, Doherty GM, et al. The role of radiologic studies in the evaluation and management of primary hyperaldosteronism. *Surgery* 2008;144:926–933.

Young WF, Stanson AW, Thompson GB, et al. Role for adrenal venous sampling in primary aldosteronism. *Surgery* 2004;136:1227–1235.

14 **Answer B.** Triphasic adrenal protocol CT is performed with three phases: unenhanced, 1 minute postcontrast, and 15 minutes postcontrast. Homogeneous adrenal nodules <4 cm that measure ≤10 Hounsfield units without macroscopic fat are consistent with lipid-rich adenomas (or adrenal cysts) and do not require postcontrast imaging for characterization. Some centers perform real-time monitoring of the unenhanced series in patients referred for adrenal nodule characterization to determine the need for contrast material administration. Delay times shorter than 15 minutes have been attempted (e.g., 10-minute delay), but these have been shown to have poorer sensitivity for adenoma compared to the traditional 15-minute delay. Shorter delay times result in a greater fraction of "indeterminate" adrenal nodules. Longer delay times have not been tested.

References: Caoili EM, Korobkin M, Francis IR, et al. Adrenal masses: characterization with combined unenhanced and delayed enhanced CT. *Radiology* 2002;222:629–633.
Sangwaiya MJ, Boland GW, Cronin CG, et al. Incidental adrenal lesions: accuracy of characterization with contrast-enhanced washout multidetector CT—10-minute delayed imaging protocol revisited in a large patient cohort. *Radiology* 2010;256:504–510.

15 **Answer D.**   In multiple series studying the ability of PET to accurately characterize adrenal nodules, activity less than that of background liver has been shown repeatedly to be a strong negative predictor for malignancy. Adrenal nodules that exhibit uptake less than background liver are almost certainly benign, while adrenal nodules that exhibit uptake substantially more than background liver are likely malignant. Those between these two extremes (i.e., uptake equal to or mild-moderately increased relative to background liver) are inconclusive by PET alone. Absolute SUV measurements have had conflicting results, with some studies showing no difference between benign and malignant lesions, and others showing clear separation (e.g., using a threshold SUV maximum of ≥3.1). The average SUV maximum of the adrenal glands is approximately 0.9 to 1.1.

References: Caoili EM, Korobkin M, Brown RK, et al. Differentiating adrenal adenomas from nonadenomas using (18)F-FDG PET/CT: quantitative and qualitative evaluation. *Acad Radiol* 2007;14:468–475.
Blake MA, Cronin CG, Boland GW. Adrenal imaging. *AJR Am J Roentgenol* 2010;194:1450–1460.
Boland GWL, Blake MA, Holalkere NS, et al. PET/CT for the characterization of adrenal masses in patients with cancer: qualitative versus quantitative accuracy in 150 consecutive patients. *AJR Am J Roentgenol* 2009;192:956–962.
Metser U, Miller E, Lerman H, et al. 18F-FDG PET/CT in the evaluation of adrenal masses. *J Nucl Med* 2006;47:32–37.

16 **Answer D.**   The clinical data suggest hypercortisolism, and the imaging findings are compatible with adrenocortical carcinoma (ACC). Open surgical resection is the best choice for management. Interventions that risk tumor spillage (e.g., percutaneous biopsy, laparoscopic resection) are not recommended because they can lead to higher rates of recurrence and an increased risk of peritoneal carcinomatosis. If the entire tumor is not removed, the disease is typically incurable. Adrenal protocol CT or MRI will not add value because the mass is heterogeneous, and there is no evident macroscopic fat; washout calculations should not be applied to heterogeneous masses. In general, operative resection is considered for most large (i.e., >4 cm) solid adrenal masses in patients without a known malignancy, regardless of lipid content or washout calculations.

References: Ayala-Ramirez M, Jasim S, Feng L, et al. Adrenocortical carcinoma: clinical outcomes and prognosis of 330 patients at a tertiary care center. *Eur J Endocrinol* 2013;23:169:891–899.
Blake MA, Cronin CG, Boland GW. Adrenal imaging. *AJR Am J Roentgenol* 2010;194:1450–1460.
Cooper AB, Habra MA, Grubbs EG, et al. Does laparoscopic adrenalectomy jeopardize oncologic outcomes for patients with adrenocortical carcinoma? *Surg Endosc* 2013;27:4026–4032.

17 **Answer D.**   Compared with traditional spin echo imaging, gradient echo imaging usually is characterized by use of a bipolar readout gradient (frequency-encoding gradient) to create an echo (as opposed to a 180-degree refocusing RF pulse), smaller flip angles (<90 degrees and often <30 degrees), greater T2* effects, and residual transverse magnetization. With smaller flip angles, shorter TRs and TEs can be used, and shorter TRs permit faster imaging. A side effect of faster imaging with smaller flip angles is the potential for persistent residual transverse (M_{xy}) magnetization. This occurs if the transverse magnetization vector is not allowed to fully relax between each excitation. Residual transverse magnetization can contribute to the MR signal and alter tissue contrast—in particular, it can contaminate T1-weighted images. One method of reducing this is through the use of RF spoiling and spoiler gradients (i.e., spoiled gradient echo). Spoiling destroys residual transverse magnetization, permitting even faster acquisition of T1-weighted images.

References: Brown MA, Semelka RC. MR imaging abbreviations, definitions, and descriptions: a review. *Radiology* 1999;213:647–662.

McRobbie DW, Moore EA, Graves MJ, et al. *MRI: From picture to proton*, 2nd ed. New York: Cambridge University Press, 2007.

18 **Answer A.** Placing the patient ipsilateral side down will restrict diaphragmatic motion, compress the ipsilateral lung, and decrease ipsilateral tidal volume. This can be a useful maneuver to minimize the risk of pneumothorax for biopsies in the upper abdomen. The risk of pneumothorax increases for patients placed in the prone or contralateral-side down positions, because both positions increase the excursion of the ipsilateral lung.

Another method that can be used to minimize the risk of pneumothorax is hydrodissection of the paraspinal space. This maintains the needle in an extrapleural position along its entire course.

References: Sharma KV, Venkatesan AM, Swerdlow D, et al. Image-guided adrenal and renal biopsy. *Tech Vasc Interv Radiol* 2010;13:100–109.

Tyng CJ, Bitencourt AGV, Martins EBL, et al. Technical note: CT-guided paravertebral adrenal biopsy using hydrodissection—a safe and technically easy approach. *Br J Radiol* 2012;85:e339–e342.

19 **Answer D.** Current evidence shows that the risk of administering intravenous low-osmolality iodinated contrast material (IV LOCM) to a patient with pheochromocytoma (regardless of active alpha- and beta-blockade) is likely no different than that of the general population. Historically, there were reports of increased circulating catecholamines and hypertensive crisis following exposure to high-osmolality iodinated contrast material (HOCM), and this led to caution for modern agents. However, several series have since shown no change in circulating catecholamines and no increase in adverse events following IV LOCM exposure in patients with known pheochromocytoma (with or without alpha- and beta-blockade).

References: Baid SK, Lai EW, Wesley RA, et al. Brief communication: radiographic contrast infusion and catecholamine release in patients with pheochromocytoma. *Ann Intern Med* 2009;6:150:27–32.

Bessell-Browne R, O'Malley ME. CT of pheochromocytoma and paraganglioma: risk of adverse events with i.v. administration of nonionic contrast material. *AJR Am J Roentgenol* 2007;188:970–974.

Mukherjee JJ, Peppercorn PD, Reznek RH, et al. Pheochromocytoma: effect of nonionic contrast medium in CT on circulating catecholamine levels. *Radiology* 1997;202:227–231.

20 **Answer A.** The images demonstrate homogeneous signal loss throughout the right adrenal nodule on opposed-phase imaging consistent with diffuse microscopic fat (i.e., "intracellular lipid"). For a homogeneous adrenal nodule <4 cm in the absence of a known confounder (e.g., clear cell renal cell carcinoma, hepatocellular carcinoma), this is diagnostic of a benign lipid-rich adrenal adenoma. Other than possible biochemical testing to determine if the nodule is secreting hormone(s), no further testing is required. The degree of signal loss required for this diagnosis varies based on the type of imaging sequence and field strength, but historically, a loss in signal of 16.5% or more is considered sufficient. Many prefer a qualitative assessment over a quantitative assessment (i.e., "obvious" loss of signal intensity without use of a numeric threshold). In fact, qualitative assessment has been shown to perform similarly to quantitative assessment in the discrimination of adenomas from metastases.

References: American Medical Association of Clinical Endocrinologists and American Association of Endocrine Surgeons: Medical Guidelines for the Management of Adrenal Incidentalomas. AACE/AAES Guidelines, 2009.

Blake MA, Cronin CG, Boland GW. Adrenal imaging. *AJR Am J Roentgenol* 2010;194:1450–1460.

Mayo-Smith WW, Lee MJ, McNicholas MM, et al. Characterization of adrenal masses (<5 cm) by use of chemical shift MR imaging: observer performance versus quantitative measures. *AJR Am J Roentgenol* 1995;165:91–95.

21 **Answer D.**   The spleen has been shown to be the best internal control on chemical shift imaging when attempting to determine the degree of signal loss within the adrenal gland. This is because the spleen does not have internal lipid content that might confound interpretation (such as is often present in the liver). However, a splenic reference standard may be complicated by the presence of secondary splenic siderosis, which will show signal loss on the longer echo time dual-echo GRE images. The pancreas is not ideal because interdigitating fat can generate India ink artifact, and the kidney is not ideal because it is uncommonly in the same plane of section as the adrenal gland(s).

References: Mayo-Smith WW, Lee MJ, McNicholas MM, et al. Characterization of adrenal masses (<5 cm) by use of chemical shift MR imaging: observer performance versus quantitative measures. *AJR Am J Roentgenol* 1995;165:91–95.

Blake MA, Cronin CG, Boland GW. Adrenal imaging. *AJR Am J Roentgenol* 2010;194:1450–1460.

22 **Answer B.**   The image demonstrates a "flattened" or "single-limbed" (pancake) adrenal gland. This appearance has a strong association with ipsilateral renal anomalies—in particular, any abnormality in which the ipsilateral kidney does not form properly in the renal fossa (e.g., renal agenesis, crossed fused ectopia, pelvic kidney). The normal "V"- or "Y"-shaped appearance of the adrenal gland appears to require the coexistence of the kidney in the renal fossa to develop.

"Single-limbed" adrenal glands have little clinical importance beyond the indication that the ipsilateral kidney is congenitally abnormal; for example, the finding is a clue that a missing kidney is congenitally absent and was not surgically removed.

References: Dyer RB, Chen MY, Zagoria RJ. Classic signs in uroradiology. *Radiographics* 2004;24(suppl 1):S247–S280.

Hoffman CK, Filly RA, Callen PW. The "lying down" adrenal sign: a sonographic indicator of renal agenesis or ectopia in fetuses and neonates. *J Ultrasound Med* 1992;11:533–536.

Kenney PJ, Robbins GL, Ellis DA, et al. Adrenal glands in patients with congenital renal anomalies: CT appearance. *Radiology* 1985;155:181–182.

23 **Answer D.**   Laboratory testing is the best next step to determine the likelihood that the mass is biochemically active. Although the mass is markedly hyperintense on T2-weighted images, this finding is neither sensitive nor specific for pheochromocytoma. In a series of 67 adrenal masses including 17 pheochromocytomas (Varghese, 1997), the positive predictive value of the T2-weighted character of an adrenal mass for the prediction of pheochromocytoma was only 65%. Surgery (Answer A) is not the best next step because the mass may be benign and nonfunctional. Biopsy (Answer C) and adrenergic blockade (Answer B) are not appropriate until it is determined whether the mass is a pheochromocytoma. Biopsy of a pheochromocytoma without first providing proper adrenergic blockade can lead to a hypertensive crisis.

References: Varghese JC, Hahn PF, Papanicolaou N, et al. MR differentiation of phaeochromocytoma from other adrenal lesions based on qualitative analysis of T2 relaxation times. *Clin Radiol* 1997;52:603–606.

Elsayes KM, Narra VR, Leyendecker JR, et al. MRI of adrenal and extraadrenal pheochromocytoma. *AJR Am J Roentgenol* 2005;184:860–867.

24 **Answer C.** Adrenal myelolipomas are characterized by the presence of macroscopic fat. Macroscopic fat can be identified with MR using a variety of techniques; among them is inversion recovery. With conventional spin echo–based inversion recovery imaging, a 180-degree preparation radiofrequency pulse is applied before a 90-degree excitation radiofrequency pulse. After a sufficient length of time has passed (the inversion recovery time [TI]: the time between the 180-degree and 90-degree pulses, equal to ln(2) of the T1 time of fat), the fat protons will recover to a point of zero net magnetization. If the 90-degree pulse is delivered at that time (the null point of fat), the fat protons will have no longitudinal magnetization to contribute to the signal.

References: Brown MA, Semelka RC. MR imaging abbreviations, definitions, and descriptions: a review. *Radiology* 1999;213:647–662.

McRobbie DW, Moore EA, Graves MJ, et al. *MRI: From picture to proton*, 2nd ed. New York: Cambridge University Press, 2007.

25 **Answer D.** The images demonstrate a 2.2-cm posterior gastric diverticulum containing gas. Posterior gastric diverticula can simulate adrenal masses, particularly when the diverticula lack internal gas. If the diagnosis is in doubt, oral contrast material can be used to distinguish the two entities. The majority (75%) of true gastric diverticula arise from the posterior fundus like this one. Most are innocuous and require no additional management; however, it is important to recognize this benign finding and distinguish it from a solid lesion.

References: Schwartz AN, Goiney RC, Graney DO. Gastric diverticulum simulating an adrenal mass: CT appearance and embryogenesis. *AJR Am J Roentgenol* 1986;146:553–554.

Anaise D, Brand DL, Smith NL, et al. Pitfalls in the diagnosis and treatment of a symptomatic gastric diverticulum. *Gastrointest Endosc* 1984;30:28–30.

26 **Answer D.** The organ at greatest risk if no precautionary measures are taken is the thyroid gland. Free radioactive iodine that has dissociated from the I[131]-MIGB complex can be taken up by the thyroid gland and remain in situ for several weeks. To prevent this from happening, patients who are scheduled to undergo radioactive MIBG scanning are given potassium iodide pills or perchlorate. The other answers are part of the normal biodistribution of I[131]-MIBG, but the spleen, myocardium, and adrenal glands are less radiosensitive than the thyroid gland. Because I[131] has a much longer half-life than I[123], many centers performing MIBG now preferentially use I[123] instead of I[131] to lessen the radiation dose and permit injection of higher activity levels. I[131] MIBG and I[123] MIBG have identical biodistributions.

References: Nakajo M, Shapiro B, Copp J, et al. The normal and abnormal distribution of the adrenomedullary imaging agent m-[I-131]iodobenzylguanidine (I-131 MIBG) in man: evaluation by scintigraphy. *J Nucl Med* 1983;672–682.

Olivier P, Colarinha P, Fettich J, et al. Guidelines for radioiodinated MIBG scintigraphy in children. Paediatric Committee of the European Association of Nuclear Medicine. *Eur J Nucl Med Mol Imaging.* 2003;30(5):B45–B50.

27 **Answer B.** The most likely diagnosis is neuroblastoma. The images demonstrate a solid mass in the right suprarenal fossa that shows uptake of I[123]-MIBG. This constellation of imaging findings raises the possibility of neuroblastoma (Answer B, most likely in this age group) and pheochromocytoma (Answer D, unlikely given the patient's age). Neuroblastoma usually occurs in young children (e.g., <5 years of age), while pheochromocytoma usually develops in adolescents and adults. If the distinction is in doubt, measurement of fractionated catecholamines and fractionated metanephrines can differentiate these two entities (fractionated levels will be elevated in only pheochromocytoma, while unfractionated levels can be elevated in both diseases). Adrenocortical carcinoma (Answer C) and sarcoma (Answer A) will not typically show uptake on I^{123}-MIBG scans.

References: Lonergan GJ, Schwab CM, Suarez ES, et al. Neuroblastoma, ganglioneuroblastoma, and ganglioneuroma: radiologic-pathologic correlation. *Radiographics* 2002;22:911–934.

Pham TH, Moir C, Thompson GB, et al. Pheochromocytoma and paraganglioma in children: a review of medical and surgical management at a tertiary care center. *Pediatrics* 2006;118:1109–1117.

28 Answer B. The organ of Zuckerkandl is located in the retroperitoneum between the inferior mesenteric artery origin and the aortic bifurcation. Like the other possible answers, the organ of Zuckerkandl is a common site of paraganglioma development.

References: Elsayes KM, Narra VR, Leyendecker JR, et al. MRI of adrenal and extraadrenal pheochromocytoma. *AJR Am J Roentgenol* 2005;184:860–867.

Lee KY, Oh YW, Noh HJ, et al. Extraadrenal paragangliomas of the body: imaging features. *AJR Am J Roentgenol* 2006;187:492–504.

29 Answer C. Neurofibromatosis type I is associated with pheochromocytoma development, in addition to café au lait spots, skin pigmentation, neurofibromas, plexiform neurofibromas, malignant peripheral nerve sheath tumors, optic gliomas, and other cancers.

Multiple endocrine neoplasia (MEN) type I (Answer A) is associated with pituitary adenomas, parathyroid adenomas, and pancreatic neuroendocrine tumors (so-called pit-para-pan). Within the MEN family, MEN type IIa and MEN type IIb are associated with pheochromocytoma. Beckwith-Wiedemann syndrome (Answer B) is associated with hemihypertrophy, macroglossia, abdominal wall defects, Wilms' tumor (nephroblastoma), hepatoblastoma, neonatal hypoglycemia, and other cancers.

Hereditary leiomyomatosis renal cell cancer (HLRCC) syndrome (Answer D) is associated with cutaneous leiomyomas, uterine leiomyomas (fibroids), and type II papillary renal cell carcinoma (an aggressive variant of papillary renal cell carcinoma).

References: Choyke PL, Glenn GM, Walther MM, et al. Hereditary renal cancers. *Radiology* 2003;226:33–46.

Grubb RL III, Franks ME, Toro J, et al. Hereditary leiomyomatosis and renal cell cancer: a syndrome associated with an aggressive form of inherited cancer. *J Urol* 2007;177:2074–2079.

Levy AD, Patel N, Dow N, et al. Abdominal neoplasms in patients with neurofibromatosis type I: radiologic-pathologic correlation. *Radiographics* 2005;25:455–480.

Scarsbrook AF, Thakker RV, Wass JAH, et al. Multiple endocrine neoplasia: spectrum of radiologic appearances and discussion of multitechnique imaging approach. *Radiographics* 2006;26:433–451.

30 Answer C. Simple calcifications without an associated mass are most commonly attributable to prior hemorrhage. Other potential etiologies include granulomatous infection (e.g., histoplasmosis, tuberculosis) and sarcoidosis. Some masses of the adrenal gland can also contain calcifications (e.g., peripherally calcified pseudocysts, adrenocortical carcinoma, specific types of metastases [mucinous adenocarcinoma, osteosarcoma, papillary thyroid cancer], pheochromocytoma, neuroblastoma), but there is no mass evident on the image from this question.

References: Hindman N, Israel GM. Adrenal gland and adrenal mass calcification. *Eur Radiol* 2005;15:1163–1167.

Johnson PT, Horton KM, Fishman EK. Adrenal imaging with MDCT: nonneoplastic disease. *AJR Am J Roentgenol* 2009;193:1128–1135.

1 Management of renal calculus disease is multifactorial, but one key component is the mineral composition of the stone(s). Pure attenuation-based methods are unreliable, but dual-energy CT has shown promise as a method of noninvasively characterizing renal stone composition. On what principle is this technique based?

   A. The likelihood of Compton scatter in unique elements imaged at differing kVp settings
   B. The difference in K-edge of unique elements imaged at differing kVp settings
   C. The change in noise levels within a particular structure imaged at differing kVp settings
   D. The change in apparent size of a particular structure imaged at differing kVp settings

2 What are the common radiographic manifestations of medullary sponge kidney?

   A. Cortical nephrocalcinosis alone
   B. Cortical nephrocalcinosis and renal tubular ectasia
   C. Medullary nephrocalcinosis alone
   D. Medullary nephrocalcinosis and renal tubular ectasia

3 Which of the following correctly describes the normal temporal progression of radiographic contrast material uptake and excretion from the kidneys?

   A. Corticomedullary, nephrographic, pyelographic
   B. Corticomedullary, pyelographic, nephrographic
   C. Nephrographic, corticomedullary, pyelographic
   D. Nephrographic, pyelographic, corticomedullary
   E. Pyelographic, corticomedullary, nephrographic
   F. Pyelographic, nephrographic, corticomedullary

4 A 65-year-old male with bladder cancer undergoes a loopogram for upper tract surveillance. Which of the following diseases is a common cause of the imaging findings in the lower pole of the left kidney?

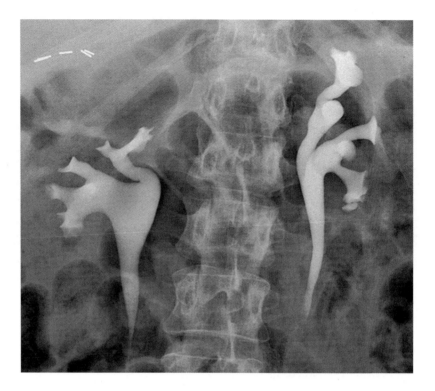

A. Tuberous sclerosis
B. Diabetes mellitus
C. Hypertension
D. Urothelial carcinoma

5 A 3-year-old boy with a congenital left ureteropelvic junction (UPJ) obstruction related to a crossing vessel undergoes MR urography. The image on the left was acquired with a repetition time (TR) of 2,000 msec and an echo time (TE) of 200 msec. The image on the right was obtained at the same level with a TR of 3.6 msec and a TE of 1.8 msec. What is the most likely cause of the hypointense material in the left renal pelvis on the right-hand image?

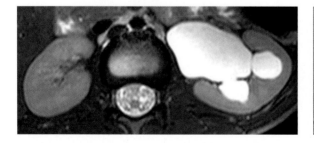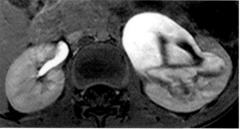

A. Hemorrhage
B. Malignancy
C. Contrast material
D. Parasitic infection
E. The etiology cannot be determined with the provided images.

6   A 25-year-old male with vesicoureteric reflux presents with right flank discomfort, and an ultrasound is obtained. The arcuate arteries are sampled within each kidney and compared to assess for symmetry. What is the formula for calculating the resistive index?

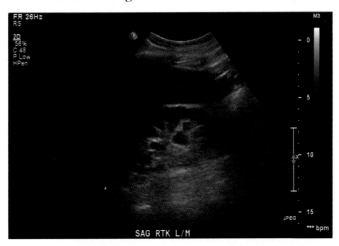 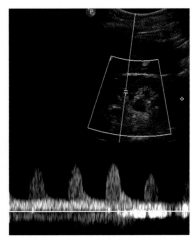

A. (Peak systolic velocity – End-diastolic velocity)/Peak systolic velocity
B. (End-diastolic velocity – Peak systolic velocity)/Peak diastolic velocity
C. (Peak systolic velocity – End-diastolic velocity)/End-systolic velocity
D. (End-diastolic velocity – Peak systolic velocity)/End-diastolic velocity
E. End-diastolic velocity/Peak systolic velocity
F. End-systolic velocity/Peak diastolic velocity
G. End-diastolic velocity/Peak diastolic velocity
H. End systolic velocity/Peak systolic velocity

7   A 62-year-old male with a 40-pack-year smoking history, chronic obstructive pulmonary disease, and hematuria presents for a CT urogram and subsequent right retrograde pyelogram. What are the two most common causes of this imaging finding?

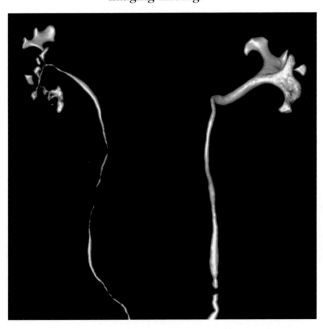 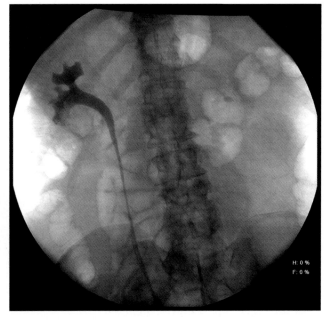

A. Urothelial cancer and *Mycobacterium tuberculosis*
B. Urothelial cancer and renal calculus disease
C. *Schistosoma haematobium* and *Proteus mirabilis*
D. *Escherichia coli* and *Proteus mirabilis*

8 A 22-year-old pregnant female in the third trimester with suspected stone disease undergoes an ultrasound examination that demonstrates moderate dilation of the proximal right collecting system and asymmetric resistive indices. The referring service requests a low-dose unenhanced renal stone protocol CT of the abdomen and pelvis. If the effective dose to the fetus is 10 mSv, what is the approximate risk of radiation-induced cancer conferred to the fetus?

A. The exact risk is speculative, but it is estimated to be roughly 1 in 250 (0.4%).
B. The exact risk is speculative, but it is estimated to be roughly 1 in 25 (4%).
C. The exact risk is speculative, but it is estimated to be roughly 1 in 5 (20%).
D. The exact risk is speculative, but it is estimated to be roughly 1 in 2 (50%).

9 A 42-year-old female with microhematuria undergoes an intravenous urogram. The only identifiable abnormality is a completely duplicated right collecting system (shown below). With respect to this finding, what does the Weigert-Meyer rule predict?

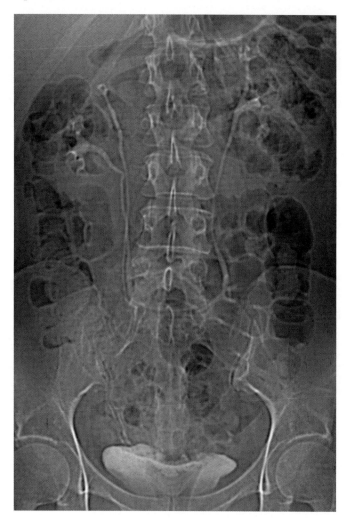

A. The upper pole moiety will insert superior and medial to the lower pole moiety.
B. The upper pole moiety will insert inferior and medial to the lower pole moiety.
C. The upper pole moiety will insert superior and lateral to the lower pole moiety.
D. The upper pole moiety will insert inferior and lateral to the lower pole moiety.

10 A 22-year-old nonsmoking female with no past medical history presents with asymptomatic microhematuria (≥3 red blood cells per high-powered field) detected during a preemployment urinalysis. A triphasic CT urogram is ordered. What is the best next step?

A. Perform the CT urogram as ordered.
B. Recommend a limited CT urogram (two of three phases).
C. Recommend an unenhanced CT.
D. Consider cancelling the test.

11 A 40-year-old male with recurrent urolithiasis undergoes an unenhanced CT of the abdomen and pelvis. The following exam card is reported by the scanner at the end of the study. What does the number 15.42 represent?

			Dose Report		
Series	Type	Scan Range (mm)	CTDIvol (mGy)	DLP (mGy–cm)	Phantom cm
1	Scout	–	–	–	–
2	Helical	14.000–1491.500	15.42	850.84	Body 32
			Total Exam DLP:	850.84	

1/1

A. It is the radiation dose delivered to the patient.
B. It is the scanner-specific radiation output.
C. It is the radiation dose delivered to a hypothetical patient.
D. It is the radiation output delivered by a hypothetical scanner.

12 A 32-year-old pregnant female in her second trimester presents with right flank pain. A retroperitoneal ultrasound is performed, demonstrating bilateral ureteral jets. Which of the following best explains the principle of color Doppler imaging?

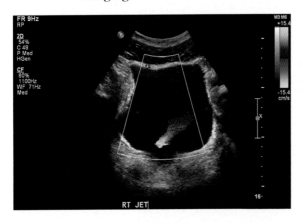 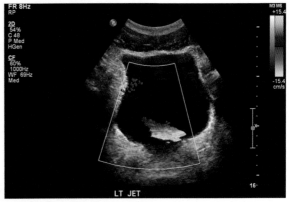

A. The reflected ultrasound frequency always increases when the ultrasound beam interacts with a structure moving toward it.
B. The reflected ultrasound wavelength always increases when the ultrasound beam interacts with a structure moving toward it.
C. Red pixels are always assigned when the ultrasound beam interacts with a structure moving toward it.
D. Blue pixels are always assigned when the ultrasound beam interacts with a structure moving toward it.

13 A 55-year-old male with gross hematuria undergoes a CT urogram consisting of unenhanced, nephrographic, and excretory phase images of the abdomen and pelvis. The following exam card is reported by the scanner at the end of the study. What is the effective dose to the patient?

Dose Report					
Series	Type	Scan Range (mm)	CTDIvol (mGy)	DLP (mGy-cm)	Phantom cm
1	Scout	–	–	–	–
2	Helical	I3.750–I381.250	4.61	203.49	Body 32
4	Helical	S38.000–I395.125	8.24	410.11	Body 32
4	Helical	S3.250–I378.000	8.20	365.29	Body 32
			Total Exam DLP:	978.89	

1/1

A. 8.24 mGy
B. 21.05 mGy
C. 978.89 mGy-cm
D. The effective dose cannot be determined with these data.

14 A 5-year-old boy with congenital orthotopic megaureter undergoes MR urography to assess anatomy and function. Three-dimensional reconstructions were performed of the coronal source data. The image on the left was obtained with a repetition time (TR) of 4,000 msec and an echo time (TE) of 200 msec. The image on the right was obtained with a TR of 3.6 msec and a TE of 1.8 msec. What is the approximate relative function of the two kidneys?

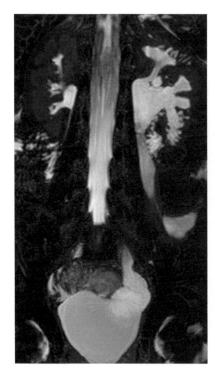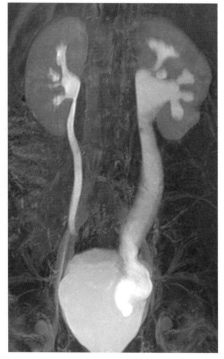

A. The right kidney is substantially less functional than is the left kidney.
B. The left kidney is substantially less functional than is the right kidney.
C. The two kidneys have grossly similar function.
D. The relative function of the kidneys cannot be estimated with these images.

15 A 52-year-old male with diabetes mellitus, fever, and leukocytosis presents with left flank pain. Vital signs are as follows: pulse 115, blood pressure 89/65, respiratory rate 22, SpO_2 98% on room air. The following ultrasound is obtained. What is the most likely diagnosis?

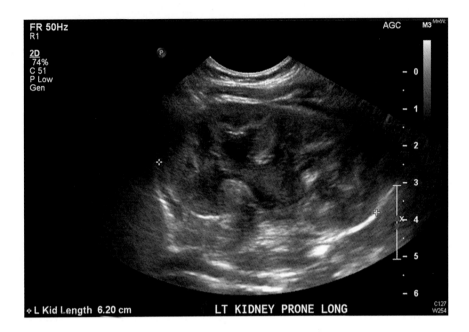

A. Pyelonephritis
B. Pyelitis
C. Pyonephrosis
D. Emphysematous pyelitis
E. Emphysematous pyelonephritis

16 A 7-year-old girl with recurrent pyelonephritis undergoes a voiding cystourethrogram (VCUG). What is the diagnosis?

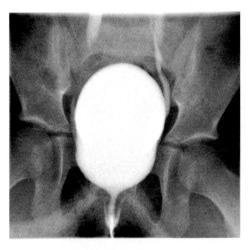
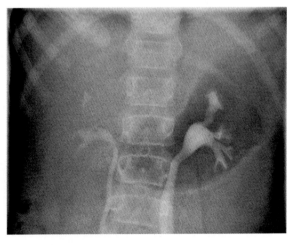

A. Normal study
B. Bilateral grade I vesicoureteric reflux
C. Bilateral grade II vesicoureteric reflux
D. Bilateral grade IV vesicoureteric reflux

17 A 70-year-old male undergoes bilateral percutaneous nephrostomy catheter placement. Which of the following best characterizes the imaging findings in the midportions of the ureters?

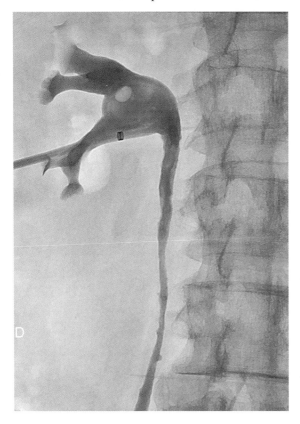
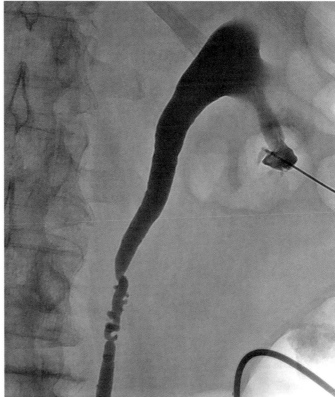

A. Malignant condition associated with urothelial carcinoma
B. Benign condition associated with urothelial carcinoma
C. Benign vascular impressions
D. Benign ureteral "kinks"

18 An 8-year-old girl with recurrent abdominal pain undergoes a retroperitoneal ultrasound. Which of the following is the best explanation for the imaging finding(s) in the left kidney?

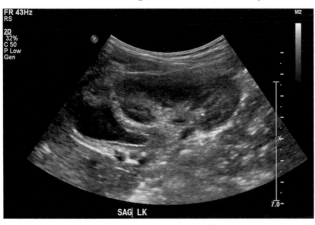
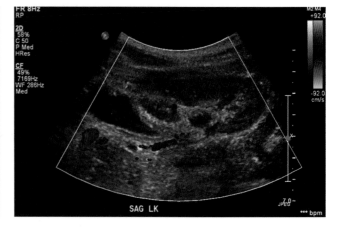

A. Multicystic dysplastic kidney
B. Autosomal dominant polycystic kidney disease
C. Acquired renal cyst
D. Obstructed ectopic ureter
E. Autosomal recessive polycystic kidney disease

19 A 55-year-old male with asymptomatic microscopic hematuria undergoes a CT urogram. Representative images below depict an abnormality in the left kidney. What is the most appropriate management for this entity?

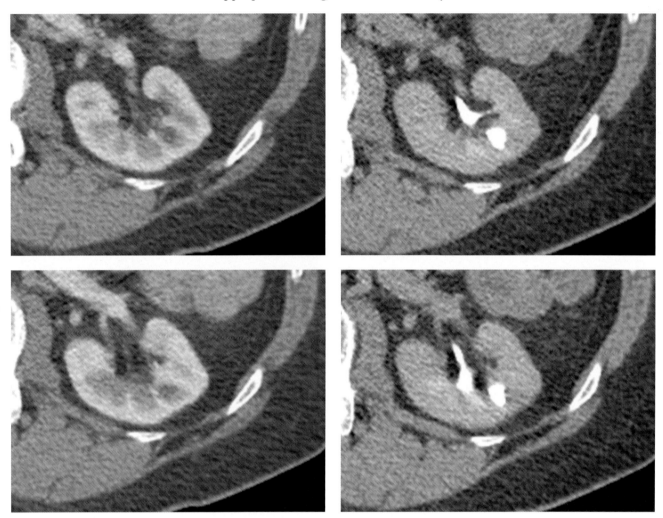

A. Ignore (benign finding)
B. Prophylactic antibiotics
C. Percutaneous aspiration
D. Embolization
E. Operative resection

20 A 50-year-old male with recurrent urolithiasis undergoes an unenhanced CT of the abdomen and pelvis with a $CTDI_{vol}$ of 14 mGy based on a 32-cm-diameter body dosimetry phantom. His effective diameter $\left[\sqrt{(\text{AP diameter} \times \text{transverse diameter})} \right]$ is 17 cm, which translates to a 1.98 f_{size}^{32cm} conversion factor, and the DLP is 700 mGy-cm (scan length: 50 cm). What is this patient's size-specific dose estimate (SSDE)?

A. 7.1 mGY
B. 27.7 mGy
C. 353.5 mGy-cm
D. 1,386 mGy-cm
E. The SSDE cannot be determined with these data.

21 A 60-year-old male with gross hematuria and a negative cystoscopy undergoes a CT urogram that demonstrates an abnormality in the left proximal collecting system. Which of the following is a correct comparison between upper tract urothelial cancer and bladder cancer?

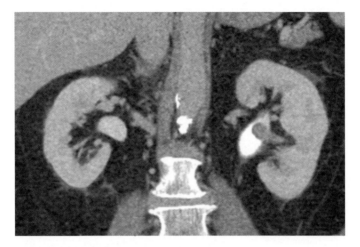

A. Upper tract urothelial cancer is more common than is bladder cancer.
B. Upper tract urothelial cancer is less likely to be invasive than is bladder cancer.
C. Smoking is a risk factor for bladder cancer but not for upper tract urothelial cancer.
D. Aromatic hydrocarbons cause both bladder cancer and upper tract urothelial cancer.

22 A 63-year-old male with a history of urothelial carcinoma of the right renal pelvis and bladder, and who is status post right nephroureterectomy, cystoprostatectomy, and ileal loop creation with an end-to-end anastomosis, undergoes a loopogram to assess for leak. How should the contrast material in the left collecting system be characterized?

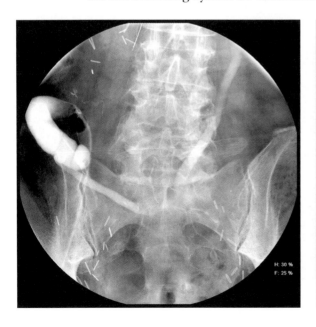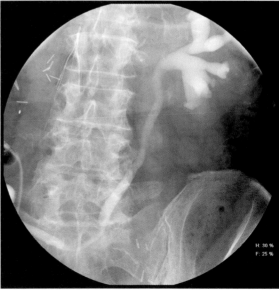

A. Abnormal spontaneous reflux, grade I
B. Abnormal spontaneous reflux, grade III
C. Abnormal spontaneous reflux, grade V
D. Expected finding

23   A 62-year-old male with hydronephrosis undergoes a right retrograde pyelogram. What is the name of this finding, and what does it imply?

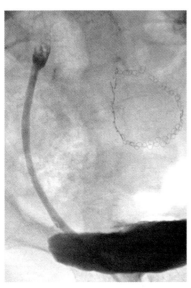
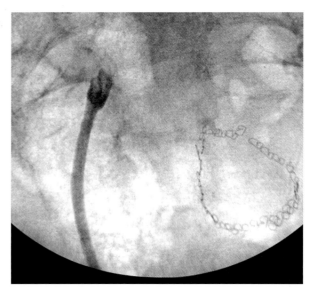

     A. Goblet sign, which supports the diagnosis of a urothelial malignancy

     B. Goblet sign, which supports the diagnosis of a ureteral calculus

     C. Comet tail sign, which supports the diagnosis of a urothelial malignancy

     D. Comet tail sign, which supports the diagnosis of a ureteral calculus

24   A 2-year-old girl with an abnormal abdominal ultrasound undergoes a voiding cystourethrogram (VCUG). What is the most likely diagnosis?

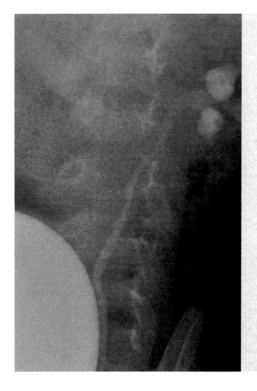
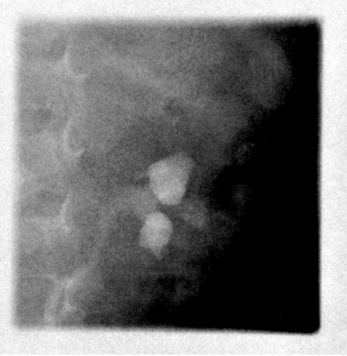

     A. Grade III reflux

     B. Grade III reflux and congenital duplication

     C. Opacification of an obstructed collecting system

     D. Opacification of a normal collecting system

25 Unnecessary renal stone CT examinations are commonly cited as a major source of radiation exposure in young patients, and efforts are underway to minimize the radiation dose from these examinations. What is the principal effect of statistical iterative reconstruction?

A. Improve image signal
B. Improve image contrast
C. Decrease radiation dose
D. Decrease image noise

26 A 25-year-old male with right lower quadrant pain and suspected appendicitis presents for a contrast-enhanced CT of the abdomen and pelvis. The effective dose is estimated to be 10 mSv. How does this compare to the typical annual natural background radiation dose for United States citizens living at sea level?

A. It is approximately five times the annual background dose of 2 mSv.
B. It is approximately 50 times the annual background dose of 0.2 mSv.
C. It is approximately 500 times the annual background dose of 0.02 mSv.
D. It is approximately 5,000 times the annual background dose of 0.002 mSv.

27 A 32-year-old female with left flank pain and hematuria undergoes an unenhanced renal stone protocol CT of the abdomen and pelvis. Which imaging sign best characterizes the more anterior calcification in the left hemipelvis, and what does it imply?

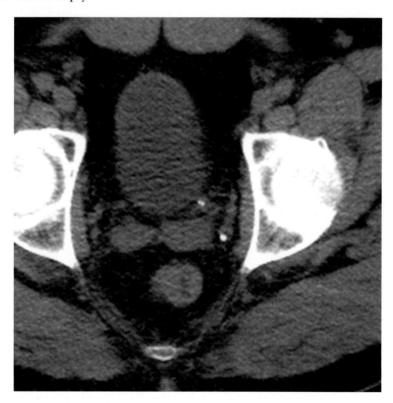

A. Comet tail sign, which supports the diagnosis of a ureteral calculus
B. Comet tail sign, which supports the diagnosis of a phlebolith
C. Soft-tissue "rim" sign, which supports the diagnosis of a ureteral calculus
D. Soft-tissue "rim" sign, which supports the diagnosis of a phlebolith

28 A 50-year-old male with recurrent urinary tract infections undergoes an
abdominal radiograph demonstrating a large calcification in the right upper
quadrant. This calcification is likely comprised of what dominant material?

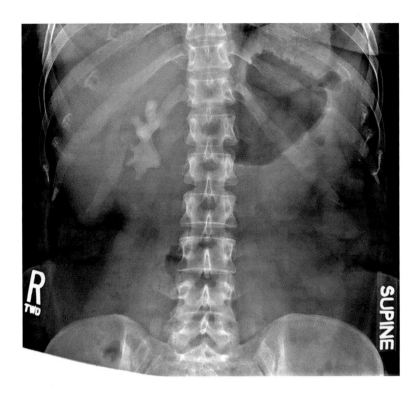

A. Calcium oxalate
B. Calcium phosphate
C. Struvite
D. Cystine
E. Uric acid

29 A radiology practice is interested in updating their abdominal CT scan protocols
to reduce the radiation dose to their patients. What effect would a lower kVp
setting (e.g., 80 kVp instead of 120 kVp) have on the resultant images?

A. Decreased image noise
B. Increased radiation dose
C. Increased attenuation of iodine
D. Decreased pseudoenhancement

30 A new imaging modality is developed for the detection of upper tract urothelial
carcinoma. Its feasibility is tested in a small patient population. The test identifies
cancer in three patients with the disease and two patients without the disease. The
test is "negative" in one patient with the disease and eight patients without the
disease. What are the sensitivity and specificity of this test based on these data?

A. Sensitivity: 75%, specificity: 20%
B. Sensitivity: 25%, specificity: 80%
C. Sensitivity: 75%, specificity: 80%
D. Sensitivity: 25%, specificity: 20%

ANSWERS AND EXPLANATIONS

1 **Answer B.**   Dual-energy CT is based on the principle of distinguishing elements that have sufficiently unique K-edges by imaging them with two different kVp settings. When an atom is struck by a photon of sufficient energy to dislodge an electron from the K-shell of that atom, the electron can be discharged and replaced by an electron from a neighboring ring. When this occurs, an x-ray photon is discharged. This phenomenon is known as the photoelectric effect.

Just above the K-shell binding energy is the K-edge, which is characterized by a sudden increase in attenuation at that energy level caused by a sudden increase in the probability of the photoelectric effect occurring. The K-edge is element specific and increases with increasing atomic number. When two elements with sufficiently unique K-edges are imaged with two different kVp settings (most commonly 80 and 140 kVp on clinical scanners), it is possible to determine the composition of those elements by the way they behave in the radiation environment. The attenuation of those elements at varying kVp settings gives information about their K-edge, and allows one to determine indirectly what they are.

Most elements that constitute the human body (e.g., carbon, hydrogen, oxygen, nitrogen) have very similar K-edges (range: 0.01 to 0.53 keV), making them unlikely candidates for dual-energy separation. However, minerals (e.g., calcium [K-edge: 4.0 keV]) and iodine (e.g., iodinated contrast material [K-edge: 33.2 keV]) are different enough from background tissue that separation is possible. Once separation is achieved, those elements can be characterized, quantified, and/or removed from the image. This forms the foundation of dual-energy characterization of renal calculi and permits the creation of "virtual unenhanced" CT.

References: Boll DT, Patil NA, Paulson EK, et al. Renal stone assessment with dual-energy multidetector CT and advanced postprocessing techniques: improved characterization of renal stone composition—Pilot study. *Radiology* 2009;250:813–820.
Heye T, Nelson RC, Ho LM, et al. Dual-energy CT applications in the abdomen. *AJR Am J Roentgenol* 2012;199:S64–S70.
Williams JC Jr, Saw KC, Paterson RF, et al. Variability of renal stone fragility in shock wave lithotripsy. *Urology* 2003;61:1092–1096.

2 **Answer D.**   Medullary sponge kidney is characterized by medullary nephrocalcinosis and renal tubular ectasia. Renal tubular ectasia is characterized by radiating parallel linear contrast arrays at the medullary tips (two examples shown below); it should be distinguished from the normal "papillary blush," which is homogeneous, vague, and nonlinear. The underlying abnormality in renal tubular ectasia is a defect in the renal tubules that results in tiny sac-like cysts that impair urine transit and predispose to stone formation. Many patients with renal tubular ectasia do not have calculi or systemic signs of renal disease; in these patients, the ectatic ducts are often thought to be an incidental finding.

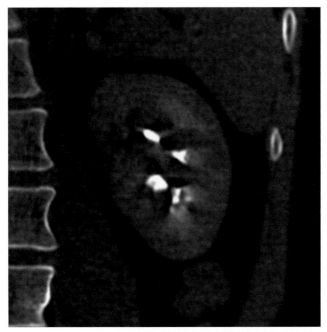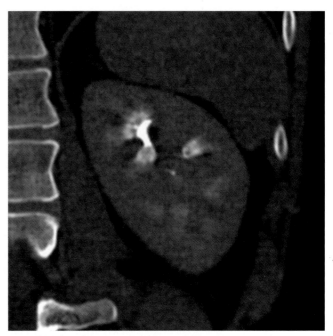

Renal tubular ectasia, characterized by radiating tubular collections at the medullary tips

The differential diagnosis for medullary nephrocalcinosis is:

- Medullary sponge kidney [common cause]
- Type I (distal) renal tubular acidosis [common cause]
- Hyperparathyroidism [common cause]
- Other causes of hypercalcinosis (e.g., hypervitaminosis D, milk–alkali syndrome)
- Sarcoidosis
- Oxaluria
- Furosemide use

The differential diagnosis for cortical nephrocalcinosis is:

- Renal cortical necrosis (secondary to severe systemic hypotension) [common cause]
- Chronic glomerulonephritis [common cause]
- Chronic pyelonephritis
- Alport syndrome
- Oxaluria

Medullary nephrocalcinosis is much more common than is cortical nephrocalcinosis.

References: Dyer RB, Chen MY, Zagoria RJ. Classic signs in uroradiology. *Radiographics* 2004;24:S247–S280.

Fabris A, Anglani F, Lupo A, et al. Medullary sponge kidney: state of the art. *Nephrol Dial Transplant* 2013;28:1111–1119.

Zagoria RJ. *Genitourinary radiology: Radiology requisites series*, 2nd ed. St. Louis: Mosby Publishing, 2004

3 **Answer A.** The normal progression of contrast material uptake and excretion from the kidneys is as follows: unenhanced (prior to contrast material uptake), arterial (20 to 25 seconds postcontrast), corticomedullary (25 to 80 seconds postcontrast), nephrographic (90 to 110 seconds postcontrast), pyelographic (starting ~3 minutes postcontrast and continuing for many minutes). The pyelographic phase is sometimes also referred to as the excretory phase.

The corticomedullary phase is most commonly imaged during routine "portal venous" phase acquisitions that are timed to optimize liver imaging. The nephrographic phase is targeted for renal mass evaluation because the homogeneous appearance of the kidneys in this phase renders it more sensitive for the detection of renal masses than the corticomedullary phase. The pyelographic phase is obtained to evaluate for abnormalities of the collecting system. Although the pyelographic phase begins earlier, most pyelographic phase images are obtained 10 to 15 minutes after contrast material administration to maximize distention of the collecting systems and minimize residual renal parenchymal uptake.

The normal pattern of uptake is important to remember because when the pattern is delayed (at an earlier stage than would be predicted based on the postcontrast timing), it indicates that a functionally significant abnormality is occurring on the affected side(s). In cases where one side is delayed and the other is not, the delayed side is the abnormal side. The generic differential diagnosis for a delayed nephrogram is as follows:

- **"Blood in"**: renal artery stenosis/thrombosis/injury
- **"Blood out"**: renal vein thrombosis
- **"Urine in"**: acute tubular necrosis, pyelonephritis, glomerulonephritis
- **"Urine out"**: collecting system obstruction

References: Dyer RB, Munitz HA, Bechtold R, et al. The abnormal nephrogram. *Radiographics* 1986;6:1039–1063.

Saunders HS, Dyer RB, Shifrin RY, et al. The CT nephrogram: implications for evaluation of urinary tract disease. *Radiographics* 1995;15:1069–1085.

Wolin EA, Hartman DS, Olson RJ. Nephrographic and pyelographic analysis of CT urography: principles, patterns, and pathophysiology. *AJR Am J Roentgenol* 2013;200:1210–1214.

Yuh BI, Cohan RH. Different phases of renal enhancement: role in detecting and characterizing renal masses during helical CT. *AJR Am J Roentgenol* 1999;173:747–755.

4 **Answer B.** The imaging findings are compatible with papillary necrosis, which manifests in a variety of ways: (a) elongated fornix, (b) "lobster claw" deformity, (c) "clubbed" calyx filled with contrast material, (d) "clubbed calyx" filled with nonenhancing debris, (e) "golf-ball-on-a-tee" deformity, and (f) a combination of the above. All of these deformities result from ischemic necrosis of the medullary papilla, often from a microangiopathic process (e.g., diabetes mellitus).

Common causes of papillary necrosis can be remembered with the mnemonic "**NSAID**," which includes

- **N**onsteroidal anti-inflammatory drugs (NSAIDs)
- **S**ickle cell disease
- **A**nalgesic abuse
- **I**nfection (Tuberculosis, fungal)
- **D**iabetes mellitus

References: Dunnick NR, Sandler CM, Newhouse JH. *Textbook of uroradiology*, 5th ed. Philadelphia: Lippincott Williams & Wilkins, 2012.

Jung DC, Kim SHK, Jung SI, et al. Renal papillary necrosis: review and comparison of findings at multi-detector row CT and intravenous urography. *Radiographics* 2006;26:1827–1836.

5 **Answer C.** The hypointense material within the left renal pelvis on the right-hand T1-weighted postcontrast image from the question is concentrated gadolinium-based contrast material (GBCM). Note the homogeneous fluid-signal intensity appearance shown within the same location on the left-hand T2-weighted image. If the material was caused by a fixed filling defect, such as hemorrhage, a mass, or a parasitic infection, the filling defect(s) would likely be visible on the T2-weighted image as well.

The principal diagnostic effect of GBCM is to indirectly shorten the T1 time of adjacent protons, but it also shortens T2 relaxation times. This effect is not noticeable on most T1-weighted images because the T1-shortening effects dominate. However, when gadolinium becomes highly concentrated (e.g., within a dilated renal pelvis, or in the dependent urinary bladder), the T2-shortening effects take over and produce a signal void. Remember that no image reflects purely T1 information or purely T2 information. MR images are a combination of both, with "weighting" toward one or the other based on the desired image contrast.

References: McRobbie DW, Moore EA, Graves MJ, et al. *MRI: From picture to proton*, 2nd ed. New York: Cambridge University Press, 2007.

Mamourian AC. *Practical MR physics*, 1st ed. New York: Oxford University Press, 2010.

6   Answer A.   The formula for calculating the renal arterial resistive index is

$$\text{Resistive Index} = (\text{Peak systolic velocity} - \text{End diastolic velocity}) / \text{Peak systolic velocity}$$

The resistive index (RI) is unit-less, and the normal value in a native kidney is 0.60 to 0.70. In elderly patients, and in patients with chronic kidney disease, it is common to have values ≥ 0.70. The utility of the resistive index is debated because it is not a sensitive marker for partial or incomplete obstruction. In a patient with a dilated system, a difference in RIs between the ipsilateral (greater RI) and contralateral (lower RI) side ≥ 0.08 to 0.10 is strongly suggestive of an acute obstruction. These changes are most commonly observed 6 to 48 hours after the inciting event.

It is important to remember that grayscale sonography only reveals anatomic information; in particular, dilation or no dilation. Collecting system dilation is not always due to obstruction. It also can be seen in patients with previous obstruction (now relieved), vesicoureteric reflux, and postsurgical change.

References: Opdenakker L, Oyen R, Vervlosessem I, et al. Acute obstruction of the renal collecting system: the intrarenal resistive index is a useful yet time-dependent parameter for diagnosis. *Eur Radiol* 1998;8;1429–1432.

Platt JF, Rubin JM, Ellis JH, et al. Duplex Doppler US of the kidney: differentiation of obstructive from nonobstructive dilation. *Radiology* 1989;171:515–517.

Tublin ME, Bude RO, Platt JF. The resistive index in renal Doppler sonography: where do we stand? *AJR Am J Roentgenol* 2003;180:885–892.

7   Answer A.   The images demonstrate an "amputated calyx," which is an infundibular stricture that results in dilation of the upstream calyces and nonvisualization of the infundibulum. It is most commonly seen in the setting of upper tract urothelial cancer and, in endemic areas, genitourinary tuberculosis.

Renal calculi (Answer B) do not typically cause this appearance. *Schistosoma haematobium* (Answer C) produces an ascending infection of the urinary tract associated with hemorrhagic cystitis, bladder wall calcifications, and squamous cell carcinoma of the bladder. Urinary strictures associated with *Schistosoma haematobium* usually concentrate in the distal ureters. *Proteus mirabilis* (Answers C and D) is a urease-producing organism that infects the urinary tract and is associated with staghorn calculi. *Escherichia coli* (Answer D) is one of the most common causes of urinary tract infection in the United States. Neither *Proteus mirabilis* nor *Escherichia coli* are common causes of urinary tract strictures.

References: Dyer RB, Chen MY, Zagoria RJ. Classic signs in uroradiology. *Radiographics* 2004;24:S247–S280.

Gupta K, Hooton TM, Naber KG, et al. International clinical practice guidelines for the treatment of acute uncomplicated cystitis and pyelonephritis in women: a 2010 update by the

Infectious Diseases Society of North America and the European Society for Microbiology and Infectious Diseases. *Clin Infect Dis* 2011;52:e103–e120.

Segura JW. Staghorn calculi. *Urol Clin North Am* 1997;24:71–80.

Shebel HM, Elsayes KM, Abou El Atta HM, et al. Genitourinary schistosomiasis: life cycle and radiologic-pathologic findings. *Radiographics* 2012;32:1031–1046.

8 **Answer A.** Stochastic effects at doses <100 mSv are speculative and based on the "linear-no-threshold" model, but the risk of cancer induction is estimated to be roughly 0.01% (1 in 1,000) for an adult patient who receives an effective dose of 10 mSv. The risk likely is higher for young adults, children, infants, and fetuses. The risk to a newborn infant is estimated to be roughly 0.4% (1 in 250) per 10 mSv dose; the risk to a fetus in the second or third trimester is likely similar, but also difficult to predict.

References: Austin LM, Frush DP. Compendium of national guidelines for imaging the pregnant patient. *AJR Am J Roentgenol* 2011;197:W737–W746.

Committee to Assess Health Risks from Exposure to Low Levels of Ionizing Radiation, Board on Radiation Effects Research, Division of Earth and Life Studies, National Research Council of the National Academies. *Health risks from exposure to low levels of ionizing radiation: BEIR VII Phase 2*. Washington, DC: National Academies Press, 2006.

Nievelstein RAJ, Frush DP. Should we obtain informed consent for examinations that expose patients to radiation? *AJR Am J Roentgenol* 2012;199:664–669.

Wagner LK, Applegate K; American College of Radiology. ACR practice guideline for imaging pregnant or potentially pregnant adolescents and women with ionizing radiation. In: *Practice guidelines and technical standards 2008 (resolution 26)*. Reston, VA: American College of Radiology, 2008.

9 **Answer B.** The Weigert-Meyer rule predicts that in a completely duplicated system, the upper pole moiety will insert inferior and medial to the lower pole moiety. Only rare exceptions to this rule exist. This rule is useful because duplicated systems have ectopic insertions; localizing these insertion sites is important for management. Ectopic ureters can insert into the bladder (most common), infrasphincteric urethra, seminal vesicles, vagina, fallopian tubes, ejaculatory ducts, and perineum. When an ectopic ureter inserts into the bladder, it often forms a ureterocele, which manifests as a so-called cobra-head deformity. "Cobra-head" describes the shape of the filling defect within the bladder caused by the distally dilated ectopic ureter.

Reference: Dunnick NR, Sandler CM, Newhouse JH. *Textbook of uroradiology*, 5th ed. Philadelphia: Lippincott Williams & Wilkins, 2012.

10 **Answer D.** The best answer is to consider cancelling the test. In a young asymptomatic female with no risk factors, the yield of a triphasic CT urogram to detect significant pathology is low. The American Urological Association recommends first completing a history and physical to assess for other potential causes of microscopic hematuria (e.g., menstruation, urinary tract infection), and then, if one or more is present, repeating the urinalysis before proceeding with other diagnostic testing. If the finding persists, a targeted assessment should be considered (e.g., unenhanced renal stone CT with or without cystoscopy, renal function testing). The benefits of performing multiphasic imaging in this patient population, which is not at risk for urothelial carcinoma, are extremely low. In patients with risk factors for urothelial malignancy (e.g., age > 35 years, male sex, smoking history, gross hematuria, etc.) workup usually consists of cystoscopy, triphasic CT urography, and renal function testing, with or without urine cytology.

References: Davis R, Jones JS, Barocas DA, et al. Diagnosis, evaluation, and follow-up of asymptomatic microhematuria (AMH) in adults: AUA guideline. *J Urol* 2012; 188(6 Suppl): 2473–2481.

Lokken RP, Sadow CA, Silverman SG. Diagnostic yield of CT urography in the evaluation of young adults with hematuria. *AJR Am J Roentgenol* 2012;198:609–615.

11 **Answer B.** The CTDI$_{vol}$ (volume CT dose index, expressed in mGy) is a measure of the scanner-specific radiation output. Because CTDI$_{vol}$ is scanner specific, it is an excellent way to compare the radiation output between scanners and scan protocols. However, it is not the dose delivered to the patient. Dose (expressed in Sv) and exposure (expressed in Gy) are related but not the same thing.

CTDI$_{vol}$ is independent of patient body size and scan length. To give a better indication of the radiation exposure to a patient, CTDI$_{vol}$ can be converted into the dose–length product, or DLP (mGy-cm), by multiplying the CTDI$_{vol}$ by the scan length. Despite the name, DLP is not an indication of patient-specific dose either; it is merely a representation of the scanner output multiplied by the scan coverage. CTDI$_{vol}$ and DLP are tools for comparison that can be used to optimize protocols and to compare scanner outputs across sites and studies (and within institutions).

References: Bankier AA, Kressel HY. Through the Looking Glass revisited: the need for more meaning and less drama in the reporting of dose and dose reduction in CT. *Radiology* 2012;265:4–8.

McCollough CH, Leng S, Yu L, et al. CT dose index and patient dose: they are not the same thing. *Radiology* 2011;259:311–316.

12 **Answer A.** The reflected ultrasound frequency always increases when the ultrasound beam interacts with a structure moving toward it. Likewise, the reflected ultrasound frequency always decreases when the ultrasound beam interacts with a structure moving away from it. This is known as the Doppler shift, and is the fundamental physical principal behind Doppler imaging. As the frequency increases, the wavelength decreases (i.e., becomes more compressed), and as the frequency decreases, the wavelength increases (i.e., becomes more elongated). Interestingly, although these properties are fixed, there must be an impedance difference between the moving structure(s) and the background fluid/tissue for a Doppler shift to be detected by the transducer (e.g., red blood cells in blood; dilute urine from the ureters entering concentrated urine in the bladder).

By convention, red pixels signify interaction with an object moving toward the transducer and blue pixels signify interaction with an object moving away from the transducer, but this is actually not a fixed property and can be altered by the ultrasound operator (Answers C and D).

Reference: Mitchell DG. Color Doppler imaging: principles, limitations, and artifacts. *Radiology* 1990;177:1–10.

13 **Answer D.** The scanner exam card does not provide sufficient information to allow calculation of the patient's effective dose. Neither the volume CT dose index (CTDI$_{vol}$) nor the dose–length product (DLP) is a measure of patient dose; rather, each is a measure of scanner and protocol-specific radiation output. To calculate an estimate of patient dose requires not only a measure of the scanner output (e.g., CTDI$_{vol}$) but also the patient's size (e.g., effective diameter), and the body area imaged (e.g., abdomen and pelvis). CTDI$_{vol}$ and DLP should not be considered as, nor reported to be, the radiation dose delivered to the patient.

References: American Association of Physicists in Medicine. *Size-specific dose estimates (SSDE) in pediatric and adult body CT examinations. Task Group 204.* College Park, MD: American Association of Physicists in Medicine, 2011.

Bankier AA, Kressel HY. Through the Looking Glass revisited: the need for more meaning and less drama in the reporting of dose and dose reduction in CT. *Radiology* 2012;265:4–8.

McCollough CH, Leng S, Yu L, et al. CT dose index and patient dose: they are not the same thing. *Radiology* 2011;259:311–316.

14 **Answer C.** Although there is a congenital megaureter and left renal scarring, the overall function of the two kidneys is grossly similar. This is evidenced by similar nephrograms and similar patterns of excretion on the excretory-phase T1-weighted right-hand image. Intravenously administered contrast media with renal-dominant excretion patterns are good indicators of glomerular filtration. Most iodinated contrast media and most gadolinium-based contrast media fit this profile.

The left-hand image is heavily T2 weighted (long TR, long TE, fast spin echo-based sequence), and the right-hand image is T1 weighted (short TR, short TE, gradient recalled echo-based sequence). Heavily T2-weighted sequences are referred to as "static-fluid" sequences because they take a long time to acquire and best depict dilated, fluid-filled structures (e.g., a congenital megaureter). Fluid has a very long T2; therefore, on a heavily T2-weighted sequence, the signal from all other structures is suppressed while the signal from fluid is preserved. This is the same principle used for MRCP imaging in the liver and pancreas.

The collecting systems are only well seen on the right-hand image because contrast material has been administered. Gadolinium-based contrast material indirectly shortens the T1 times of adjacent protons, rendering them hyperintense on T1-weighted images. On MR urography, heavily T2-weighted images are used for anatomic depiction of the collecting systems (in particular, when dilated), and postcontrast T1-weighted images are used to assess function and to detect pathologic enhancement.

References: Leyendecker JR, Barnes CE, Zagoria RJ. MR urography: techniques and clinical applications. *Radiographics* 2008;28:23–46.
O'Connor OJ, McLaughlin P, Maher MM. MR urography. *AJR Am J Roentgenol* 2010;295: W201–W206.

15 **Answer C.** The constellation of findings (echogenic material within a dilated collecting system in the setting of sepsis) is compatible with pyonephrosis, which should be managed with intravenous antibiotic therapy and emergent decompression of the collecting system. Often this is achieved with an antegrade percutaneous nephrostomy. Delay in or failure to decompress the collecting system can result in severe sepsis and loss of the renal unit. Pyelonephritis (Answer A) is a renal parenchymal infection without collecting system dilation, pyelitis (Answer B) is infection or inflammation of a nondilated collecting system, emphysematous pyelitis (Answer D) is infection of the collecting system by one or more gas-producing organism(s), and emphysematous pyelonephritis (Answer E) is infection of the renal parenchyma by one or more gas-producing organism(s).

References: Gupta K, Hooton TM, Naber KG, et al. International clinical practice guidelines for the treatment of acute uncomplicated cystitis and pyelonephritis in women: a 2010 update by the Infectious Diseases Society of North America and the European Society for Microbiology and Infectious Diseases. *Clin Infect Dis* 2011;52:e103–e120.
Wessells H. *Urological emergencies: a practical approach*, 2nd ed. New York: Humana Press, 2013.

16 **Answer C.** The images demonstrate reflux into the pelvicalyceal systems without dilation. Therefore, this is grade II reflux. This study cannot be normal because the contrast material was instilled retrograde. In a native system, it is not normal for fluid to enter the upper tracts in a retrograde fashion. Vesicoureteric reflux grading has high interrater agreement (weighted kappa: 0.93 to 0.94) and is performed using the following scale:

- Grade I: Reflux into the ureter(s) only
- Grade II: Reflux into the pelvicalyceal system(s) without dilation
- Grade III: Reflux into the pelvicalyceal system(s) with mild dilation

- Grade IV: Reflux into the pelvicalyceal system(s) with moderate dilation
- Grade V: Reflux into the pelvicalyceal system(s) with severe dilation

References: Craig JC, Irwig LM, Lam A, et al. Variation in the diagnosis of vesicoureteric reflux using micturating cystourethrography. *Pediatr Nephrol* 1997;11:455–459.

Lebowitz RL, Olbing H, Parkkulainen KV, et al. International system of radiographic grading of vesicoureteric reflux. International reflux study in children. *Pediatr Radiol* 1985;15:105–109.

Williams G, Fletcher JT, Alexander SI, et al. Vesicoureteral reflux. *JASN* 2008;19:847–862.

17 **Answer B.**   The images demonstrate numerous contrast-filled pseudodiverticula arising from the ureteral walls consistent with ureteral pseudodiverticulosis. This uncommon condition is associated with chronic urinary tract infection, and it has a strong association with urothelial malignancy (up to 45% of affected patients will develop a urothelial malignancy). Routine surveillance of the upper and lower urinary tracts is recommended in these patients. Despite the location of the pseudodiverticula, urothelial carcinoma of the bladder remains more common than urothelial carcinoma of the upper tracts (as it is in the general population). When urothelial carcinoma does develop, it usually does so 2 to 10 years after the pseudodiverticula are initially identified. Benign vascular impressions (Answer C) and benign ureteral "kinks" (Answer D) can distort the ureter, but they do not cause outpouchings to extend beyond the normal luminal contour. Only the left ureter from the question has extrinsic impressions that might reflect "kinks" or vascular impressions; therefore Answer C and Answer D are not the best choices.

References: Dunnick NR, Sandler CM, Newhouse JH. *Textbook of uroradiology*, 5th ed. Philadelphia: Lippincott Williams & Wilkins, 2012.

Smith AD, Preminger G, Badlani G, et al. *Smith's textbook of endourology*, 3rd ed. Hoboken: Wiley-Blackwell Publishing, 2012.

Wasserman NF, Zhang G, Posalaky IP, et al. Ureteral pseudodiverticula: frequent association with uroepithelial malignancy. *AJR Am J Roentgenol* 1991;157:69–72.

Wasserman NF, La Pointe S, Posalaky IP. Ureteral pseudodiverticulosis. *Radiology* 1985;155:561–566.

18 **Answer D.**   The imaging findings are compatible with an obstructed upper pole moiety in a complete congenital duplication. A single dominant upper pole "cyst" with no or minimal surrounding cortex in a young patient is strongly suggestive of this diagnosis. In a complete duplication, the upper pole moiety tends to obstruct because of the ectopic insertion of the upper pole ureter upon the bladder or a nearby structure, often with associated ureterocele formation. The lower pole moiety, which is prone to vesicoureteric reflux and recurrent infection, typically inserts at or near the normal location at the bladder trigone.

Multicystic dysplastic kidney (Answer A) is characterized by a congenitally nonfunctional kidney replaced by noncommunicating cysts and minimal parenchymal volume. Autosomal dominant polycystic kidney disease (Answer B, ADPCKD) usually does not present this early in life. ADPCKD can be diagnosed in young patients 15 to 39 years of age if there are three or more unilateral or bilateral cysts with a confirmed family history. This is in contradistinction to autosomal recessive polycystic kidney disease (Answer E, ARPCKD), which typically presents in young children with innumerable tiny cysts replacing both kidneys. The cysts in this condition (ARPCKD) are so small that they can actually appear echogenic on ultrasound. Acquired renal cysts (Answer C) of this size are rare in young children and should not affect the cortical volume.

References: Avni FE, Garel C, Cassart M, et al. Imaging and classification of congenital cystic renal diseases. *AJR Am J Roentgenol* 2012;198:1004–1013.

Pei Y, Obaji J, Dupuis A, et al. Unified criteria for ultrasonographic diagnosis of ADPKD. *J Am Soc Nephrol* 2009;20:205–212.

Schaffer RM, Shih YH, Becker JA. Sonographic identification of collecting system duplications. *J Clin Ultrasound* 1983;11:309–312.

19 Answer A. The images demonstrate a well-demarcated fluid-filled peripherally based structure that accumulates contrast material on excretory-phase imaging compatible with a calyceal diverticulum. Calyceal diverticula require no management unless they become complicated. Because they predispose to local urinary stasis, they carry a risk of recurrent infection and stone disease. Recurrent infection and stone disease are complications associated with all causes of urinary stasis (e.g., urethral diverticula, bladder outlet obstruction).

References: Canales B, Monga M. Surgical management of the calyceal diverticulum. *Curr Opin Urol* 2003;13:255–260.

Chong TW, Bui MHT, Fuchs GJ. Calyceal diverticula: ureteroscopic management. *Urol Clin North Am* 2000;27:647–654.

Wulfsohn MA. Pyelocaliceal diverticula. *J Urol* 1980;123:1–8.

20 Answer B. The correct answer is 27.7 mGy ($14 \times 1.98 = 27.7$). The size-specific dose estimate (SSDE, expressed in mGy) takes into account the patient's size (i.e., diameter or effective diameter), as well as the radiation output of the scanner ($CTDI_{vol}$), to provide an estimate of the patient-specific radiation dose. The units are mGy (not mSv) because this is an estimate based on exposure; it is not a true dose. The formula for calculating SSDE is as follows:

$$f_{size}^{32cm} \times CTDI_{vol}^{32cm} = SSDE$$

f_{size} is a conversion factor based on the patient's body diameter that is determined using a look-up table produced by the American Association of Physicists in Medicine Task Group 204 (2011). The f_{size} is contingent on the phantom size that was used in the $CTDI_{vol}$ determination (32 cm or 16 cm), and can be determined with a variety of diameter measurements (lateral + AP diameter, lateral diameter, AP diameter, or effective diameter). Effective diameter is calculated with the following equation:

$$\left[\sqrt{(AP\,diameter \times transverse\,diameter)} \right] = Effective\,diameter$$

References: American Association of Physicists in Medicine. *Size-specific dose estimates (SSDE) in pediatric and adult body CT examinations. Task Group 204.* College Park, MD: American Association of Physicists in Medicine, 2011.

Bankier AA, Kressel HY. Through the Looking Glass revisited: the need for more meaning and less drama in the reporting of dose and dose reduction in CT. *Radiology* 2012;265:4–8.

McCollough CH, Leng S, Yu L, et al. CT dose index and patient dose: they are not the same thing. *Radiology* 2011;259:311–316.

21 Answer D. Industrial aromatic hydrocarbons, such as those associated with aniline dyes, textiles, petrochemicals, and coal increase the risk of both bladder cancer and upper tract urothelial cancer by approximately eight times. Smoking is a leading cause of both upper tract and lower tract malignancy. Upper tract urothelial cancer is much less common than is bladder cancer, with approximately 90% to 95% of urothelial cancers arising in the bladder. When diagnosed, upper tract urothelial cancers are more likely to be muscle invasive (60% vs. 15% to 25%). Patients with urothelial carcinoma of either the upper tract or lower tract are considered to have "at-risk" urothelium, and typically undergo annual surveillance for local recurrence, metastatic disease, and/or metachronous malignancies.

References: Colin P, Koenig P, Ouzzane A, et al. Environmental factors involved in carcinogenesis of urothelial cell carcinomas of the upper tract. *BJU Int* 2009;104:1436–1440.

Roupret M, Babjuk E, Comperat R, et al. *Guidelines on urothelial carcinomas of the upper urinary tract.* European Association of Urology, 2013.

22 Answer D. It is often normal to see spontaneous ureteric reflux after an ileal loop creation. This is because the submucosal tunnel of the ureter through the bladder wall, which helps prevent reflux from occurring in the native system, is no longer present. In some cases, antirefluxing surgical techniques are applied to the ureteroenteric anastomoses to minimize the risk of high-volume reflux. In this case, a refluxing end-to-end anastomosis was created. Absence of reflux in this setting is actually an indirect sign of pathology (e.g., benign stricture [most common], obstructing mass) at the level of the anastomosis. The normal pattern of reflux seen after ileal loop creation can be exploited during a loopogram to monitor the upper tract(s) for metachronous urothelial carcinoma recurrence.

References: Applbaum YN, Diamond AB, Rappoport AS. Retrograde ureteral catheterization via the ileal conduit. *AJR Am J Roentgenol* 1986;146:61–63.

Jude JR, Lusted LB, Smith RR. Radiographic evaluation of the urinary tract following urinary diversion to ileal bladder. *Cancer* 1959;12:1134–1141.

Onur MR, Sidhu R, Dogra VS. Imaging of urinary diversion and neobladder. In: Dogra VS and MacLennan GT (eds). *Genitourinary radiology: Male genital tract, adrenal, and retroperitoneum*. London: Springer, 2013:327–342.

Sudakoff GS, Guralnick M, Langenstroer P, et al. CT urography of urinary diversions with enhanced CT digital radiography: preliminary experience. *AJR Am J Roentgenol* 2005;184: 131–138.

23 Answer A. The images demonstrate a "goblet sign," which is associated with urothelial carcinoma of the ureter. It is caused by slow expansion of a mass within the lumen of the ureter that grows slowly enough to allow the segment to distend and accommodate its growth pattern. It can also be seen with other slowly growing processes (e.g., ureteral metastasis, ureteral endometriosis). The combined features of a central ureteral filling defect with a tapered lumen caudal to it produce the shape of a goblet (i.e., wine glass). Interestingly, there is a second sign on the images that favors urothelial carcinoma of the ureter: the "stipple sign." This sign, described in 1979, is characterized by entrapment of contrast material within the lucent papillary projections of a urothelial malignancy.

The "comet tail" sign (Answers C and D) is a finding on CT in which a calcification (the "comet") is at the tip of a linear soft tissue attenuation structure (a vein) without a surrounding rim. When seen, it favors that the calcification is a phlebolith (i.e., a benign venous calcification) and not a calcification in the ureter.

References: Dunnick NR, Sandler CM, Newhouse JH. *Textbook of uroradiology, 5th ed.* Philadelphia: Lippincott Williams & Wilkins, 2012.

Dyer RB, Chen MY, Zagoria RJ. Classic signs in uroradiology. *Radiographics* 2004;24:S247–S280.

McLean GK, Pollack HM, Banner MP. The "stipple sign"—urographic harbinger of transitional cell neoplasms. *Urol Radiol* 1979;1:77–79.

24 Answer B. The images demonstrate grade III vesicoureteric reflux (reflux associated with mild collecting system dilation) and a "drooping lily" sign, indicative of reflux into the lower pole moiety of a duplicated collecting system. The "drooping lily" sign refers to the morphology of the lower pole calyces and lower pole infundibula, and their appearance in the setting of a nonvisualized upper pole. The upper pole moiety is not identified on this study and cannot be evaluated. In the setting of a completely duplicated collecting system, the upper pole moiety is associated with obstruction, and the lower pole moiety is associated with reflux and infection. The upper pole moiety typically inserts ectopically inferior and medial to the lower pole moiety (Weigert-Meyer rule). A VCUG is a retrograde study; therefore, an obstructed system (Answer C) would not be visible with this technique.

References: Dunnick NR, Sandler CM, Newhouse JH. *Textbook of uroradiology*, 5th ed. Philadelphia: Lippincott Williams & Wilkins, 2012.

Dyer RB, Chen MY, Zagoria RJ. Classic signs in uroradiology. *Radiographics* 2004;24:S247–S280.

Callahan MJ. The drooping lily sign. *Radiology* 2001;219:226–228.

25 **Answer D.** The primary function of statistical iterative reconstruction methods (ASIR, IRIS, SAFIRE, iDose) is to reduce image noise. This is accomplished by matching a simulated CT projection to the acquired CT projection in an iterative (repeated) fashion to better model the image noise. Reduced image noise can translate into radiation dose savings, but the effect is indirect: one can obtain noisier images with less radiation exposure, and then "clean up" the noisy images with statistical iterative reconstruction after they are acquired. Most statistical iterative reconstruction algorithms allow a blend of filtered back projection and iterative reconstruction data. Greater iterative reconstruction equates to less noise and greater image smoothing. Images reconstructed with 100% statistical iterative reconstruction can have a waxy, surreal appearance. The ideal blend varies based on the desired appearance, imaging protocol, and intended spatial resolution.

References: Kaza RK, Platt JF, Goodsitt MM, et al. Emerging techniques for dose optimization in abdominal CT. *Radiographics* 2014;34:4–17.

Silva AC, Lawder JH, Hara A, et al. Innovations in CT dose reduction strategy: application of the adaptive statistical iterative reconstruction algorithm. *AJR Am J Roentgenol* 2010;194:191–199.

26 **Answer A.** The average annual natural background radiation dose is 2 to 3 mSv. A CT examination with an effective dose of 10 mSv is roughly four to five times this. No deterministic effects of radiation exposure (e.g., erythema, CNS abnormalities) occur at this dose level. Stochastic effects below 100 mSv are speculative and based on the "linear-no-threshold" model, but the risk of fatal cancer induction is estimated to be roughly 0.01% (1 in 1,000) for an adult patient who receives an effective dose of 10 mSv. Because a large fraction of people (about 1 in 5, or 20%) will be diagnosed with some form of cancer in their lifetime, the incremental risk is quite small (i.e., increasing from 20% to 20.01%). Decisions about imaging should include a consideration of the risks of imaging (e.g., the risk of a contrast reaction, the risk of radiation exposure), the benefits of imaging (e.g., diagnosis, prognosis), and the risks of not imaging (e.g., failure to diagnose).

References: Committee to Assess Health Risks from Exposure to Low Levels of Ionizing Radiation, Board on Radiation Effects Research, Division of Earth and Life Studies, National Research Council of the National Academies. *Health risks from exposure to low levels of ionizing radiation: BEIR VII Phase 2*. Washington, DC: National Academies Press, 2006.

Nievelstein RAJ, Frush DP. Should we obtain informed consent for examinations that expose patients to radiation? *AJR Am J Roentgenol* 2012;199:664–669.

Katayama H, Yamaguchi K, Kozuka T, et al. Adverse reactions to ionic and nonionic contrast media. A report from the Japanese Committee on the Safety of Contrast Media. *Radiology*. 1990;175:621–628.

U. S. Food and Drug Administration. What are the risks from CT? http://www.fda.gov/ radiation-emittingproducts/radiationemittingproductsandprocedures/medicalimaging/ medicalx-rays/ucm115329.htm. Updated 6, August, 2009. Accessed January 26, 2014.

27 **Answer C.** The images demonstrate a soft-tissue "rim" sign, which supports the diagnosis of a ureteral calculus. This sign is caused by mural edema surrounding a ureteral calculus. It is useful for differentiating a suspected ureteral calculus from a phlebolith (i.e., a benign venous calcification) because phleboliths are chronic and generally do not cause thickening of the vein wall. When a soft-tissue "rim" sign is detected, the positive predictive value for a ureteral calculus is high. Not all ureteral calculi demonstrate the soft-tissue "rim" sign. It is more frequently absent with larger calculi and those lodged at the ureterovesical junction (UVJ).

The comet tail sign is less reliable; its presence somewhat supports the diagnosis of a phlebolith over a ureteral calculus. With the comet tail sign, the calcification (the "comet") is at the tip of a linear soft tissue attenuation structure (a vein, the "tail") without a surrounding rim. An example of the comet tail sign is on the same image (the more posterior calcification in the left hemipelvis).

References: Bell TV, Fenlon HM, Davison BD, et al. Unenhanced helical CT criteria to differentiate distal ureteral calculi from pelvic phleboliths. *Radiology* 1998;207:363–367.
Dyer RB, Chen MY, Zagoria RJ. Classic signs in uroradiology. *Radiographics* 2004;24: S247–S280.
Guest AR, Cohan RH, Korobkin M, et al. Assessment of the clinical utility of the rim and comet-tail signs in differentiating ureteral stones from phleboliths. *AJR Am J Roentgenol* 2001;177:1285–1291.
Heneghan JP, Dalrymple NC, Verga M, et al. Soft-tissue "rim" sign in the diagnosis of ureteral calculi with use of unenhanced helical CT. *Radiology* 1997;202:709–711.

28 **Answer C.** Staghorn calculi usually are composed of struvite, a mineral (magnesium ammonium phosphate) that forms in alkaline urine, though they may often be admixed with variable amounts of calcium or other minerals. Staghorn calculi are strongly associated with urease-producing bacteria such as *Proteus mirabilis*. Urease splits uric acid and alkalinizes the urine. The following table details the basic characteristics of common minerals found in renal calculi. Note that many stones are formed from a combination of these minerals, and that the raw attenuation of many stones overlap (prohibiting classification by simple CT attenuation measurements alone).

Mineral	Visible on Radiography	Visible on CT	HU Range	Associations
Calcium oxalate	Often	Yes	800–1,000	Most common (~80%)
Calcium phosphate	Often	Yes	800–1,000	
Struvite	Often	Yes	330–900	Staghorn calculi
Cystine	Often	Yes	200–880	Congenital cystinuria
Uric acid	No	Yes	150–500	Invisible on plain x-ray
"Indinavir stones"	No	No	<100	HIV therapy, invisible on CT

References: Becknell B, Carpenter AR, Bolon B, et al. Struvite urolithiasis and chronic urinary tract infection in a murine model of urinary diversion. *Urology* 2013;81:943–948.
Brant WE, Helms CA. *Fundamentals of diagnostic radiology*, 3rd ed. Philadelphia: Lippincott Williams & Wilkins, 2006.
Segura JW. Staghorn calculi. *Urol Clin North Am* 1997;24:71–80.
Segura JW, Preminger GM, Assimos DG, et al. Nephrolithiasis clinical guidelines panel summary report on the management of staghorn calculi. The American Urological Association Nephrolithiasis Clinical Guidelines Panel. *J Urol* 1994;151:1648–1651.

29 **Answer C.** Decreasing kVp decreases the average and peak energy of the x-ray beam, which increases image noise, decreases radiation dose, increases the attenuation of iodine, and decreases pseudoenhancement effects. kVp has a quadratic relationship with radiation dose, while mA has a linear relationship with radiation dose. Therefore, lowering kVp will have a greater effect on radiation dose than does lowering mA. However, changes in kVp have a greater effect on the resulting image (kVp affects noise as well as attenuation, while mA only affects noise).

Pseudoenhancement is common with multidetector CT scanners and is primarily related to a computational error that fails to appropriately correct for beam hardening. As the beam energy approaches the K-edge of iodine (33.2 keV), the likelihood of the photoelectric effect will increase with respect to Compton interactions, thereby reducing non-linearity errors due to scattered radiation. Additionally, use of a lower kVp will permit a reduction in the necessary volume of iodinated contrast material while maintaining the same degree of attenuation. This reduction will decrease the beam hardening effects of iodine, which will decrease the incidence and magnitude of pseudoenhancement.

References: Kaza RK, Platt JF, Goodsitt MM, et al. Emerging techniques for dose optimization in abdominal CT. *Radiographics* 2014;34:4–17.

Patel J, Davenport MS, Khalatbari S, et al. In vivo predictors of renal cyst pseudoenhancement at 120 kVp. *AJR Am J Roentgenol* 2014;202:336–342.

Wang ZJ, Coakley FV, Fu Y, et al. Renal cyst pseudoenhancement at multidetector CT: what are the effects of number of detectors and peak tube voltage? *Radiology* 2008; 248:910–916.

30 **Answer C.** The sensitivity is 75%, and the specificity is 80%. Unlike positive (PPV) and negative (NPV) predictive values, which vary with the disease prevalence, sensitivity and specificity are fixed characteristics of the test. Sensitivity indicates the probability that the test will be positive in a patient with the disease (true positive rate), while specificity indicates the probability that the test will be negative in a patient without the disease (true negative rate). Most clinical decisions do not rely on sensitivity and specificity because usually it is unknown whether the patient has the disease; most clinical decisions instead rely on positive and negative predictive value, which are the probabilities that the patient has (PPV) or does not have (NPV) the disease given that the test is positive (PPV) or negative (NPV). To calculate these parameters, it is helpful to organize the data into a 2 × 2 table, as follows:

	Disease Present	Disease Absent	Predictive Value*
Test Positive	3	2	PPV = 3/(3+2) = 0.60
Test Negative	1	8	NPV = 8/(8+1) = 0.89
Sens./Spec.	Sens. = 3/(1+3) = 0.75	Spec.: 8/(2+8) = 0.80	

As mentioned, the positive and negative predictive values depend on the prevalence of disease in the population; therefore, the PPV and NPV will be different if the test is applied to a population with different disease prevalence.

Reference: Weinstein S, Obuchowski NA, Lieber ML. Clinical evaluation of diagnostic tests. *AJR Am J Roentgenol* 2005;184:14–19.

Lower Tract (Bladder and Urethra)

QUESTIONS

1   A 32-year-old male is involved in a snowmobile accident. Pelvic fluid and pelvic fractures are identified on a trauma protocol venous-phase CT of the abdomen and pelvis (left). Delayed images obtained 15 minutes after the administration of contrast material are also obtained (right). How should the bladder be characterized?

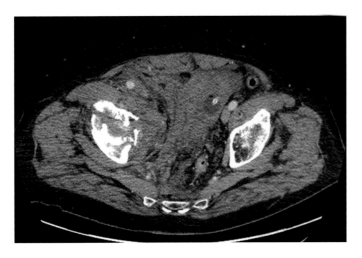
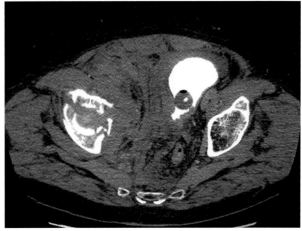

  A. There is an intraperitoneal bladder rupture.
  B. There is an extraperitoneal bladder rupture.
  C. There is no bladder injury.
  D. The bladder is nondiagnostic.

2   A 40-year-old nursing home resident with neurocognitive deficits and urinary retention is found to have bladder cancer attributable to a chronic indwelling Foley catheter. Which of the following risk factors for bladder cancer is classically associated with the same malignant cell type?

  A. Smoking history
  B. Urachal remnant
  C. *Schistosoma haematobium* infection
  D. Polycyclic aromatic hydrocarbon exposure

3 A 60-year-old male with a 50-pack-year smoking history presents with pelvic pain and gross hematuria. A CT is performed demonstrating a left anterolateral bladder mass that is later confirmed to be urothelial carcinoma. Based on the TNM classification system and below imaging findings, what is the T stage of this tumor?

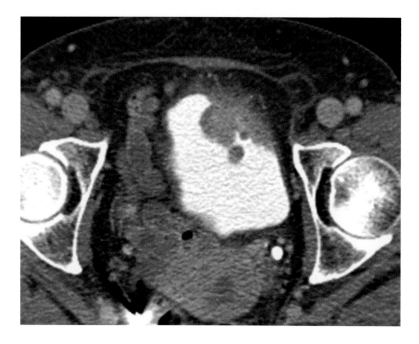

A. T1

B. T2

C. T3

D. T4

E. The T stage cannot be reliably determined.

4 A 30-year-old female with postvoid dribbling undergoes pelvic MR to localize a suspected urethral diverticulum. She has questions about the safety of MRI. What is the maximum allowed whole-body specific absorption rate for an otherwise healthy patient based on FDA guidelines?

A. 2 W/kg every 15 minutes

B. 4 W/kg every 15 minutes

C. 8 W/kg every 15 minutes

D. 16 W/kg every 15 minutes

5 A 25-year-old female with recurrent urinary tract infections undergoes a fluoroscopic voiding cystourethrogram (VCUG). If the analog spatial resolution of this study is 4 lp/mm, what is the pixel spacing required to preserve this resolution in a digital format?

A. 0.125 mm

B. 0.250 mm

C. 0.375 mm

D. 0.500 mm

6 Where along the male urethra are the glands of Littre?

A. Dorsal surface of the anterior urethra

B. Ventral surface of the anterior urethra

C. Dorsal surface of the posterior urethra

D. Ventral surface of the posterior urethra

7   A 42-year-old male with type 1 diabetes mellitus presents with abdominal pain and systemic inflammatory response syndrome (SIRS). A urine specimen is obtained with a Foley catheter, and a CT of the abdomen and pelvis is performed (below). What is the most appropriate management?

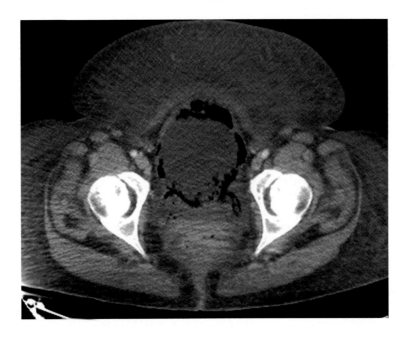

A. Ignore (incidental finding)
B. Suprapubic catheter
C. Antibiotics
D. Urgent cystectomy

8   A 72-year-old male inpatient with congestive heart failure, atrial fibrillation, and sepsis presents with hematuria. A CT urogram is performed demonstrating a mass in the urinary bladder, and an image representative of the entire abnormality is shown below. Which of the following risk factors would best explain the imaging findings?

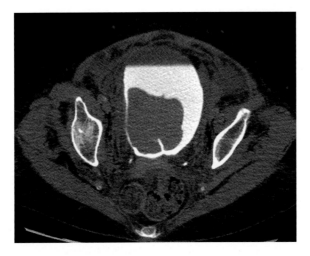

A. A 40-pack-year smoking history
B. Warfarin therapy
C. Hyperparathyroidism
D. Diabetes mellitus type 1

9 A 55-year-old male with benign prostatic hyperplasia presents with palpitations and fainting spells during micturition. A CT is performed demonstrating an enlarged prostate gland and a small 1-cm mass along the left lateral bladder wall. Which of the following bladder tumors is classically associated with this history?

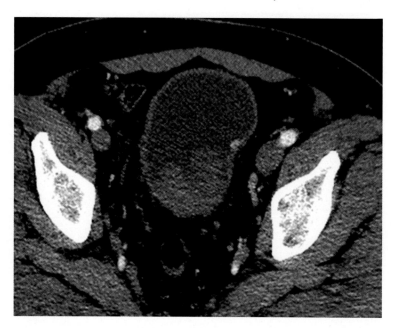

    A. Metastatic melanoma
    B. Urothelial cancer
    C. Paraganglioma
    D. Squamous cell carcinoma
    E. Adenocarcinoma

10 A 25-year-old male suffers severe pelvic trauma and develops a type II urethral injury. Which of the following mechanisms is most strongly associated with this injury pattern?

    A. Blunt anterior injury
    B. Shearing injury
    C. Anterior penetrating injury
    D. Straddle injury

11 A 55-year-old male with squamous cell carcinoma of the urethra presents for an MR of the penis to determine local disease extent. Which of the following TE and flip angle combinations will produce the most T1 weighting on a gradient echo pulse sequence using a TR of 50 msec?

    A. TE: 40 msec; flip angle: 70 degrees
    B. TE: 40 msec; flip angle: 20 degrees
    C. TE: 10 msec; flip angle: 70 degrees
    D. TE: 10 msec; flip angle: 20 degrees

12 A 28-year-old radiology resident in her 22nd week of pregnancy is scheduled to perform fluoroscopic voiding cystourethrograms (VCUG) while on the genitourinary radiology service. What is the regulatory radiation dose limit for her fetus once she declares her pregnancy?

    A. 0.05 mSv
    B. 0.5 mSv
    C. 5 mSv
    D. 50 mSv

13 A 14-year-old male is involved in an equestrian accident and presents with blood at the urethral meatus. He undergoes a retrograde urethrogram. How would you classify this urethral injury?

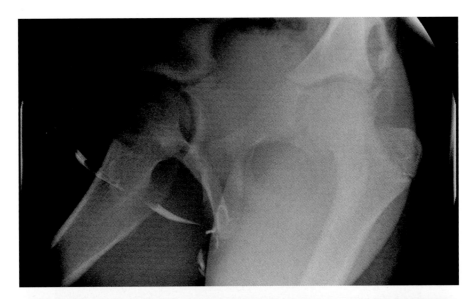

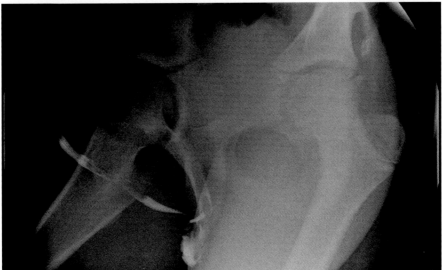

A. Type I
B. Type II
C. Type III
D. Type IV/IVa
E. Type V

14 A 32-year-old male with no relevant past medical history was involved in a motor vehicle collision and sustained pelvic trauma. A retrograde urethrogram was performed and is shown below. What best characterizes the findings in the posterior urethra?

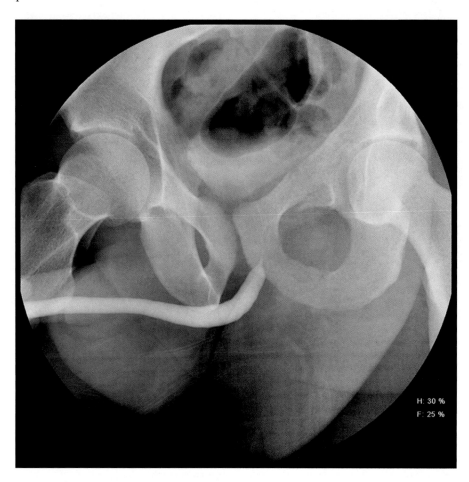

A. Normal

B. Stricture of the bulbar urethra

C. Stricture of the bulbar and membranous urethra

D. Stricture of the bulbar, membranous, and prostatic urethra

15 A 20-year-old male trauma victim presents with blood at the urethral meatus. What is the best next step to evaluate this patient's suspected injury?

A. Retrograde urethrogram

B. Foley catheter placement

C. CT cystogram

D. CT urogram

16 An 85-year-old male with asymptomatic microhematuria undergoes a CT urogram and is noted to have an unusually shaped bladder. What is the etiology of this finding?

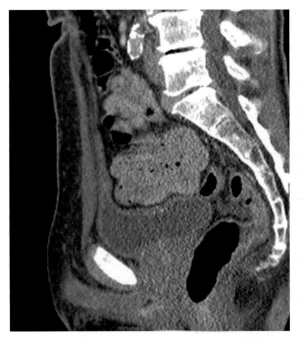 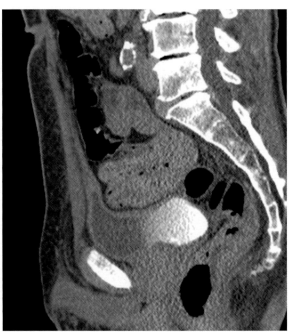

A. Obliterated median umbilical ligament
B. Obliterated medial umbilical ligament
C. Incomplete closure of the median umbilical ligament
D. Incomplete closure of the medial umbilical ligament

17 A 50-year-old female with recurrent urinary tract infections undergoes a CT urogram. Which of the following risk factors best explains her recurrent infections?

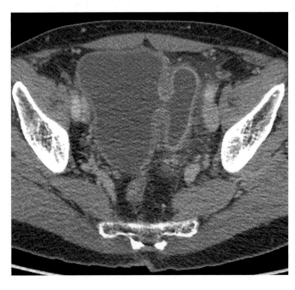 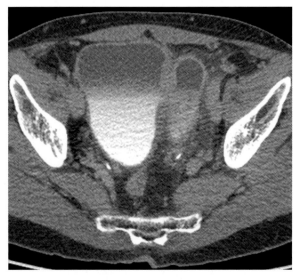

A. Urinary stasis
B. Bladder calculi
C. Vesicoureteric reflux
D. Colovesical fistula
E. Vesicovaginal fistula

18 A 57-year-old female with leukemia undergoes an unenhanced CT for gross hematuria. Which of the following chemotherapeutics is the most likely cause of the imaging findings?

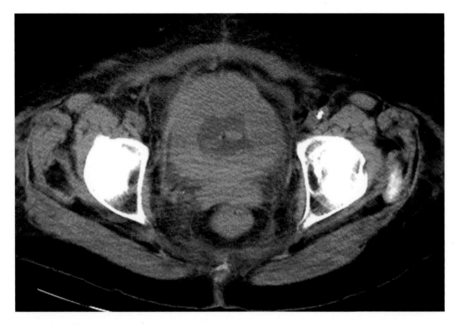

A. Etoposide
B. Methotrexate
C. Cyclophosphamide
D. Cytarabine
E. Vincristine

19 A 65-year-old male has multiple urinary tract infections 5 years after prostatectomy and salvage radiotherapy for T3a prostate cancer. A cystogram is performed. What is the most likely cause of his symptoms?

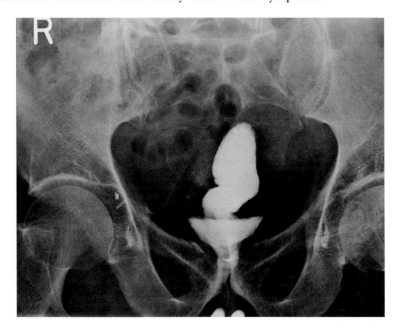

A. Urinary stasis
B. Vesicoureteric reflux
C. Colovesical fistula
D. Enterovesical fistula

20   A 52-year-old female with a 40-pack-year smoking history presents with urinary incontinence. An intravenous urogram is performed. What is the most likely diagnosis?

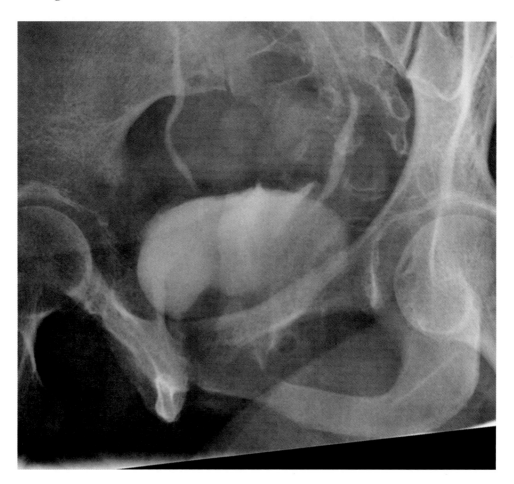

   A. Neurogenic bladder
   B. Patent urachus
   C. Urachal adenocarcinoma
   D. Vesicovaginal fistula
   E. Vesicoureteric reflux

21   What visible anatomic landmark most reliably signifies the junction between the anterior and posterior urethra on retrograde urethrography?

   A. Inferior margins of the obturator foramina
   B. Superior margins of the obturator foramina
   C. Cone-shaped end of the bulbar urethra
   D. Cone-shaped end of the membranous urethra

22   A 69-year-old male undergoes radical prostatectomy for Gleason sum 7 prostate cancer. A cystogram is performed 2 weeks later. What best describes the imaging findings?

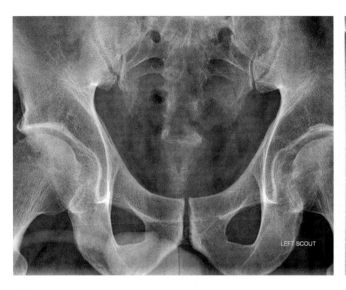
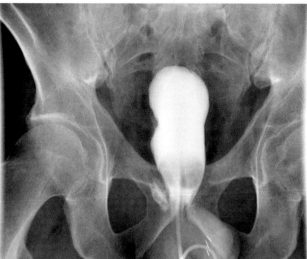

LEFT SCOUT

   A. Normal study
   B. Coloenteric fistula
   C. Colovesical fistula
   D. Anastomotic leak

23   A 60-year-old male with bladder cancer and a hip replacement undergoes contrast-enhanced MR of the pelvis with both extracellular gadolinium-based contrast material and ultrasmall iron oxide particles (USPIO). Match the materials with the corresponding class of susceptibility.

A. Metal hip arthroplasty	1. Diamagnetic
B. Bladder wall	2. Paramagnetic
C. Ultrasmall iron oxide particles	3. Superparamagnetic
D. Gadolinium-based contrast material	4. Ferromagnetic

24   What is a "watering can perineum"?
   A. Postinfectious perineal fistulas
   B. Gangrenous perineal abscesses
   C. Severe perineal edema
   D. Postoperative perineal ulcers

25 A 50-year-old male with history of *Chlamydia trachomatis* infection and difficulty with urination undergoes a retrograde urethrogram. What best describes the imaging findings?

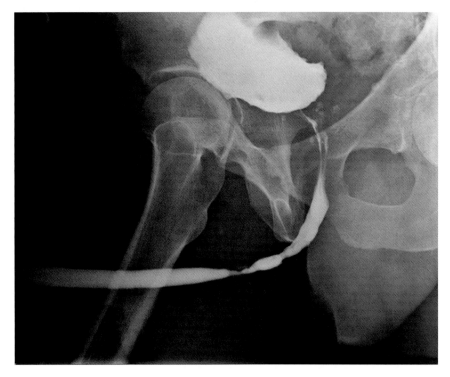

A. Normal study
B. Strictures of the anterior urethra
C. Strictures of the posterior urethra
D. Strictures of both the anterior and posterior urethra

26 A 29-year-old female with right flank pain and a dilated right collecting system undergoes a CT urogram. What is likely the underlying cause of this patient's collecting system dilation?

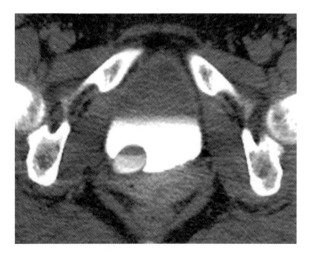

A. Renal calculus
B. Congenital duplication
C. Vesicoureteric reflux
D. Prune belly syndrome

27   A 33-year-old female with pelvic discomfort and a soft palpable mass along the anterior vaginal wall undergoes pelvic MR. Representative T2-weighted images with and without fat saturation are shown below. What is the most likely diagnosis?

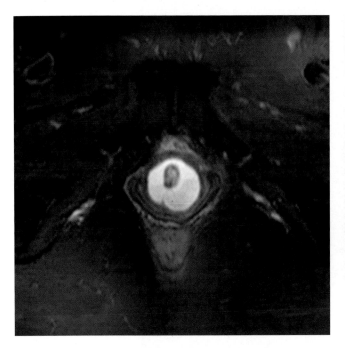
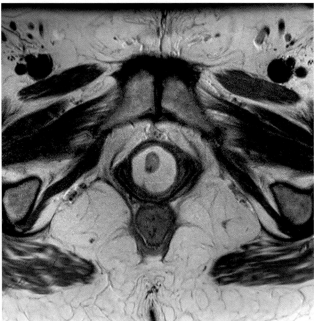

A. Normal study
B. Gartner duct cyst
C. Bartholin gland cyst
D. Urethral diverticulum

28   Where is the verumontanum?

A. Seminal vesicles
B. Bladder
C. Prostatic urethra
D. Membranous urethra

29 A 70-year-old male undergoes a postoperative cystogram. What is the best explanation for the appearance of the bladder?

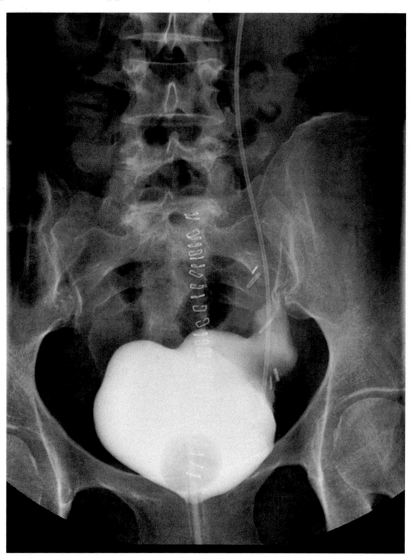

A. Psoas hitch
B. Contained bladder rupture
C. Malpositioned ureteral stent
D. Congenital megaureter

30 A 66-year-old male with fevers undergoes a retroperitoneal ultrasound demonstrating gas in the bladder wall. What is the cause of the so-called "dirty shadowing" posterior to the gas?

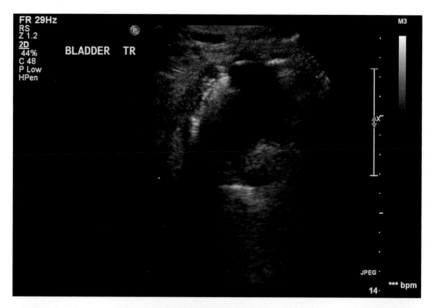

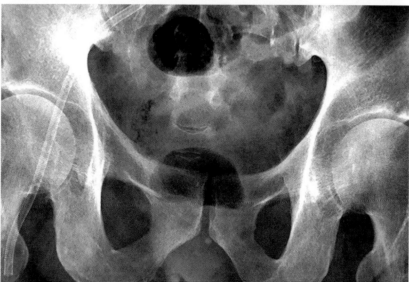

A. Reverberation artifact
B. Mirror-image artifact
C. Twinkling artifact
D. Comet tail artifact
E. Side lobe artifact

ANSWERS AND EXPLANATIONS

1 **Answer D.**   Venous-phase CT is typically unable to diagnose bladder injury because the kidneys have not yet excreted contrast material. In some cases, delayed-phase (i.e., excretory phase) CT can demonstrate a bladder leak if there is extraluminal contrast material. However, delayed-phase CT is not sensitive for this abnormality. Therefore, venous- and delayed-phase CT imaging of the bladder are insufficient to exclude a bladder injury. Cystography is required (either fluoroscopic or CT cystography). This is because the bladder must be distended with sufficient pressure to "stress" the wall and reveal small defects. The typical volume that must be instilled in an adult patient is 300 to 400 mL, although that varies based on several factors, including patient age, patient size, prior operations, prior pelvic radiation, and the size of the defect (if any). The amount instilled is often driven by patient symptoms.

Examples of intraperitoneal (on left) and extraperitoneal (on right) bladder injury are shown below. Discriminating between the two major types of bladder injury is important because the management differs. Intraperitoneal bladder injuries are managed operatively, and extraperitoneal bladder injuries are managed with Foley catheter decompression.

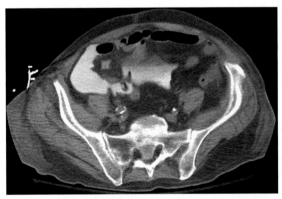
Intraperitoneal bladder rupture

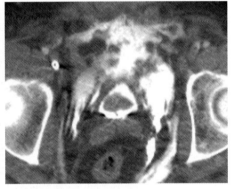
Extraperitoneal bladder rupture

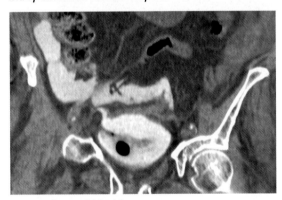
Intraperitoneal bladder rupture

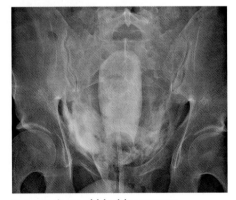
Extraperitoneal bladder rupture

References: Mee SL, McAnnich JW, Federle MP. Computerized tomography in bladder rupture: diagnostic limitations. *J Urol* 1987;137:207–209.

Pao DM, Ellis JH, Cohan RH, et al. Utility of routine trauma CT in the detection of bladder rupture. *Acad Radiol* 2000;7:317–324.

Vaccaro JP, Brody JM. CT cystography in the evaluation of major bladder trauma. *Radiographics* 2000;20:1373–1381.

2   **Answer C.**   Patients with chronic indwelling Foley catheters are at risk for squamous cell carcinoma of the bladder. This cell type represents the minority of bladder cancers in the United States (<5%) but is more common worldwide due to *Schistosoma haematobium* infection in endemic areas. Squamous cell carcinoma of the bladder occurs in the setting of chronic bladder wall inflammation; both chronic Foley catheter use and *Schistosoma haematobium* infection result in this. Smoking (Answer A) and exposure to industrial chemicals (Answer D) are dominant risk factors for urothelial carcinoma, which is the most common type of bladder cancer in the United States. "Urothelial carcinoma" is the new name applied to "transitional cell carcinoma," because although it is usually composed predominantly of transitional cell neoplasia, it often has a blend of cell types. Congenital urachal remnant abnormalities (Answer B) are associated with adenocarcinoma of the bladder.

References: Kaufman DS, Shipley WU, Feldman AS. Bladder cancer. *Lancet* 2009;374:239–249.
Shokeir AA. Squamous cell carcinoma of the bladder: pathology, diagnosis, and treatment. *BJU Int* 2004;93:216–220.

3   **Answer E.**   CT is unreliable for the local staging of bladder cancer. In particular, it is unable to accurately discriminate muscle-invasive ($\geq$T2) from noninvasive ($\leq$T1) bladder cancer or discriminate muscle-invasive (T2) from extravesical ($\geq$T3) bladder cancer. Accurate staging of bladder cancer is important because management decisions (e.g., radical cystectomy vs. transurethral resection [TURBT], use of neoadjuvant chemotherapy) are made based on the T stage of the tumor. Although MR is superior to CT for T staging, both have difficulty, and neither is widely used. T staging is usually clinical based on cystoscopy and cystoscopic biopsy (to assess for muscle invasion), and this staging is in many cases erroneous.

The T staging of bladder cancer can be summarized in the following fashion:

T stage	Description
TX	T stage cannot be evaluated
T0	No primary tumor
Ta	Noninvasive papillary carcinoma
Tis	Carcinoma in situ
T1	Tumor invades bladder wall connective tissue (nonmuscular invasion)
T2	Tumor invades bladder wall muscle (muscular invasion)
T3	Tumor extends outside the bladder wall (extravesical disease)
T4	Tumor invades the abdominal wall or adjacent organ

References: Beyersdorff D, Zhang J, Schoder H, et al. Bladder cancer: can imaging change patient management? *Curr Opin Urol* 2008;18:98–104.
Dutta SC, Smith JA, Shappell SB, et al. Clinical under staging of high risk nonmuscle invasive urothelial carcinoma treated with radical cystectomy. *J Urol* 2001;166:490–493.
Verma S, Rajesh A, Prasad SR, et al. Urinary bladder cancer: role of MR imaging. *Radiographics* 2012;32:371–387.
Zhang J, Gerst S, Lefkowitz RA, et al. Imaging of bladder cancer. *Radiol Clin North Am* 2007;45:183–205.

4 Answer B. The specific absorption rate (SAR) is a measure of the radiofrequency energy deposition within the body per unit mass and is typically expressed in Watts/kilogram. High SAR levels can result in tissue heating and occasionally burns. Therefore, the FDA has established a 4 W/kg-per 15 minute limit for whole-body average exposure in patients with normal thermoregulatory function. As parameters are adjusted on the scanner, the computer calculates the estimated effect of those adjustments on SAR and will notify the operator if the SAR limit is reached. Accurate calculations require that an accurate weight for the patient has been entered into the scanner before scanning commences. SAR is affected by pulse sequence selection and field strength. Multi–spin-echo and multislice acquisitions tend to increase SAR, and doubling the field strength (e.g., increasing from 1.5 T to 3.0 T) quadruples SAR (if the pulse sequences are left unchanged at the higher field strength). Decreasing the flip angle can lower SAR, but this also can affect tissue contrast (i.e., decreasing the flip angle often results in less T1 weighting). In general, stretching out the pulse sequences and delivering RF pulses less frequently will decrease SAR.

References: Bottomley PA. Turning off the heat on MRI. *J Am Coll Radiol* 2008; 5:853–855. FDA guidance document. A primer on medical device interactions with magnetic resonance imaging systems. http://www.fda.gov/MedicalDevices/DeviceRegulationandGuidance/GuidanceDocuments/ucm107721.htm. Published 1997, Updated 2009, Accessed February, 2014.

5 Answer A. If the analog spatial resolution is 4 line pairs (lp) per mm, then that information must be sampled at a frequency at least twice that (eight samples, or pixels, per mm) to preserve the integrity of the data. If there are eight samples, or pixels, per mm (8 pixels/mm), then the pixel spacing is 1/8, or 0.125 mm. This means that a new pixel occurs every 0.125 mm; this is another way of saying that there are 8 pixels/mm.

Before analog data can be displayed in a digital format, it must first be converted to digital data using an "analog-to-digital" converter (ADC). The sampling frequency (f_s) of the ADC must be at least twice that of the analog frequency to preserve the integrity of the data. The analog frequency that is equal to half the sampling frequency (f_s) is known as the Nyquist frequency (f_N). This can be expressed like so:

$$f_N = 0.5 \times f_s$$

This information can be used to calculate the amount of storage space required to archive an analog image in a digital format. For example, if a chest radiograph has a spatial resolution of 4 lp/mm and is 30 cm × 50 cm, what is the digital storage space required to preserve this image at the same resolution if each pixel is encoded with 8 bits (2^8 = 1 byte) of grayscale information? Let us calculate this in a stepwise fashion:

1. Radiograph dimensions = 30 cm × 50 cm
2. Convert radiograph dimensions to mm = 300 mm × 500 mm
3. Analog spatial resolution = 4 lp/mm
4. Minimum required sampling frequency is twice the analog resolution = 8 pixels/mm
5. Calculating digital pixel density: 300 mm × 8 pixels/mm and 500 mm × 8 pixels/mm
6. Pixel density = 2,400 pixels × 4,000 pixels
7. Digital storage (bytes) = 2,400 pixels × 4,000 pixels × 1 byte/pixel = 9,600,000 bytes
8. 1 kilobyte = 2^{10} bytes (1,024 bytes)
9. Digital storage (kbytes) = 9,600,000 bytes × (1 kbyte/1,024 bytes) = 9,375 kilobytes

10. 1 megabyte = 2^{10} kilobytes (1,024 kilobytes)
11. Digital storage (Mbytes) = 9,375 kilobytes × (1 Mbyte/1,024 kbytes) = 9.16 megabytes

Reference: Huda W. *Review of radiologic physics*, 3rd ed. Philadelphia: Lippincott Williams & Wilkins, 2010.

6 **Answer A.**   The glands of Littre are located on the dorsal surface of the anterior male urethra. They express secretions designed to lubricate the urethra and are not usually visible on retrograde urethrography. In patients with chronic stricture disease and certain inflammatory sexually transmitted infections (e.g., *Neisseria gonorrhoeae, Chlamydia trachomatis*), they dilate and become evident. Unlike the Cowper glands and ducts, which are a normal finding near the ventral bulbomembranous junction, visualization of the glands of Littre is always abnormal.

The image below demonstrates the glands of Littre along the dorsal aspect of the anterior urethra (short arrows) and Cowper gland and duct along the ventral urethra (long arrows). The Cowper duct originates from the bulbar urethra, and the Cowper gland is located near the level of the membranous urethra.

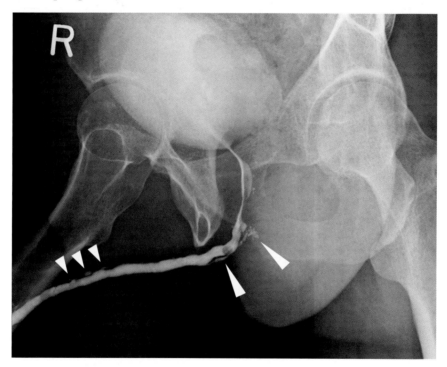

References: Brant WE, Helms CA. *Fundamentals of diagnostic radiology*, 3rd ed. Philadelphia: Lippincott Williams & Wilkins, 2006.
Currarino G, Fuqua F. Cowper's glands in the urethrogram. *Am J Roentgenol Radium Ther Nucl Med* 1972;116:838–842.

7 **Answer C.**   The appropriate management for emphysematous cystitis is antibiotic therapy. Emphysematous cystitis is characterized by gas in the urinary bladder wall secondary to a urinary tract infection. *Escherichia coli* is the most common offending organism, and diabetes mellitus is a known risk factor. Although gas-forming infections in the kidney parenchyma (i.e., emphysematous pyelonephritis) are primarily treated with operative or percutaneous debridement, emphysematous cystitis and emphysematous pyelitis (gas in the upper tract without involvement of the renal parenchyma) often can be managed effectively with antibiotics alone.

Gas within the bladder or upper tract(s) can often be seen following catheterization. This benign gas can be distinguished from that of infectious gas based on its location: iatrogenic gas typically does not localize to the bladder wall or renal parenchyma. When the gas is purely intraluminal, it can be either iatrogenic or infectious. Rarely, gas within the urinary bladder lumen can indicate fistula formation.

References: Amano M, Shimizu T. Emphysematous cystitis: a review of the literature. *Intern Med* 2014;53:79–82.

Thomas AA, Lane BR, Thomas AZ, et al. Emphysematous cystitis: a review of 135 cases. *BJR Int* 2007;100:17–20.

8   **Answer B.**   The most likely cause of this large intraluminal mass is a blood clot. Of the answers, warfarin therapy related to the patient's atrial fibrillation is the best choice (Answer B). The mass shows no connection with the bladder wall, and it has retractile, concave margins. Smoking (Answer A) is a risk factor for bladder cancer; bladder cancer would be expected to arise from the wall and not be solely intraluminal. Hyperparathyroidism (Answer C) is a risk factor for calculus disease; though bladder calculi can be quite large, they would not "float" in urine or be so low in attenuation. Diabetes mellitus type 1 (Answer D) is a risk factor for papillary necrosis; filling defects from sloughed papillae would not be this large.

A generic differential diagnosis for a filling defect in the urinary tract includes blood, pus, stone, mass, sloughed papilla, and fungus ball.

References: Dunnick NR, Sandler CM, Newhouse JH. *Textbook of uroradiology*, 5th ed. Philadelphia: Lippincott Williams & Wilkins, 2012.

O'Connor OJ, Maher MM. CT urography. *AJR Am J Roentgenol* 2010;195:W320–W324.

Silverman SG, Cohan RH. *CT urography: An atlas*, 1st ed. Philadelphia: Lippincott Williams & Wilkins, 2006.

9   **Answer C.**   Bladder wall paragangliomas are associated with the classic history of "fainting with micturition." In patients with this condition, symptoms (e.g., palpitations, headaches, fainting) are caused by stimulated release of sympathetic hormones from the tumor during bladder wall contraction. However, few bladder wall paragangliomas are hormonally active; most are detected incidentally during biopsy for presumed urothelial malignancy.

Paragangliomas can occur anywhere along the sympathetic chain from the skull base to the pelvis. They are associated with multiple genetic syndromes. Examples include (1) hereditary paraganglioma and pheochromocytoma syndrome (many variants exist), (2) von Hippel-Lindau syndrome, (3) multiple endocrine neoplasia type 2 (MEN-2a and MEN-2b), and (4) neurofibromatosis type I.

References: Das S, Bulusu NV, Lowe P. Primary vesical pheochromocytoma. *Urology* 1983;21:20–25.

Ingram M, Barber B, Bano G, et al. Radiologic appearance of hereditary adrenal and extraadrenal paraganglioma. *AJR Am J Roentgenol* 2011;197:W687–W695.

10   **Answer B.**   Type II posterior urethral injuries (partial or complete tear of the posterior urethra without disruption of the urogenital diaphragm) are often caused by shearing injuries that result in avulsion of the posterior urethra from the relatively fixed bulbomembranous junction. The membranous urethra is a short segment of the urethra that courses through the urogenital diaphragm. As a result, it is relatively immobile and can act as a fixed point about which the more mobile prostatic urethra can torque.

Blunt (Answer A) and penetrating (Answer C) anterior mechanisms often cause isolated anterior (type V) or combined-type (type III) urethral injuries. Straddle injuries (Answer D) often result in type V urethral injuries.

References: Goldman SM, Sandler CM, Corriere JN, et al. Blunt urethral trauma: a unified, anatomical mechanical classification. *J Urol* 1997;157:85–89.

Rosenstein DI, Alsikafi NF. Diagnosis and classification of urethral injuries. *Urol Clin North Am* 2006;73–85.

11 **Answer C.** T1-weighted gradient echo images often have short echo times (<20 msec) and flip angles >45 degrees. Short echo times (TE) minimize T2 (T2*) contrast because when the TE is short, there is insufficient time for spin–spin relaxation to occur, and so therefore all substances, regardless of their T2 time, will appear similar. Large flip angles promote T1 weighting by converting a large fraction of longitudinal magnetization into transverse magnetization. This allows differences in T1 times to become evident during spin–lattice relaxation. Small flip angles retain a large fraction of the longitudinal magnetization, causing substances with different T1 times to remain clustered in signal intensity and prohibiting differentiation on the basis of T1.

References: Mamourian AC. *Practical MR physics*, 1st ed. New York: Oxford University Press, 2010.
McRobbie DW, Moore EA, Graves MJ, et al. *MRI: from picture to proton*, 2nd ed. New York: Cambridge University Press, 2007.

12 **Answer C.** According to the United States Nuclear Regulatory Commission, the cumulative dose to the fetus cannot exceed 5 mSv. This is intentionally greater than the dose limit set for the general public (1 mSv/year) to permit women of child-bearing age to be radiation workers. Pregnant women who do not declare their pregnancy have the same dose limits as nonpregnant radiation workers (total effective dose: 50 mSv/year).

References: Huda W. *Review of radiologic physics*, 3rd ed. Philadelphia: Lippincott Williams & Wilkins, 2010.
United States Nuclear Regulatory Commission. Part 20: Standards for protection against radiation. Updated January, 2014. Accessed February, 2014. http://www.nrc.gov/reading-rm/doc-collections/cfr/part020/full-text.html

13 **Answer E.** The images demonstrate complete disruption of the anterior urethra with no involvement of the posterior urethra compatible with a type V urethral injury. This injury pattern is often caused by a straddle-type mechanism (e.g., falling on a metal bar) or a direct impaction injury on the perineum (e.g., groin kick). Complete anterior urethral disruptions caused by blunt trauma are usually managed by suprapubic tube placement and delayed repair, while complete anterior urethral disruptions caused by penetrating trauma are often repaired primarily. The following table outlines an accepted classification system of urethral injuries in males stratified by injury location:

Injury Type	Description of Urethral Injury (Male Patients)
I	Stretching injury of the posterior urethra without partial or complete tear
II	Partial or complete tear of the posterior urethra above the urogenital diaphragm
III	Partial or complete tear of the anterior and posterior urethra above and below the urogenital diaphragm
IV	Bladder neck injury involving the urethra
IVa	Bladder base injury without urethral involvement mimicking a true type IV injury; type IV and type IVa injuries may be indistinguishable radiographically
V	Partial or complete tear isolated to the anterior urethra

References: Goldman SM, Sandler CM, Corriere JN, et al. Blunt urethral trauma: a unified, anatomical mechanical classification. *J Urol* 1997;157:85–89.

Martinez-Pineiro L, Djakovic N, Pla E, et al. EAU guidelines on urethral trauma. *Eur Urol* 2010;57:791–803.

Rosenstein DI, Alsikafi NF. Diagnosis and classification of urethral injuries. *Urol Clin North Am* 2006;73–85.

14 **Answer A.** The image demonstrates a normal appearance of the posterior urethra, with the cone of the bulbar urethra tapering to a point just below the urogenital diaphragm. The inferior margins of the obturator foramina serve as useful fixed anatomic landmarks for the level of the urogenital diaphragm at the junction of the anterior and posterior urethra. This permits identification of the approximate junction between the anterior and posterior urethra without reliance on the luminal contour of the urethra. This is especially helpful in the setting of bulbar urethral strictures in which strictured segments can resemble the cone of the bulbar urethra. The clue to the pathology in the setting of stricture disease is an abnormally positioned "cone" well below the inferior margins of the obturator foramina.

References: Kawashima A, Sandler CM, Wasserman NF, et al. Imaging of urethral disease: pictorial review. *Radiographics* 2004;24:S195–S216.

McCallum RW. The adult male urethra: normal anatomy, pathology, and method of urethrography. *Radiol Clin North Am* 1979;17:227–244.

15 **Answer A.** In trauma patients with blood at the urethral meatus, injury of the urethra should be suspected. The best next step is a retrograde urethrogram. In this setting, Foley catheter placement (Answer B) should not preempt urethrography because if the urethra is disrupted, catheter placement could create a false passage. CT cystogram (Answer C) and CT urography (Answer D) do not directly assess the urethra and are not the best next step.

References: Goldman SM, Sandler CM, Corriere JN, et al. Blunt urethral trauma: a unified, anatomical mechanical classification. *J Urol* 1997;157:85–89.

Martinez-Pineiro L, Djakovic N, Pla E, et al. EAU guidelines on urethral trauma. *Eur Urol* 2010;57:791–803.

Rosenstein DI, Alsikafi NF. Diagnosis and classification of urethral injuries. *Urol Clin North Am* 2006;73–85.

16 **Answer C.** The images depict a tubular partially fluid-filled structure arising from the anterior-superior bladder midline coursing toward the umbilicus without umbilical patency compatible with a urachal diverticulum. This is one of four major types of urachal remnant abnormalities caused by incomplete obliteration of the median umbilical ligament. The median umbilical remnant

Urachal Remnant	Description
Urachal diverticulum	Bladder diverticulum arising at the anterior-superior bladder midline extending anterior-superior toward the umbilicus
Urachal sinus	Incomplete sinus tract arising at the umbilicus extending inferior-posterior toward the bladder
Urachal cyst	Fluid-filled cyst along the otherwise obliterated median umbilical ligament without communication to the umbilicus or bladder lumen
Patent urachus	Complete patent tract extending from the anterior-superior bladder midline to the umbilicus (causes symptomatic umbilical discharge)

(single midline structure, remnant of the cloaca and allantois, location of urachal abnormalities) should be distinguished from the paired medial umbilical ligaments (off-midline structures, remnants of the obliterated umbilical arteries).

Patients with urachal remnant disease are at risk for recurrent infection and urachal adenocarcinoma. Urachal adenocarcinoma arises in the urachal remnant and spreads in the retroperitoneal perivesical space; therefore, it is usually asymptomatic until locally advanced. The table details the four major types of urachal remnant abnormalities:

References: Moore KL. The urogenital system. In: Moore KL, eds. *The developing human*, 3rd ed. Philadelphia, PA: Saunders, 1982.

Yu JS, Kim KW, Lee HJ, et al. Urachal remnant diseases: spectrum of CT and US findings. *Radiographics* 2001;21:451–461.

17 Answer A.   The images demonstrate a large inflamed bladder diverticulum. When large, bladder diverticula promote stasis of urine, and urinary stasis is a risk factor for urinary tract infection and calculus disease. Other risk factors for recurrent urinary tract infection include calculus disease, vesicoureteric reflux, urinary catheterization, fistula formation, sexual intercourse, female sex, and spermicide use.

References: Hooton TM, Bradley SF, Cardenas DD, et al. Diagnosis, prevention, and treatment of catheter-associated urinary tract infection in adults: 2009 International Practice Guidelines from the Infectious Diseases Society of America. *Clin Infect Dis* 2010;50:625–663.

Rao NP, Preminger GM, Kavanagh JP. *Urinary tract stone disease*. London: Springer Publishing, 2011.

Scholes D, Hooton TM, Roberts PL, et al. Risk factors for recurrent urinary tract infection in young women. *J Infect Dis* 2000;182:1177–1182.

18 Answer C.   The image demonstrates a markedly thick-walled urinary bladder with high-attenuation intraluminal filling defects compatible with hemorrhagic cystitis. Of the listed agents, cyclophosphamide (specifically, its metabolite acrolein) has the strongest association with this disease. In addition to causing hemorrhagic cystitis, the acrolein metabolite of cyclophosphamide is also considered a risk factor for bladder cancer. The toxic effects of acrolein can be mitigated by the compound mesna (sodium 2-sulfanylethanesulfonate) if mesna is coadministered with cyclophosphamide. Other risk factors for hemorrhagic cystitis other than chemotherapeutics include pelvic radiation, infection (e.g., BK virus), and stem cell transplantation.

References: Cannon J, Linke CA, Cos LR. Cyclophosphamide-associated carcinoma of the urothelium: modalities for prevention. *Urology* 1991;38:413–416.

Riachy E, Krauel L, Rich BS, et al. Risk factors and predictors of severity score and complications of pediatric hemorrhagic cystitis. *J Urol* 2014;191:186–192.

Stillwell TJ, Benson RC. Cyclophosphamide-induced hemorrhagic cystitis. A review of 100 patients. *Cancer* 1988;61:451–457.

19 Answer C.   The cystogram demonstrates opacification of both the bladder and rectum consistent with a colovesical fistula. Colovesical fistulae are most commonly caused by diverticulitis, although pelvic radiation, surgery, trauma, and malignancy are alternative etiologies. Urinary stasis (Answer A) is not the correct answer because it does not explain the contrast material in the rectum. Vesicoureteric reflux (Answer B) would be off-midline and confined to the collecting system. The image does not support a diagnosis of enterovesical fistula (Answer D) because the opacified rectum is vertically oriented and midline; small bowel loops would be smaller and in a different location.

Reference: Brant WE, Helms CA. *Fundamentals of diagnostic radiology*, 3rd ed. Philadelphia: Lippincott Williams & Wilkins, 2006.

Zagoria R. *Genitourinary radiology: Radiology requisites series*, 2nd ed. Maryland Heights: Mosby Publishing, 2004.

20 Answer D. The intravenous urogram demonstrates a "double density" in the midline pelvis, with contrast material filling the bladder and vagina. Vaginal opacification during an antegrade urogram is not normal under most circumstances and is suggestive of a fistula (although occasionally reflux through the vaginal introitus can occur in the absence of a fistula in patients with urinary incontinence). Vesicovaginal fistulae are usually caused by pelvic radiation, surgery (e.g., hysterectomy), inflammatory bowel disease, or obstructed labor.

Neurogenic bladder (Answer A) is associated with increased bladder capacity, bladder wall trabeculations, bladder wall thickening, and incomplete voiding. A patent urachus (Answer B) is a midline congenital abnormality between the anterior-superior bladder wall and umbilicus related to incomplete obliteration of the median umbilical ligament. Urachal adenocarcinoma (Answer C) is an aggressive neoplasm that often arises in urachal remnants and would be associated with a filling defect, not a double density. Although there is opacification of the ureters on the image, vesicoureteric reflux (Answer E) is not correct because an intravenous urogram is an antegrade study; opacification of the ureters is a normal finding.

References: Lewis A, Kaufman MR, Wolter CE, et al. Genitourinary fistula experience in Sierra Leone: review of 505 cases. *J Urol* 2009;181:1725–1731.

Narayanan P, Nobbenhuis M, Reynolds KM, et al. Fistulas in malignant gynecologic disease: etiology, imaging, and management. *Radiographics* 2009;29:1073–1083.

Rovner ES. Vesicovaginal and urethrovaginal fistulas. *AUA Update Series* 2006:46–55.

21 Answer A. An imaginary line drawn across the inferior margins of the obturator foramina is a useful landmark to signify the approximate location of the urogenital diaphragm and, by extension, the membranous urethra and bulbomembranous junction. Remember that the anterior urethra is composed of the penile (pendulous) urethra and bulbar urethra, and the posterior urethra is composed of the membranous urethra and prostatic urethra. Localizing the urogenital diaphragm is important because the inferior aspect of the urogenital diaphragm separates the anterior from the posterior urethra. Failure to identify this landmark can lead to confusion on retrograde urethrography between urethral stricture disease and the normal cone of the bulbar urethra.

References: Kawashima A, Sandler CM, Wasserman NF, et al. Imaging of urethral disease: pictorial review. *Radiographics* 2004;24:S195–S216.

McCallum RW. The adult male urethra: normal anatomy, pathology, and method of urethrography. *Radiol Clin North Am* 1979;17:227–244.

22 Answer D. The images demonstrate a small volume of extraluminal contrast material near the bladder–urethral anastomosis compatible with a small, contained anastomotic leak. This is the most common location for a urine leak after prostatectomy, and it is typically managed with prolonged Foley catheter placement (i.e., several weeks or more). Small leaks such as this one can delay catheter removal and delay recovery of urinary continence, but often do not have a long-term effect on urinary continence (i.e., by 12 months, patients with or without a small leak have similar continence rates).

In addition to the anastomotic leak, note the concave margins of the lateral bladder walls. Although not the primary abnormality in this case, this appearance is typically associated with external mass effect upon the bladder from one or more objects along the pelvic sidewall. The classic differential diagnosis for concave displacement of the lateral bladder wall(s) includes extraperitoneal hemorrhage (such as might be present in the recent postoperative state), pelvic lymph node enlargement, iliac artery aneurysm(s), pelvic lipomatosis, and other pelvic masses. In cases where the cause is not obvious, a pelvic CT scan can clarify the differential diagnosis.

References: Brant WE, Helms CA. *Fundamentals of diagnostic radiology*, 3rd ed. Philadelphia: Lippincott Williams & Wilkins, 2006.
Patil N, Krane L, Javed K, et al. Evaluating and grading cystographic leakage: correlation with clinical outcomes in patients undergoing robotic prostatectomy. *BJR Int* 2009;103:1108–1110.
Williams TJ, Longoria OJ, Asselmeier S, et al. Incidence and imaging appearance of urethrovesical anastomotic urinary leaks following da Vinci robotic prostatectomy. *Abdom Imaging* 2008;33:367–370.

23 **Answer A-4, B-1, C-3, D-2.** Susceptibility reflects the tendency of an object to become magnetized when placed into an external magnetic field. There are four major categories:

Susceptibility Type	Example	Additional Information
Diamagnetic	Barium sulfate	Diamagnetism is the weakest form of susceptibility. Diamagnetic materials have no inherent magnetism, but when placed into an external magnetic field, they gain a weak negative magnetic field that causes signal loss.
Paramagnetic	Gadolinium	Paramagnetism is more susceptible than diamagnetism. Unlike diamagnetic substances, when paramagnetic substances are placed into an external magnetic field, they tend to align with the field and strengthen it.
Superparamagnetic	Iron oxide particles	Superparamagnetism is more susceptible than paramagnetism. Unlike paramagnetism, when superparamagnetic materials are placed into an external magnetic field, the material aligns with the field on a whole-structure level, not just an atomic level.
Ferromagnetic	Metal hardware	Ferromagnetism is more susceptible than superparamagnetism. Ferromagnetic materials may be magnetized irrespective of an external magnetic field. They create severe artifacts on MR that are exaggerated with gradient echo and echo planar imaging.

References: Mamourian AC. *Practical MR physics*, 1st ed. New York: Oxford University Press, 2010.
McRobbie DW, Moore EA, Graves MJ, et al. *MRI: from picture to proton*, 2nd ed. New York: Cambridge University Press, 2007.

24 **Answer A.** A "watering can perineum" is perineal fistulous disease resulting from chronic inflammatory strictures. It most commonly develops in patients with advanced infection from *Neisseria gonorrhoeae* or *Mycobacterium tuberculosis*.

An example is shown below:

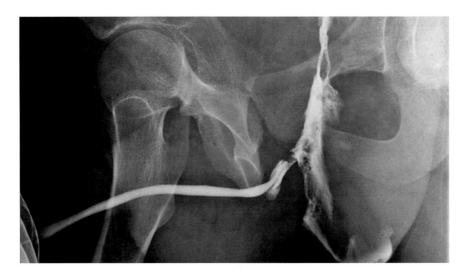

References: Mungadi IA, Ntia IO. Management of "watering-can" perineum. *East Afr Med J* 2007;84:283–286.

Sharfi AR, Elarabi YE. The "watering-can" perineum: presentation and management. *Br J Urol* 1997;80:933–936.

25 **Answer B.** The retrograde urethrogram demonstrates multiple strictures of the bulbar urethra. The bulbar urethra is a segment of the anterior urethra. There is no evidence of stricture disease involving the posterior urethra.

The midline lucency within the prostatic urethra corresponds to the verumontanum. The anterior urethra is composed of the penile (pendulous) urethra and bulbar urethra, and the posterior urethra is composed of the membranous urethra and prostatic urethra. An imaginary line drawn across the inferior margins of the obturator foramina should be used as the anatomic landmark to differentiate the anterior from the posterior urethra. The endoluminal appearance of the urethra should not be used because it is not reliable in patients with urethral pathology.

The normal posterior urethra is narrower than the normal anterior urethra. This is because unlike the anterior urethra, the segments of the posterior urethra are more tightly encircled by adjacent tissue (the membranous urethra by the urogenital diaphragm, and the prostatic urethra by the prostate). In some patients, it may be difficult to opacify the posterior urethra on retrograde urethrography due to sphincter spasm. Slow, steady injection pressure can occasionally overcome this. Stricture disease of the posterior urethra would result in distortion of the pressurized urethra distal to the stricture.

References: Kawashima A, Sandler CM, Wasserman NF, et al. Imaging of urethral disease: pictorial review. *Radiographics* 2004;24:S195–S216.

McCallum RW. The adult male urethra: normal anatomy, pathology, and method of urethrography. *Radiol Clin North Am* 1979;17:227–244.

26 **Answer B.** The image demonstrates a thin-walled ureterocele inserting near the right ureterovesical junction (UVJ). Such ureteroceles are usually associated with the insertion of an upper pole moiety in the setting of a complete congenital duplication and can be classified as "orthotopic" or "ectopic." Orthotopic ureteroceles insert at the expected location of the UVJ, while ectopic ureteroceles insert elsewhere, either at an atypical location on the bladder wall or on another organ. Thin-walled ureteroceles associated with congenital duplication should be distinguished from thick-walled pseudoureteroceles associated with ureteral filling defects such as calculi or urothelial cancer. A pseudoureterocele due to multiple impacted distal right ureteral calculi is shown below.

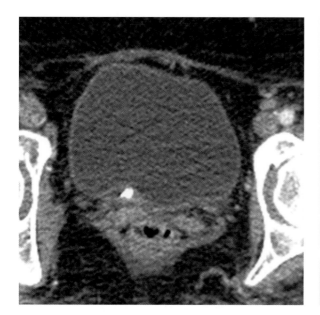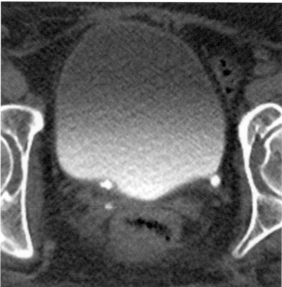

References: Dyer RB, Chen MY, Zagoria RJ. Classic signs in uroradiology. *Radiographics* 2004;24:S247–S280.

Rowell AC, Sangster GP, Caraway JD, et al. Genitourinary imaging: Part 1, Congenital urinary anomalies and their management. *AJR Am J Roentgenol* 2012;199:W545–W553.

27 **Answer D.** The images demonstrate a urethral diverticulum circumferentially encasing the female urethra. Urethral diverticula can have a varied appearance: single or multiple; saccular, horseshoe shaped, or circumferential; one or more "necks"; simple or complicated (stones, urothelial cancer, debris); anterior or posterior; lateral or medial; or a combination of the above. High-resolution thin-section T2-weighted imaging can depict with a high degree of accuracy the size, location, and type of the urethral diverticulum. MR imaging also can distinguish this entity from other fluid-filled pathologic structures in the lower pelvis and perineum. Identifying the location and number of diverticular "necks" (i.e., site(s) of communication of the diverticulum with the urethral lumen) is important for surgical planning because failure to resect one or more "necks" can result in recurrence of the diverticulum.

A simplified differential diagnosis for common "cystic lesions of the lower female pelvis" is summarized in the following table. This table is not all-inclusive. Rare entities have been intentionally excluded (e.g., müllerian remnant cysts, epidermal inclusion cysts).

Location	Entity	Notes
Above the inferior margin of the symphysis pubis	Urethral diverticulum	Midline, encircles the urethra, can be single or multiple, complicated or simple
	Gartner duct cyst	Usually singular, off-midline oval-shaped cyst in the anterolateral vaginal wall
	Periurethral collagen injection	Iatrogenic bulking agent injected near the proximal urethra to promote continence; round with variable signal intensity
At or below the inferior margin of the symphysis pubis	Bartholin gland cyst	Usually singular, medial to the labia in the posterolateral vaginal wall
	Skene gland cysts	Paired, periurethral cysts along the lateral aspect of the lower third of urethra near the external meatus

References: Hahn WY, Israel GM, Lee VS. MRI of female urethral and periurethral disorders. *AJR Am J Roentgenol* 2004;182:677–682.

Hosseinzadeh K, Furlan A, Torabi M. Pre- and postoperative evaluation of urethral diverticulum. *AJR Am J Roentgenol* 2008;190:165–172.

28 Answer C.   The verumontanum is located at the level of the prostatic urethra, is the entry site for the ejaculatory ducts into the urethral lumen, and is the site of the prostatic utricle. On retrograde urethrography, it is identifiable as an ovoid filling defect. On MR, the verumontanum is identifiable as a posterior impression upon the prostatic urethra at the site of ejaculatory duct entry.

References: Hansford BG, Peng Y, Jiang Y, et al. Revisiting the central gland anatomy via MRI: dose the central gland extend below the level of the verumontanum? *J Magn Reson Imaging* 2014;39:167–171.

Kawashima A, Sandler CM, Wasserman NF, et al. Imaging of urethral disease: pictorial review. *Radiographics* 2004;24:S195–S216.

McCallum RW. The adult male urethra: normal anatomy, pathology, and method of urethrography. *Radiol Clin North Am* 1979;17:227–244.

29 Answer A.   The image demonstrates the postoperative appearance of a psoas hitch, which is a procedure used to relieve tension on the distal ureter after a distal ureterectomy. Distal ureterectomy shortens the ureter. If no precautions are taken, anastomosing the shortened ureter to the bladder can create tension that threatens the anastomosis. A psoas hitch procedure addresses this by suturing the ipsilateral bladder to the psoas muscle. This effectively holds the bladder in place and relieves the tension on the ureter. It is important to recognize this normal postoperative appearance and not mistake it for a contained leak.

Reference: Matthews R, Marshall FF. Versatility of the adult psoas hitch ureteral reimplantation. *J Urol* 1997;158:2078–2082.

30 **Answer A.**   So-called "dirty shadowing" is caused by a type of reverberation artifact that develops along smooth surfaces or surfaces with a large radius of curvature (i.e., "flat" objects). It is often seen posterior to gas-containing structures because the surface of gas is smooth, and gas tends to collect along structures with a large radius of curvature (e.g., bowel lumen). Gas that is trapped in small objects with a small radius of curvature (e.g., pneumobilia) can produce "clean shadows," such as those more often seen posterior to bone or calcification.

The mechanism of "dirty shadowing" relates to the coherence of the reflected ultrasound beam. When the ultrasound beam is released from the transducer, the sound waves are "in phase." When the beam strikes a smooth surface (e.g., a collection of gas), it is reflected back to the transducer with the beam coherence intact. As the reflected coherent beam interacts with other objects on its path back to the transducer, it creates additional reflections; because the reflected beam is coherent (i.e., reflected with the phase coherence intact), the reflections are able to produce a measurable (though artifactual) signal.

These reflections are mapped by the ultrasound device posterior to the original object, creating a "dirty shadow." This occurs because object depth is mapped by the ultrasound machine based on the length of time it takes for the beam to return to the transducer, as a function of the speed of sound. Multiple reflections delay the ultrasound beam, giving the machine the false impression that the object is deeper than it actually is. Depending on the depth and number of reflections, reverberation artifact can create multiple copies of an object or create nonsensical noise of varying depth posterior to the actual location of an object in space.

"Clean shadowing," commonly seen posterior to bone or calcification, occurs because the ultrasound beam reflected from a rough object (or an object with a small radius of curvature) loses its coherence. Therefore, interactions of the incoherent beam with other objects on its path back to the transducer will produce no coherent signal.

References: Rubin JM, Adler RS, Bude RO, et al. Clean and dirty shadowing at US: a reappraisal. *Radiology* 1991;181:231–236.

Sommer FG, Taylor KJW. Differentiation of acoustic shadowing due to calculi and gas collections. *Radiology* 1980;135:399–403.

6 Male Genital (Prostate, Penis, and Scrotum)

QUESTIONS

1 A 65-year-old male with an elevated prostate-specific antigen (PSA, 16.4 ng/mL) and a palpable prostate nodule undergoes prostate MRI. The images demonstrate a 2.5-cm mass at the left base with extracapsular extension (axial image on left) and ipsilateral seminal vesicle invasion (coronal image on right). The apparent diffusion coefficient (ADC) is 700×10^{-6} mm^2/s. What is the T stage of this prostate cancer?

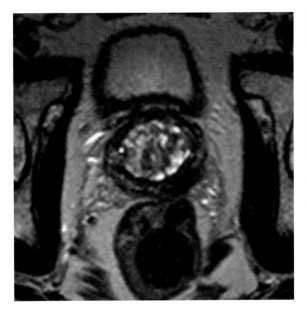 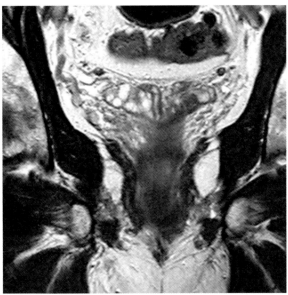

A. T2c
B. T3a
C. T3b
D. T4a

2   A 57-year-old asymptomatic male with no past medical history presents with an elevated prostate-specific antigen (PSA, 7.2 ng/mL). What is the reported sensitivity of transrectal grayscale ultrasound for the detection of clinically significant prostate cancer?

A. <1%

B. 10%

C. 50%

D. 90%

3   A 33-year-old male with acute scrotal pain undergoes Doppler ultrasound of his testicles with a linear 12-MHz transducer. How do high-frequency ultrasound transducers compare to low-frequency ultrasound transducers with respect to imaging depth and spatial resolution?

A. High-frequency transducers have less penetration and greater spatial resolution.

B. High-frequency transducers have more penetration and greater spatial resolution.

C. High-frequency transducers have less penetration and less spatial resolution.

D. High-frequency transducers have more penetration and less spatial resolution.

4   A 30-year-old male with scrotal swelling and scrotal pain undergoes Doppler ultrasound. What is the clinical significance of the findings in the left scrotal sac?

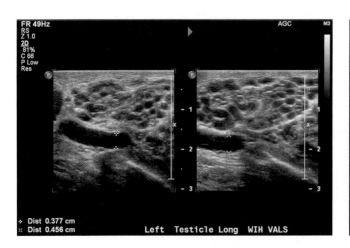 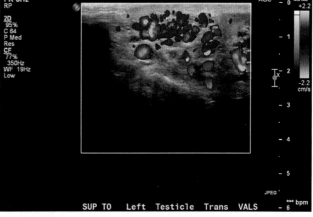

A. Benign finding of no clinical significance

B. Risk factor for infertility

C. Risk factor for testicular cancer

D. Risk factor for sexually transmitted infection

5   Modern multiparametric prostate MRI incorporates multiple advanced anatomic and functional pulse sequences. Which of the following pulse sequences utilize strong bipolar gradients to differentiate moving from stationary spins?

A. Fast spin echo and spin echo

B. Spin echo and balanced gradient echo

C. Balanced gradient echo and echo planar imaging

D. Echo planar imaging and phase contrast

6 A 60-year-old male with an elevated prostate-specific antigen (PSA, 10.5 ng/mL) and two negative prostate biopsies undergoes prostate MRI. The following images were obtained. What type of pulse sequence was most likely used for these single-shot acquisitions?

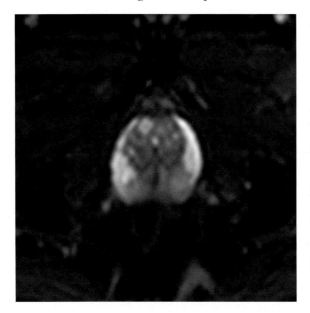 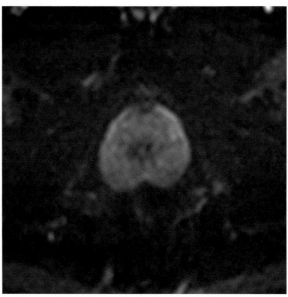

A. T2-weighted fast spin echo
B. T2*-weighted gradient-recalled echo
C. Balanced gradient-recalled echo
D. Echo planar imaging

7 A 50-year-old trauma victim presents with groin pain. A Doppler ultrasound is performed, and an abnormality is identified in his right testicle. What is the most likely diagnosis?

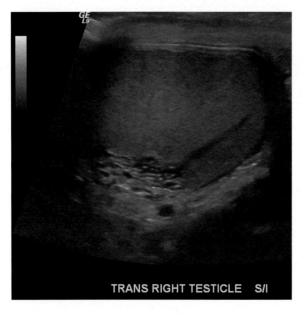 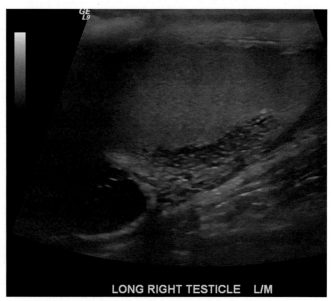

A. Benign finding (ignore)
B. Contained rupture
C. Germ cell tumor
D. Vascular malformation

8 A 32-year-old male presents with scrotal pain, and a Doppler ultrasound is performed. Which of the following risk factors is most likely related to the imaging findings?

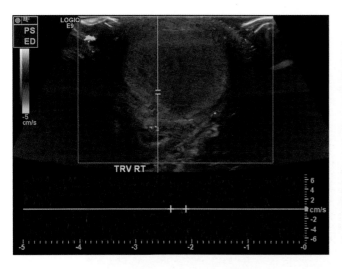 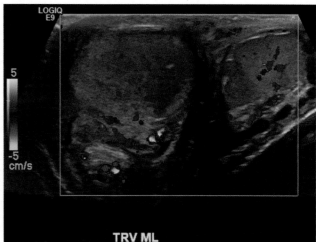

A. Testicular microlithiasis
B. "Bell clapper" deformity
C. *Neisseria gonorrhoeae* infection
D. Human immunodeficiency virus infection

9 A 32-year-old male presents with scrotal swelling. A Doppler ultrasound is performed. Which of the following is a strong risk factor for this disease?

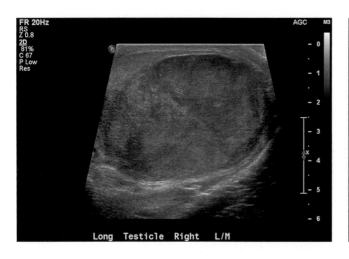 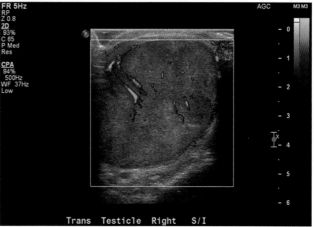

A. Cryptorchidism
B. Prior vasectomy
C. *Neisseria gonorrhoeae* infection
D. Renal agenesis

10 A 42-year-old male presents with a palpable finding in his left scrotum. An ultrasound is performed demonstrating a solid mass. What imaging finding is most helpful for determining whether this mass is benign or malignant?

A. Presence of calcifications
B. Degree of vascularity
C. Echogenicity
D. Location in or outside the testicle

11 A 60-year-old male with a palpable prostate nodule undergoes transrectal ultrasound (TRUS)-guided sextant biopsy. The pathology returns consistent with multifocal bilateral Gleason 4 + 4 = 8 prostate cancer. A bone scan is performed. How should the images be interpreted?

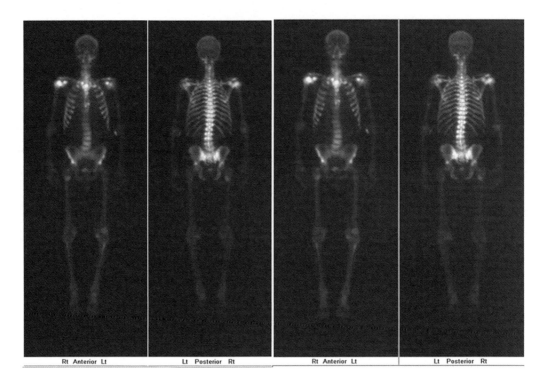

Rt Anterior Lt   Lt Posterior Rt   Rt Anterior Lt   Lt Posterior Rt

A. Normal study
B. Degenerative change
C. Hyperparathyroidism
D. Widespread metastases

12 A 25-year-old male notices a palpable lump in his scrotum. An ultrasound is performed. What is the most likely diagnosis?

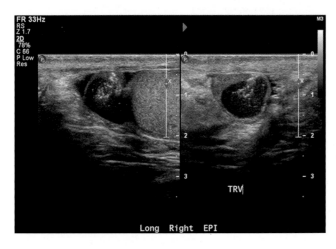
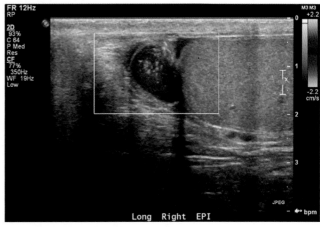

A. Spermatocele
B. Adenomatoid tumor
C. Varicocele
D. Seminoma

13 A 30-year-old male with abdominal pain and weight loss undergoes an abdominopelvic CT examination. Multiple enlarged lymph nodes are identified suggestive of metastatic disease. What is the typical nodal drainage of the male gonads?

A. Inguinal and external iliac lymph nodes
B. Obturator and internal iliac lymph nodes
C. Paracaval and para-aortic lymph nodes
D. Paraceliac and gastrohepatic lymph nodes

14 A 50-year-old female with multiple cardiovascular risk factors and congestive heart failure presents with left perineal swelling, warmth, and erythema. What is the definitive management for this condition?

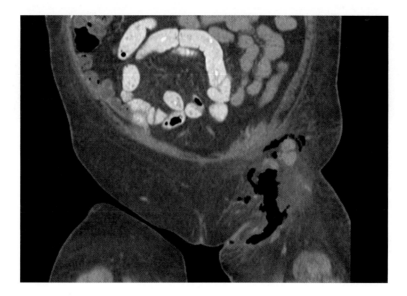

A. Observation
B. Diuretic therapy
C. Needle aspiration
D. Operative debridement

15 A 19-year-old male with von Hippel-Lindau syndrome presents with bilateral scrotal masses. Which tumors of the scrotal sac are associated with this disease?

A. Seminoma
B. Embryonal cell carcinoma
C. Epididymal cystadenoma
D. Spermatic cord liposarcoma

16 A 60-year-old asymptomatic male with an elevated prostate-specific antigen (PSA, 9.7 ng/mL) is diagnosed with Gleason 3 + 4 = 7 prostate cancer in 3 of 12 sextant core biopsies. What is the likelihood that this patient will have osseous metastatic disease detectable on imaging?

A. <1%
B. 5%
C. 20%
D. 50%

17   A 5-year-old male with scrotal swelling undergoes a scrotal ultrasound demonstrating bowel in the left scrotal sac. The bowel is followed cephalad along a superolateral course to the level of the inferior epigastric artery, where it is seen to wrap lateral to the artery and enter the peritoneal cavity. What type of hernia does this most likely represent?

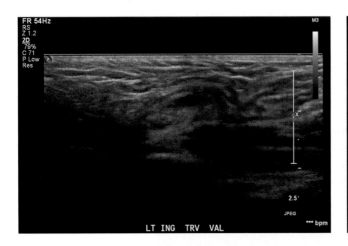 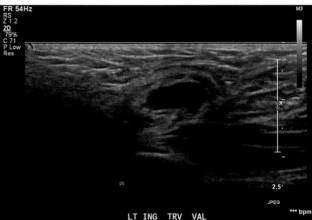

A. Direct inguinal hernia
B. Indirect inguinal hernia
C. Femoral hernia
D. Obturator hernia

18   A 43-year-old male with HIV presents with a large verrucous growth on his scrotum and perineum as shown on the coronal contrast-enhanced CT image below. He is diagnosed with Buschke-Löwenstein disease. This is strongly associated with what entity?

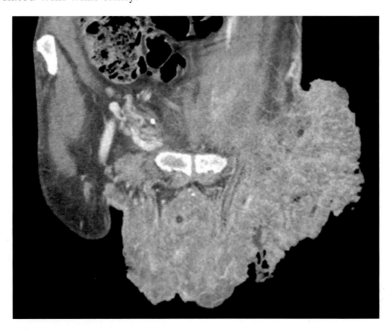

A. Adenocarcinoma
B. Squamous cell carcinoma
C. Melanoma
D. Basal cell carcinoma

19 A 55-year-old male with an elevated prostate-specific antigen (PSA, 8.9 ng/mL) and a prior negative prostate biopsy undergoes prostate MRI. A nodule is identified in the anterior transition zone with an apparent diffusion coefficient (ADC) value of 700×10^{-6} mm²/s. What does the ADC map represent?

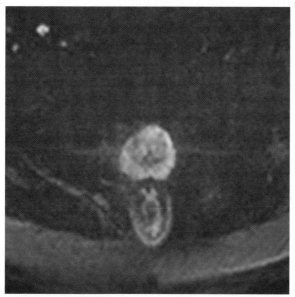
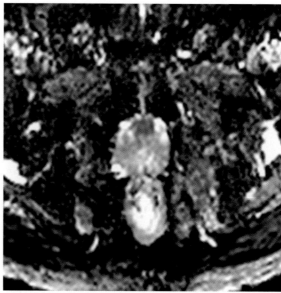

DWI (b = 800 s/mm²)   *ADC map*

A. An inverted pixel-by-pixel map of signal intensity (SI) at the highest acquired b value

B. An inverted pixel-by-pixel map of SI at the lowest acquired b value

C. A pixel-by-pixel map of the slope of SI measured across different acquired b values

D. A pixel-by-pixel map of the slope of ln(SI) measured across different acquired b values

20 A 19-year-old male presents with scrotal swelling after a straddle injury. A Doppler ultrasound is performed. What is the best next step?

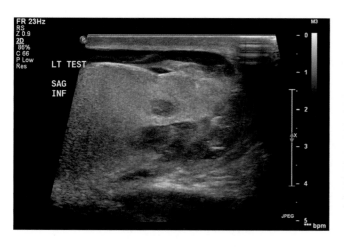
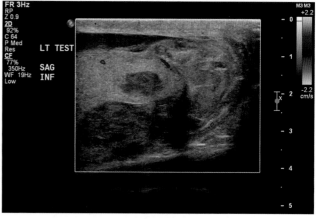

A. Imaging follow-up

B. Intravenous antibiotics

C. Percutaneous biopsy

D. Operative management

21 A 75-year-old male with a palpable prostate nodule undergoes a transrectal ultrasound (TRUS)-guided prostate biopsy demonstrating multifocal Gleason 4 + 5 = 9 prostate cancer throughout the right gland. A multiparametric prostate MRI is performed that demonstrates a large mass in the right anterior transition zone. Which of the following is an accepted specific sign of extracapsular disease?

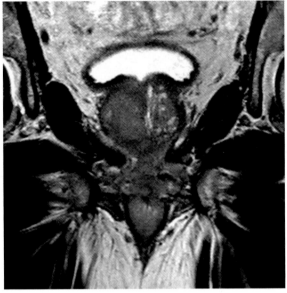 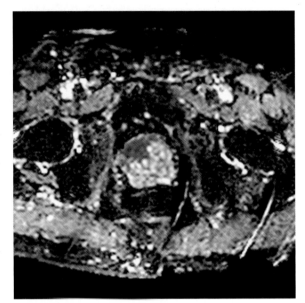

Coronal 2D T2-Weighted Fast Spin Echo   *Axial ADC map*

A. Focal capsular bulge
B. ADC <800 × 10^{-6} mm^2/s
C. ≥5 mm of capsular abutment
D. Nonvisible T2-hypointense capsule

22 MR spectroscopy has been explored as a method of improving detection of prostate cancer. What is the characteristic spectroscopic pattern of prostate cancer?

A. Elevated citrate:choline ratio
B. Elevated citrate:creatine ratio
C. Elevated choline:citrate ratio
D. Elevated creatine:citrate ratio

23 A 33-year-old male with priapism undergoes Doppler imaging of his penis. Which of the following correctly describes the flow detection characteristics of color and power Doppler imaging?

A. Power Doppler imaging is velocity dependent and color Doppler imaging is not.
B. Power Doppler imaging is less sensitive to slow flow than is color Doppler imaging.
C. Power Doppler imaging is direction independent and color Doppler imaging is not.
D. Power Doppler imaging is more affected by aliasing than is color Doppler imaging.

24   A 60-year-old male with elevated prostate-specific antigen (PSA, 7.1 ng/mL) undergoes a transrectal ultrasound-guided prostate biopsy. Four days later, he presents with scrotal pain and swelling. A Doppler ultrasound is performed. What is the best next step?

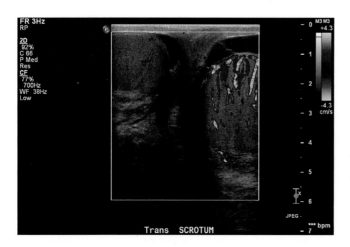 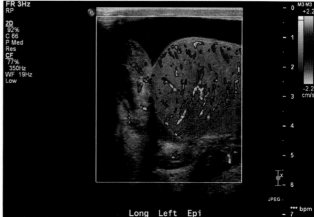

A. Observation
B. Antibiotic therapy
C. Surgical detorsion
D. Prostatectomy

25   A 50-year-old male with T3aNxMx Gleason 4 + 4 = 8 prostate cancer undergoes an In-111 capromab pendetide (ProstaScint) scan. What is the most appropriate interpretation of the imaging findings?

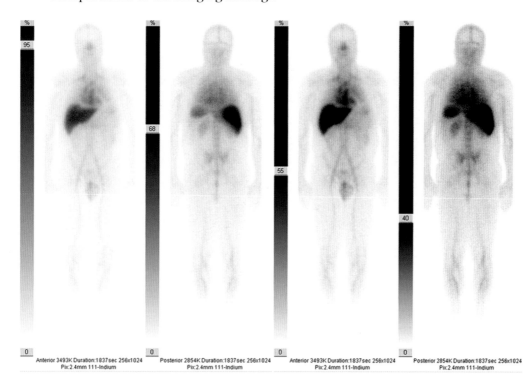

A. Normal study
B. Hepatic metastatic disease
C. Osseous metastatic disease
D. Pulmonary metastatic disease

26   A 16-year-old male with groin pain undergoes a scrotal ultrasound. Multiple masses are identified in both testicles. Which of the following diseases is associated with this imaging finding?

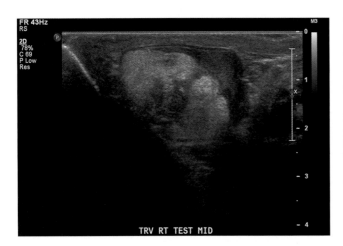 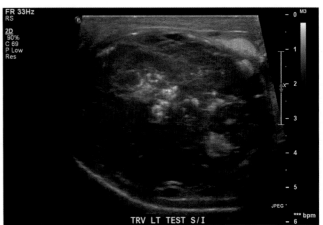

A. Multiple endocrine neoplasia type 2
B. Congenital adrenal hyperplasia
C. von Hippel-Lindau syndrome
D. Autosomal dominant polycystic kidney disease

27   A 20-year-old male with a suspected hernia and no relevant history undergoes a scrotal ultrasound. What is the most appropriate management for this imaging finding?

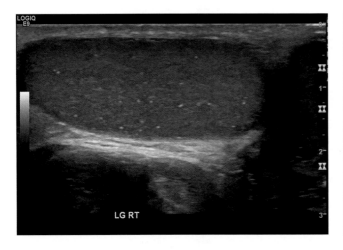 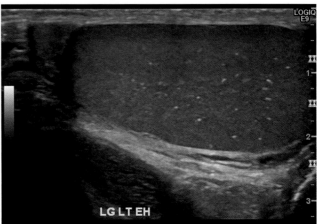

A. Ignore (benign incidental finding)
B. Regular scrotal self-examination
C. Follow-up ultrasound every 6 months
D. Prophylactic bilateral orchiectomy

28   A 60-year-old male with T2bN0Mx Gleason 3 + 4 = 7 prostate cancer undergoes prostatectomy. Two years later, his prostate-specific antigen (PSA, 1.2 ng/mL) becomes detectable. Dynamic contrast-enhanced T1-weighted gradient echo imaging is performed (on left), and subtractions are generated (on right). What is the best next step?

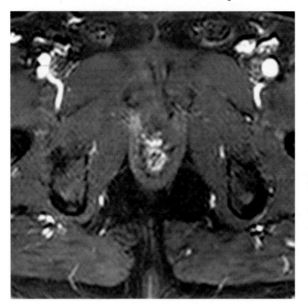 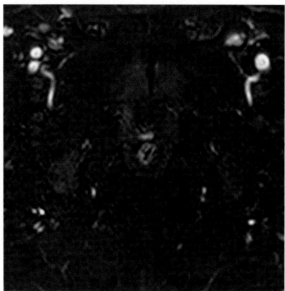

A. Observation with PSA monitoring
B. Observation with serial prostate MRI
C. Antibiotic therapy and drain placement
D. Salvage radiotherapy

29   A 69-year-old male with an elevated prostate-specific antigen (PSA, 18.4 ng/mL) and a prior negative prostate biopsy undergoes prostate MRI. Diffusion-weighted imaging is performed. Which of the following has been shown to correlate with high Gleason score prostate cancer?

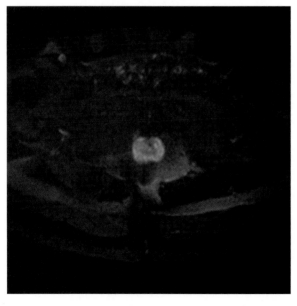 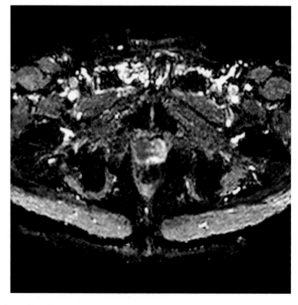

A. Signal intensity on trace b = 800 s/mm^2 diffusion images >800
B. Signal intensity on trace b = 800 s/mm^2 diffusion images <800
C. Signal intensity on ADC map >850 × 10^{-6} mm^2/s
D. Signal intensity on ADC map <850 × 10^{-6} mm^2/s

30 A 55-year-old male with right lower quadrant pain undergoes a CT of the abdomen and pelvis. Plaque-like calcifications are identified within the penis. What is most likely calcified?

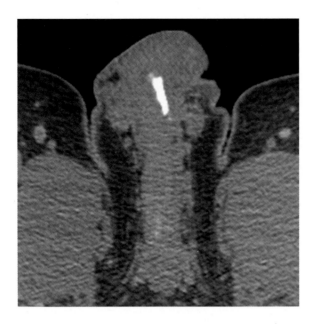
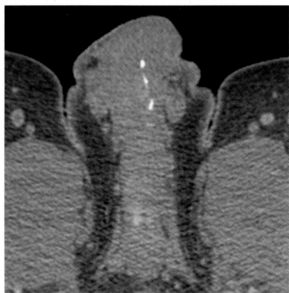

A. Arteries of the corpora cavernosa
B. Veins of the corpora cavernosa
C. Tunica albuginea
D. Tunica vaginalis

ANSWERS AND EXPLANATIONS

1 **Answer C.**   Seminal vesicle invasion signifies T3b disease according to the AJCC 2010 TNM classification system. The various T stages of prostate cancer are shown below. Of these, the most important to memorize for the radiologist is T2 versus T3.

T Stage	Description
T0	No evidence of prostate cancer
Nonpalpable, nonvisible tumor, confined to the prostate	
T1a	Cancer incidentally detected in ≤5% of resected tissue (e.g., TURP)
T1b	Cancer incidentally detected in >5% of resected tissue (e.g., TURP)
T1c	Cancer detected by needle biopsy (e.g., PSA-triggered biopsy)
Palpable or visible tumor, confined to the prostate	
T2a	Unilateral involvement (one lobe involved), ≤50% lobe volume
T2b	Unilateral involvement (one lobe involved), >50% lobe volume
T2c	Bilateral involvement (both lobes involved)
Tumor extends outside the prostate	
T3a	Extracapsular extension
T3b	Seminal vesicle invasion
T4	Invasion of adjacent structures other than the seminal vesicles (e.g., bladder)

Reference: Prostate. In: Edge SB, Byrd DR, Compton CC, et al. (eds). *AJCC cancer staging manual*, 7th ed. New York, NY: Springer, 2010: 457–468.

2 **Answer C.**   The sensitivity of grayscale transrectal ultrasound for the detection of clinically significant prostate cancer is reported to be approximately 50%, though even this is probably an overestimation. Grayscale ultrasound is not a reliable method of detecting primary prostate cancer. Ultrasound is primarily used to guide transrectal ultrasound (TRUS)-guided biopsies. TRUS-guided biopsies are usually nontargeted and randomly directed (i.e., sextant biopsy). Sampling during a random TRUS-guided biopsy usually consists of 12 or more core biopsy specimens obtained using a template approach, with intentional oversampling of the peripheral zone. The anterior gland and transition zone are often undersampled or not sampled at all.

References: Carter HB, Hamper UM, Sheth S, et al. Evaluation of transrectal ultrasound in the early detection of prostate cancer. *J Urol* 1989;142:1008–1010.
Terris MK, Freiha FS, McNeal JE, et al. Efficacy of transrectal ultrasound for identification of clinically undetected prostate cancer. *J Urol* 1991;146:78–83.

3 **Answer A.** High-frequency transducers have less penetration and greater spatial resolution than do low-frequency transducers. This is why superficial structures (e.g., testicles, thyroid) are preferentially imaged with high-frequency transducers. It is also why, when applicable, endocavitary probes are preferred over transcutaneous probes (e.g., transvaginal vs. transabdominal ultrasound). In general, linear transducers are higher frequency transducers than are curved transducers. You can tell which probe has been used by the superficial shape of the image: a linear transducer will have a flat superficial edge, and a curved transducer will have a curved superficial edge. Examples of images obtained with high-frequency linear (left) and low-frequency curved (right) transducers are shown below demonstrating an epididymal head cyst and a normal gallbladder, respectively. Note the relationship between the shape of the transducer and the shape of the image. The linear transducer is set at a depth of 4.5 cm and has a frequency of 14 MHz; the curved transducer is set at a depth of 15 cm and has a frequency of 4 MHz.

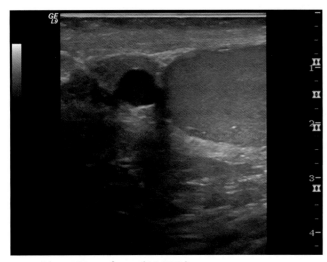 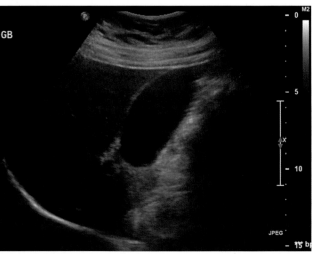

Linear Transducer (14 MHz)   *Curved Transducer (4 MHz)*

Reference: Rumack CM, Wilson SR, Charboneau JW, et al. *Diagnostic ultrasound, 2-volume set,* 4th ed. Philadelphia: Mosby, 2011.

4 **Answer B.** Dilated veins within the pampiniform plexus of the spermatic cord ≥3 mm in caliber are specific (90%+) for the diagnosis of a varicocele. Associated findings include a tangled congested venous network and increasing venous distention with Valsalva.

Surgical removal of a varicocele (varicocelectomy) is an accepted treatment for male infertility with a high technical success rate. Many patients who receive this therapy will experience improved sperm density and improved sperm quality. However, only a minority (~2.5%) will achieve a successful pregnancy without additional reproductive assistance.

References: Chiou RK, Anderson JC, Wobig RK, et al. Color Doppler ultrasound criteria to diagnose varicoceles: correlation of a new scoring system with physical examination. *Urology* 1997;50:953–956.
Lee R, Li PS, Goldstein M, et al. A decision analysis of treatments for nonobstructive azoospermia associated with varicocele. *Fertil Steril* 2009;92:188–196.
Masson P, Branningan RE. The varicocele. *Urol Clin North Am* 2014;41:129–144.
Petros JA, Andriole GL, Middleton WD, et al. Correlation of testicular color Doppler ultrasonography, physical examination and venography in the detection of left varicoceles in men with infertility. *J Urol* 1991;145:785–788.

5   **Answer D.**   Strong bipolar gradients are used in echo planar imaging and phase-contrast imaging to differentiate moving from stationary spins. When bipolar gradients are activated in succession, they induce a phase shift in moving spins because the moving spins are affected differently by the two equal gradient pulses. Moving spins will have moved to a different location along the gradient by the time the second gradient pulse is activated, so the phase accumulated from the first gradient pulse is not cancelled by the second gradient pulse. This phase shift is related to the velocity of the moving spins and can be used to determine the speed of a moving structure (e.g., flow across a stenotic valve). Stationary spins (i.e., precessing protons in immobile tissue) will be equally affected by both gradients resulting in zero phase shift because the stationary spins will not have moved between the times of gradient activation.

References: Lee VS. *Cardiovascular MR imaging: physical principles to practical protocols*, 1st ed. Philadelphia, PA: Lippincott Williams & Wilkins, 2005.

McRobbie DW, Moore EA, Graves MJ, et al. *MRI: from picture to proton*, 2nd ed. New York: Cambridge University Press, 2007.

6   **Answer D.**   Diffusion-weighted imaging is most commonly performed with echo planar imaging (EPI) using single-shot acquisitions (multishot EPI is possible but has technical limitations). Echo planar imaging is an extremely fast imaging modality that can acquire images in <100 msec. It is used for diffusion-weighted imaging, perfusion imaging, and functional MRI (e.g., BOLD [**B**lood **O**xygen **L**evel-**D**ependent] imaging). The speed of the technique is such that gross patient motion is essentially eliminated. Speed is important for diffusion-weighted imaging because diffusion-weighted imaging attempts to measure subvoxel Brownian motion. Any superimposed gross patient motion can destroy the sequence. A disadvantage of echo planar imaging is that it is exceptionally prone to susceptibility artifacts.

References: McRobbie DW, Moore EA, Graves MJ, et al. *MRI: from picture to proton*, 2nd ed. New York: Cambridge University Press, 2007.

Poustchi-Amin M, Mirowitz SA, Brown JJ, et al. Principles and applications of echo-planar imaging: a review for the general radiologist. *Radiographics* 2001;21:767–779.

7   **Answer A.**   The images demonstrate cystic dilation of the rete testis, which is a benign finding of little clinical significance. It can be seen incidentally or after vasectomy. It is important to distinguish this from an intratesticular neoplasm. Unlike neoplasms, dilation of the rete testis does not have solid elements. Dilated rete testes are characterized by small (1 to 3 mm) adjacent fluid-filled sacs and tubes that develop along or replace the mediastinum testis. They should show absent Doppler flow. If Doppler flow is present within the anechoic sacs without evidence of solid tissue, the diagnosis is likely an intratesticular varicocele (much rarer).

References: Dogra VS, Gottlieb RH, Rubens DJ, et al. Benign intratesticular cystic lesions: US features. *Radiographics* 2001;21:S273–S281.

Older RA, Watson LR. Tubular ectasia of the rete testis: a benign condition with a sonographic appearance that may be misinterpreted as malignant. *J Urol* 1994;152:477–478.

8   **Answer B.**   The images demonstrate absent flow within the right testicle consistent with testicular torsion. Testicular torsion is often associated with a congenital "bell clapper" deformity in which the tunica vaginalis (the serous covering around the testicles, outside the tunica albuginea) extends too high along the posterior wall and attaches to the spermatic cord instead of the testicle. Normally, the inferior aspect of the tunica vaginalis inserts upon the testicle, anchoring it and preventing it from rotating. In the "bell clapper" state, the tunica vaginalis does not insert upon the testicle, but rather higher up, permitting the testicle to freely rotate in the space this creates.

Testicular microlithiasis (Answer A) is associated with testicular malignancy; *Neisseria gonorrhoeae* infection is associated with epididymo-orchitis (Answer C); and human immunodeficiency virus infection (Answer D) is associated with testicular lymphoma and opportunistic infections.

References: Aso C, Enriquez G, Fite M, et al. Gray-scale and color Doppler sonography of scrotal disorders in children: an update. *Radiographics* 2005;25:1197–1214.
Avery LL, Scheinfeld MH. Imaging of penile and scrotal emergencies. *Radiographics* 2013;33:721–740.

9 **Answer A.** The images demonstrate a solid mass in the right testicle compatible with testicular malignancy, for which cryptorchidism (Answer A) is a strong risk factor. Although orchiopexy cannot eliminate this risk, early orchiopexy is performed to prevent other complications (subfertility) and permit surveillance. Uncomplicated undescended testicles are generally not removed because despite the increased risk, the vast majority of patients with cryptorchidism will not go on to develop testicular cancer.

Vasectomy (Answer B) and *Neisseria gonorrhoeae* infection (Answer C) do not have a strong association with testicular malignancy. *Neisseria gonorrhoeae* is associated with infectious orchitis, but the images demonstrate a solid intratesticular mass, not an inflamed testicle (note the normal parenchyma "claw sign" in the upper left-hand corner and the lack of hypervascularity). Although renal agenesis (Answer D, as well as other urinary malformations) is associated with a variety of congenital genital conditions, it does not have a direct role in the development of testicular cancer.

References: Albers P, Albrecht W, Algaba F, et al. EAU guidelines on testicular cancer: 2011 update. *Eur Urol* 2011;60:304–319.
Hutson JM, Clarke MC. Current management of the undescended testicle. *Semin Pediatr Surg* 2007;16:64–70.

10 **Answer D.** The most important factor predicting malignancy within an intrascrotal mass is whether the mass is within (very likely cancer) or outside (unlikely cancer) the testicle. Of course, exceptions to both rules exist (e.g., benign "onion-skinned" testicular epidermoid, malignant inguinal canal liposarcoma), but the trend is strong enough to help govern management. The presence of calcification (Answer A), the degree of vascularity (Answer B), and the echogenicity (Answer C) of a solid intrascrotal mass are much less helpful.

References: Aso C, Enriquez G, Fite M, et al. Gray-scale and color Doppler sonography of scrotal disorders in children: an update. *Radiographics* 2005;25:1197–1214.
Beccia DJ, Krane RJ, Olsson CA. Clinical management of non-testicular intrascrotal tumors. *J Urol* 1976;116:476–479.
Woodward PJ, Schwab CM, Sesterhann IA. Extratesticular scrotal masses: radiologic-pathologic correlation. *Radiographics* 2003;23:215–240.

11 **Answer D.** The bone scan images show diffuse osseous uptake with lack of or faint renal uptake (so-called "superscan" appearance) consistent with diffuse metastatic disease. A "superscan" can be caused by a variety of pathologic conditions, including diffuse sclerotic metastatic disease, metabolic derangements (e.g., hyperparathyroidism), and myeloproliferative disorders. It is caused by consumptive hypermetabolic bone scavenging radiotracer away from the urinary system. The CT images below were taken from the same patient on the same day. They demonstrate extensive sclerotic bone lesions consistent with metastases. Although hyperparathyroidism (Answer C) is also capable of producing a superscan, it would not be the most likely diagnosis in the setting of multifocal high-grade prostate cancer. A normal study (Answer A), or a study with simple degenerative change (Answer B), would be expected to have more conspicuous uptake within the urinary system.

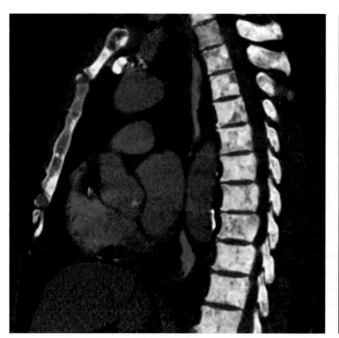 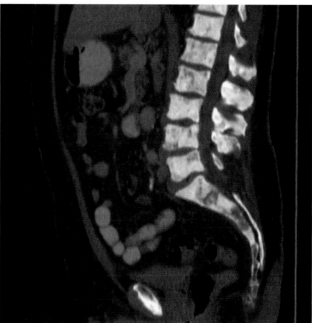

References: Buckley O, O'Keeffe S, Geoghegan T, et al. 99mTc bone scintigraphy superscans: a review. *Nucl Med Commun* 2007;28:521–527.
Constable AR, Cranage RW. Recognition of the superscan in prostatic bone scintigraphy. *Br J Radiol* 1981;54:122–125.

12   **Answer A.**   The images demonstrate a heterogeneous cystic structure within the right epididymal head containing small echogenic foci and no internal Doppler flow signal. This likely represents a benign spermatocele containing nonviable sperm. Spermatoceles can also be anechoic and resemble epididymal head cysts (epididymal cysts do not contain sperm), but both have similar clinical management, and therefore differentiating the two on imaging is not required.

    Adenomatoid tumors (Answer B) are common, often benign, extratesticular masses. Both adenomatoid tumors and varicoceles (Answer C) typically would show flow on Doppler imaging. Seminoma (Answer D) is an intratesticular mass, not an extratesticular mass.

References: Erikci V, Hosgor M, Aksoy N, et al. Management of epididymal cysts in childhood. *J Pediatr Surg* 2013;48:2153–2156.
Sista AK, Filly RA. Color Doppler sonography in evaluation of spermatoceles: the "falling snow" sign. *J Ultrasound Med* 2008;27:141–143.
Woodward PJ, Schwab CM, Sesterhann IA. Extratesticular scrotal masses: radiologic-pathologic correlation. *Radiographics* 2003;23:215–240.

13   **Answer C.**   The gonadal lymphatics follow the gonadal veins. The right gonadal vein drains into the inferior vena cava below the level of the right renal vein(s) (i.e., paracaval), and the left gonadal vein drains into the left renal vein (i.e., para-aortic). These landing zones are important to remember because the nodal spread of testicular cancer is different from that of many other pelvic malignancies. Testicular cancer does not typically spread to the pelvic lymph nodes (Answers A and B). Incidentally detected lymph node enlargement near the insertion of one or both gonadal veins should prompt a scrotal ultrasound to determine if the lymph node enlargement is secondary to a testicular malignancy.

References: Albers P, Albrecht W, Algaba F, et al. EAU guidelines on testicular cancer: 2011 update. *Eur Urol* 2011;60:304–319.

Dunnick NR, Sandler CM, Newhouse JH. *Textbook of uroradiology*, 5th ed. Philadelphia, PA: Lippincott Williams & Wilkins, 2012.

14 **Answer D.** Gas within the inguinal and perineal soft tissues in the setting of cellulitis is suggestive of Fournier gangrene, which is a surgical emergency. This rapidly progressive necrotizing infection can result in severe morbidity or death if not managed aggressively (Answers A, B, and C are incorrect). It is most commonly associated with immune-compromised states (e.g., diabetes mellitus).

CT is the most sensitive modality for detection of soft tissue gas. Gas on ultrasound may produce a so-called "dirty shadow." The differential diagnosis for pelvic soft tissue gas includes Fournier gangrene, enterocutaneous fistula, sinus tract, abscess, a recent operation or percutaneous procedure, and inferiorly tracking subcutaneous emphysema from a pneumothorax or pneumomediastinum.

References: Eke N. Fournier's gangrene: a review of 1726 cases. *Br J Surg* 2000;87:718–728.

Levenson RB, Singh AK, Novelline RA. Fournier gangrene: role of imaging. *Radiographics* 2008;28:519–528.

15 **Answer C.** von Hippel-Lindau syndrome is associated with epididymal cystadenoma, central nervous system and retinal hemangioblastoma, pancreatic neuroendocrine tumors, pancreatic cysts, renal cell carcinoma, and pheochromocytoma.

Reference: Choyke PL, Glenn GM, Walther MM, et al. von Hippel-Lindau disease: genetic, clinical, and imaging features. *Radiology* 1995;194:629–642.

16 **Answer A.** In patients with prostate cancer and a prostate-specific antigen (PSA) level <10 ng/mL, the likelihood of osseous metastatic disease is <1%. This information can be useful in managing incidental isolated small sclerotic osseous lesions detected in asymptomatic patients with prostate cancer and is the basis for prostate cancer staging guidelines. Indications for metastatic disease screening in patients with prostate cancer include bone pain, T3/T4 disease, Gleason score ≥8, high-volume Gleason score 7, and/or PSA ≥20 ng/mL.

References: Huncharek M, Muscat J. Serum prostate-specific antigen as a predictor of radiographic staging studies in newly diagnosed prostate cancer. *Cancer Invest* 1995;13:31–35.

Oesterling JE, Martin SK, Bergstralh EJ, et al. The use of prostate-specific antigen in staging patients with newly diagnosed prostate cancer. *JAMA* 1993;269:57–60.

17 **Answer B.** Indirect inguinal hernias enter the inguinal canal from the deep inguinal ring lateral to the inferior epigastric vasculature and course inferomedially into the scrotal sac (Answer B). Direct inguinal hernias (Answer A) bulge anteriorly, arising medial to the inferior epigastric vasculature. Femoral hernias (Answer C) enter the femoral canal along an inferolateral course and often compress the ipsilateral femoral vein. Obturator hernias (Answer D) enter the obturator fossa cephalad to the obturator internus. Examples of these hernias are provided below. All are presented in the coronal plane except for the obturator hernia (axial plane).

Note the location of the inferior epigastric vasculature in relation to the direct and indirect hernias. Direct hernias arise medial to the vessels, and indirect hernias arise lateral to the vessels.

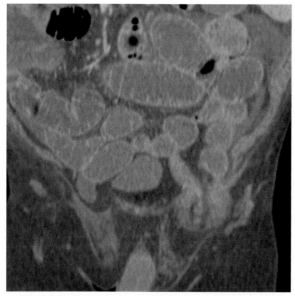

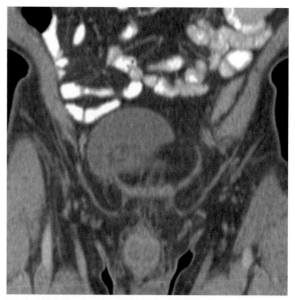

Indirect Inguinal Hernia (left indirect and right direct, with bowel)

Direct Inguinal Hernia (bilateral, right hernia contains bladder)

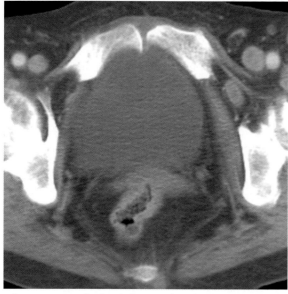

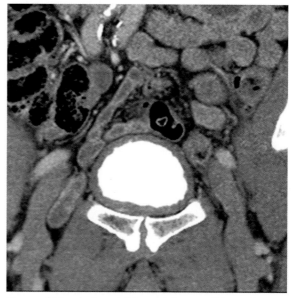

Obturator Hernia (on left, contains decompressed small bowel)

Femoral Hernia (on right, contains small bowel)

References: Aguirre DA, Santosa AC, Casola G, et al. Abdominal wall hernias: imaging features, complications, and diagnostic pitfalls at multi-detector row CT. *Radiographics* 2005;25:1501–1520.

Burkhardt JH, Arshanskiy Y, Munson JL, et al. Diagnosis of inguinal region hernias with axial CT: the lateral crescent sign and other key findings. *Radiographics* 2011;31:E1–E12.

18 Answer B. Buschke-Löwenstein disease is characterized by massive condylomata secondary to human papillomavirus (HPV), often HPV 6. It is locally aggressive and strongly associated with squamous cell carcinoma. Detection of enlarged or necrotic nodes is a clue that the disease has become invasive. Patients with human immunodeficiency virus (HIV) are at greater risk of invasive disease.

References: Boshart M, zur Hausen H. Human papillomaviruses in Buschke Löwenstein tumors: physical state of the DNA and identification of a tandem duplication in the noncoding region of a human papillomavirus 6 subtype. *J Virol* 1986;58:963–966.

Chu QD, Vezeridis MP, Libbey NP, et al. Giant condyloma acuminatum (Buschke Löwenstein tumor) of the anorectal and perianal regions. Analysis of 42 cases. *Dis Colon Rectum* 1994;37:950–957.

19 Answer D.   The apparent diffusion coefficient (ADC) map is a pixel-by-pixel map of the slope of the plot of the natural logarithm of signal intensity (ln[SI]) measured on trace diffusion-weighted images with different b values. The formula used to calculate ADC is

$$S = S_0 \times e^{-b \times ADC}$$

Where

S is the signal intensity at a given b value (b)

S_0 is the signal intensity when b = 0 s/mm^2

Therefore, ADC is the slope of the plot ln(SI) at various b values.

References: Kim CK, Park BK, Kim B. Diffusion-weighted MRI at 3 T for the evaluation of prostate cancer. *AJR Am J Roentgenol* 2010;194:1461–1469.

Schaefer PW, Grant PE, Gonzalez RG. Diffusion-weighted MR imaging of the brain. *Radiology* 2000;217:331–345.

20 Answer D.   The images demonstrate disruption of the tunica albuginea along the inferior margin of the left testicle, with hemorrhage and herniation of testicular contents into the scrotal sac compatible with testicular rupture. The best next step is operative organ salvage. Delays in operative management can result in loss of the testicle, which can have an effect on potency, cosmesis, and hormonal status. Prompt diagnosis and repair result in excellent salvage rates (>80%). Ultrasound has excellent test characteristics for the diagnosis of testicular rupture (>90% sensitivity and specificity). The key imaging finding is loss of the normal circumscribed margin around the testicle indicative of tunica albuginea disruption.

References: Buckley JC, McAninch JW. Diagnosis and management of testicular ruptures. *Urol Clin North Am* 2006;33:111–116.

Buckley JC, McAninch JW. Use of ultrasonography for the diagnosis of testicular injuries in blunt scrotal trauma. *J Urol* 2006;175:175–178.

21 Answer A.   Specific signs of extracapsular disease include focal capsular bulge (Answer A), loss of the rectoprostatic angle, soft tissue ingrowth into the neurovascular bundle(s), and measurable extraprostatic extension. Low ADC values (Answer B) moderately correlate with high Gleason scores, and high Gleason score tumors are more likely to have extracapsular extension, but low ADC value(s) alone are not specific for extracapsular disease. Broad capsular contact (Answer C) and capsular obscuration (Answer D) are suggestive but not specific signs of extracapsular disease.

References: Barentsz JO, Richenberg J, Clements R, et al. ESUR prostate MR guidelines 2012. *Eur Radiol* 2012;22:746–757.

Bloch BN, Genega EM, Costa DN, et al. Prediction of prostate cancer extension with high spatial resolution dynamic contrast-enhanced 3-T MRI. *Eur Radiol* 2012;22:2201–2210.

22 Answer C.   Elevated choline:citrate ratio (Answer C) and elevated choline + creatine:citrate ratio are spectroscopic indicators of prostate cancer. Choline is a marker of cellular proliferation because it is incorporated into cell walls. Citrate is a marker of normal prostate tissue and benign prostatic hyperplasia. The spectroscopic peak of creatine is often inseparable from the spectroscopic peak of choline, and so they are often summed together (choline + creatine:citrate ratio). Elevated citrate:choline ratio (Answer A) and elevated citrate:creatine ratio (Answer B) are benign spectroscopic patterns. An elevated creatine:citrate ratio (Answer D) has no particular significance.

Although MR spectroscopy has been shown to improve prostate cancer detection over anatomic imaging alone, it is often eschewed in the United States in favor of diffusion-weighted imaging (DWI) and dynamic contrast-enhanced imaging (DCE-MRI). This is because MR spectroscopy is time intensive, demanding, and prone to artifact. Additionally, the current value added beyond the combination of anatomic imaging, DWI, and DCE-MRI is small.

References: Barentsz JO, Richenberg J, Clements R, et al. ESUR prostate MR guidelines 2012. *Eur Radiol* 2012;22:746–757.

Leake JL, Hardman R, Ojili V, et al. Prostate MRI: access to and current practice of prostate MRI in the United States. *J Am Coll Radiol* 2014;11:156–160.

Murphy G, Haider M, Ghai S, et al. The expanding role of MRI in prostate cancer. *AJR Am J Roentgenol* 2013;201:1229–1238.

Verma S, Rajesh A, Futterer JJ, et al. Prostate MRI and 3D MR spectroscopy: how we do it. *AJR Am J Roentgenol* 2010;194:1414–1426.

23 Answer C. Power Doppler imaging is direction independent, and color Doppler imaging is not (Answer C). Power Doppler imaging is more sensitive to slow flow than is color Doppler imaging, and unlike color Doppler imaging, it is not affected by aliasing (because unlike color Doppler imaging, power Doppler imaging is a magnitude-only, directionless expression). Power Doppler imaging is related to the amplitude of the echo (which is proportional to the number of flowing particles), while color Doppler imaging is related to the frequency of the echo (which contains information about the Doppler shift, and hence, direction of flow).

Aliasing with color Doppler imaging occurs when the pulse repetition frequency is too low to accurately measure the velocity being sampled and results in an underestimation of the measured velocity. Aliasing with color Doppler imaging can be reduced by increasing the pulse repetition frequency. According to the Nyquist theorem, the maximum frequency that can be accurately sampled is equal to half the sampling frequency ($N_f = 0.5 \times$ sampling frequency). In this context, the sampling frequency is the pulse repetition frequency, and the Nyquist frequency (N_f) is the maximum velocity of flowing blood that can be accurately measured. Why not always maximize the pulse repetition frequency? Two reasons: (1) low pulse repetition frequencies are more sensitive to slow flow (e.g., venous blood), and (2) the pulse repetition frequency is limited by the depth of the object being measured (it takes a longer time to receive an echo from a deeper structure, and so it can be difficult to increase the sampling rate).

Power Doppler imaging is useful for differentiating slow flow from absent flow and for the detection of flow in small vessels. Slow flow can mimic thrombus with both color and power Doppler imaging, but it is more likely to occur with color Doppler imaging.

Because the strength of the power Doppler signal relates to the number of moving particles in the sample, including nonmoving structures (e.g., adjacent soft tissue) in the sample will decrease the effective strength of the signal.

References: McDicken WN, Anderson T. The difference between colour Doppler velocity imaging and power Doppler imaging. *Eur J Echocardiogr* 2002;3:240–244.

Rumack CM, Wilson SR, Charboneau JW, et al. *Diagnostic ultrasound, 2-volume set*, 4th ed. Philadelphia: Mosby, 2011.

24 Answer B. Acute epididymo-orchitis is characterized on Doppler ultrasound by hypervascularity and enlargement of the testicle and ipsilateral epididymis. It is best managed with antibiotics (Answer A). Common causes include sexually transmitted infections (e.g., *Neisseria gonorrhoeae*, *Chlamydia trachomatis*) and

Escherichia coli infection. It is a known complication of transrectal ultrasound (TRUS)-guided prostate biopsy. Occasionally, testicular hypervascularity can be seen soon after a torsion–detorsion episode, but that is much less common. Grayscale images can be used to ensure that the hypervascularity is not due to a solid testicular mass.

References: Aso C, Enriquez G, Fite M, et al. Gray-scale and color Doppler sonography of scrotal disorders in children: an update. *Radiographics* 2005;25:1197–1214.
Avery LL, Scheinfeld MH. Imaging of penile and scrotal emergencies. *Radiographics* 2013;33:721–740.

25 **Answer A.** The images demonstrate physiologic uptake of In-111 capromab pendetide (ProstaScint, murine [mouse] monoclonal antibody), which can include liver, spleen, bone marrow, and blood pool. It is excreted into the bowel and urinary tract. In-111 capromab pendetide has been explored as an adjunct to CT and bone scan for the detection of metastatic prostate cancer, but its use has been limited by suboptimal positive predictive value and suboptimal specificity. In the United States, it is not part of any routine staging protocol, but it is sometimes used for problem solving in tertiary care centers.

References: Mettler FA, Guiberteau MJ. *Essentials of nuclear medicine imaging*, 6th ed. Philadelphia: Saunders, 2012.
Schuster DM, Savir-Baruch B, Nieh PT, et al. Detection of recurrent prostate carcinoma with anti-1-amino-3-18 F-fluorocyclobutane-1-carboxylic acid PET/CT and 111In-capromab pendetide SPECT/CT. *Radiology* 2011;259:852–861.

26 **Answer B.** Congenital adrenal hyperplasia can result in adrenal rest tumors that develop within the retroperitoneum and testicles. Intratesticular adrenal rest tumors can have a varied appearance but are usually hypoechoic and eccentrically located. It is important to recognize the association between congenital adrenal hyperplasia and adrenal rest tumors because adrenal rest tumors are benign, and most other intratesticular masses are malignant. A short differential diagnosis for bilateral testicular masses includes lymphoma, metastatic disease, bilateral germ cell tumors, granulomatous infection, and adrenal rest tumors.

Multiple endocrine neoplasia type 2 (Answer A) is divided into two subtypes: (IIa) medullary thyroid cancer, pheochromocytoma, and parathyroid adenoma and (IIb) medullary thyroid cancer, pheochromocytoma, mucosal neuromas, and other manifestations.

von Hippel-Lindau syndrome (Answer C) is associated with epididymal cystadenoma, central nervous system and retinal hemangioblastoma, pancreatic neuroendocrine tumors, pancreatic cysts, renal cell carcinoma, and pheochromocytoma.

Autosomal dominant polycystic disease (Answer D) is associated with bilateral renal cysts, nephromegaly, hepatic cysts, intracranial aneurysms, hypertension, and urinary tract infections.

References: Choyke PL, Glenn GM, Walther MM, et al. von Hippel-Lindau disease: genetic, clinical, and imaging features. *Radiology* 1995;194:629–642.
Dogra V, Nathan J, Bhatt S. Sonographic appearance of testicular adrenal rest tissue in congenital adrenal hyperplasia. *JUM* 2004;979–981.
Rozenfeld MN, Ansari SA, Shaibani A, et al. Should patients with autosomal dominant polycystic kidney disease be screened for cerebral aneurysms? *AJNR Am J Neuroradiol* 2014;35(1):3–9.
Scarsbrook AF, Thakker RV, Wass JA, et al. Multiple endocrine neoplasia: spectrum of radiologic appearances and discussion of a multitechnique imaging approach. *Radiographics* 2006;26:433–451.

27 **Answer B.** Testicular microlithiasis has been associated with testicular cancer in both adults and children. As a result, current guidelines advocate routine testicular self-examinations in asymptomatic patients with this condition. The cost-effectiveness of serial imaging follow-up (Answer C) has been questioned and is not universally recommended. Prophylactic orchiectomy (Answer D) is not indicated because the majority of patients with testicular microlithiasis will not develop a testicular malignancy. Although benign and incidental in the majority of patients, it is not an ignorable finding (Answer A).

References: Albers P, Albrecht W, Algaba F, et al. EAU guidelines on testicular cancer: 2011 update. *Eur Urol* 2011;60:304–319.

Cooper ML, Kaefer M, Fan R, et al. Testicular microlithiasis in children and associated testicular cancer. *Radiology* 2014;270:857–863.

DeCastro BJ, Peterson AC, Costabile RA. A 5-year followup study of asymptomatic men with testicular microlithiasis. *J Urol* 2008;179:1420–1423.

28 **Answer D.** The images demonstrate a small solid enhancing nodule anterior to the rectum near the urethral anastomosis. A solid enhancing nodule near the urethral anastomosis in a patient with a newly detectable prostate-specific antigen (PSA) level after radical prostatectomy likely represents recurrent prostate cancer. The best next step is salvage radiotherapy (Answer D). The PSA level is expected to be undetectable after radical prostatectomy; if the PSA level becomes detectable or is rising during the follow-up period, it indicates recurrent disease. Imaging is often performed to differentiate a local recurrence (as in this case) from metastatic disease. If a local recurrence is present, salvage local therapy is performed. If there is no local recurrence, systemic therapy is pursued instead.

References: Ray GR, Bagshaw MA, Freiha F. External beam radiation salvage for residual or recurrent local tumor following radical prostatectomy. *J Urol* 1984;132:926–930.

Trock BJ, Han M, Freedland SJ, et al. Prostate cancer-specific survival following salvage radiotherapy vs observation in men with biochemical recurrence after radical prostatectomy. *JAMA* 2008;299:2760–2769.

29 **Answer D.** Gleason score has been shown to have a significant moderate inverse correlation with ADC; in other words, low ADC is associated with higher Gleason score. This relationship is strongest for cancers in the peripheral zone.

Although there is overlap at any given ADC, ADC $<850 \times 10^{-6}$ mm²/s has been shown to be a reliable predictor of Gleason sum ≥ 7 prostate cancer. ADC values between 850×10^{-6} mm²/s and 1150×10^{-6} mm²/s are indeterminate, and ADC values $>1150 \times 10^{-6}$ mm²/s are either benign or predict a lower Gleason score histology.

Any MR-based quantitative measurement (e.g., ADC, DCE-MRI) is subject to variation across MR systems, vendors, and practice sites, though ADC has been shown to be fairly repeatable. The coefficient of variation (which is equal to the standard deviation divided by the mean) for ADC repeatability is around 15% to 20%.

References: Braithwaite AC, Dale BM, Boll DT, et al. Short- and midterm reproducibility of apparent diffusion coefficient measurements at 3.0-T diffusion-weighted imaging of the abdomen. *Radiology* 2009;250:459–465.

Donati OF, Mazaheri Y, Afaq A, et al. Prostate cancer aggressiveness: assessment with whole-lesion histogram analysis of the apparent diffusion coefficient. *Radiology* 2014;271(1):143–152.

Jung SI, Donati OF, Vargas HA, et al. Transition zone prostate cancer: incremental value of diffusion-weighted endorectal MR imaging in tumor detection and assessment of aggressiveness. *Radiology* 2013;269:493–503.

Somford DM, Hambrock T, Hulsbergen-van de Kaa CA, et al. Initial experience with identifying high-grade prostate cancer using diffusion-weighted MR imaging (DWI) in patients with a Gleason score $\leq 3 + 3 = 6$ upon schematic TRUS-guided biopsy: a radical prostatectomy correlated series. *Invest Radiol* 2012;47:153–158.

30 **Answer C.**   The calcified plaques that occur in the setting of Peyronie disease develop along the tunica albuginea. They are associated with penis pain and penis deformity and are difficult to treat. On imaging, it is important to distinguish these calcified plaques from other causes of penile calcification (discussed below, e.g., urethral calculus). The incidence of Peyronie disease ranges from 1% to 20% depending on the definition applied. The disease is believed to result from microtrauma to the penis such as that might occur during sexual intercourse. Treatment is difficult and often not successful.

Other causes of penile calcification include calcification of the dorsal penile artery due to microvascular disease (e.g., diabetes mellitus, calciphylaxis), urethral calcification related to a migrating urinary calculus, soft tissue calcification related to systemic sclerosis (i.e., CREST syndrome), and dystrophic calcification related to a prior insult.

References: Jalkut M, Gonzalez-Cadavid N, Rajfer J. Peyronie's disease: a review. *Rev Urol* 2003;5:142–148.
Kuehhas FE, Weibl P, Georgi T, et al. Peyronie's disease: nonsurgical therapy options. *Rev Urol* 2011;13:139–146.

Female Genital I (Uterus and Cervix)

QUESTIONS

1   A 70-year-old female presents with postmenopausal bleeding. No biopsy has been performed. What is the best imaging test for this patient?

A. Hysterosalpingogram
B. Transvaginal ultrasound
C. Computed tomography
D. Magnetic resonance imaging
E. FDG PET

2   A 30-year-old female with menorrhagia undergoes a pelvic MRI. What is the most likely diagnosis?

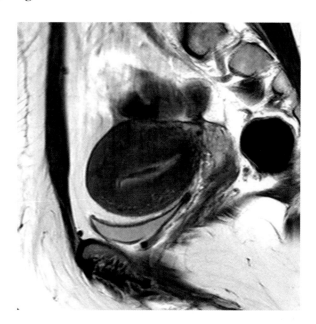

A. Normal study
B. Leiomyoma
C. Adenomyosis
D. Endometrial cancer
E. Cesarean-section scar

3 A 57-year-old female with postmenopausal bleeding undergoes a transvaginal ultrasound. How should the endometrial stripe measurement be made?

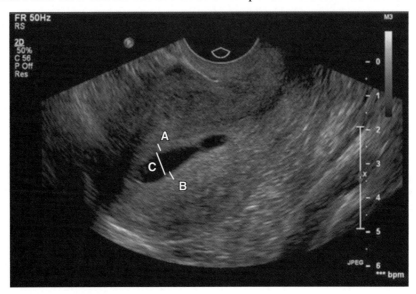

A. Line A + Line B
B. Line A + Line B + Line C
C. Line A + Line B – Line C
D. Line A
E. Line B
F. Line C

4 A 70-year-old female with postmenopausal bleeding undergoes a transvaginal pelvic ultrasound. What endometrial stripe measurement is an indication for endometrial biopsy?

A. ≥3 mm
B. ≥4 mm
C. ≥5 mm
D. ≥6 mm

5 A 22-year-old female with pelvic pain and a serum hCG of 1,200 mIU/mL undergoes a transvaginal pelvic ultrasound. The ovaries are normal, and no adnexal mass is identified. How should the imaging findings be reported?

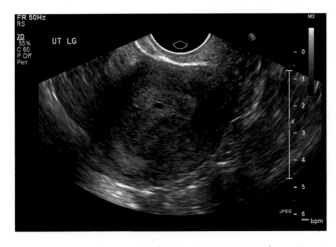
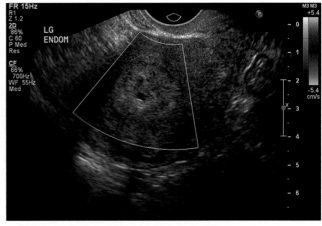

A. Findings consistent with an intrauterine pregnancy, no follow-up required
B. Findings consistent with a pseudogestational sac, treat for ectopic pregnancy
C. Findings likely an intrauterine pregnancy, follow-up to confirm
D. Findings likely a pseudogestational sac, admit for possible ectopic pregnancy

6   A 28-year-old female with primary infertility undergoes a hysterosalpingogram. Which of the following maneuvers will reduce the radiation dose delivered to the patient?

A. Changing from 5 to 3 pulses per second
B. Placing a lead apron on the operator
C. Moving the image intensifier away from the patient
D. Opening the collimation

7   A 56-year-old female with pelvic pain undergoes a pelvic examination, and biopsy demonstrates cervical cancer. MRI of the pelvis is performed. What stage is this neoplasm?

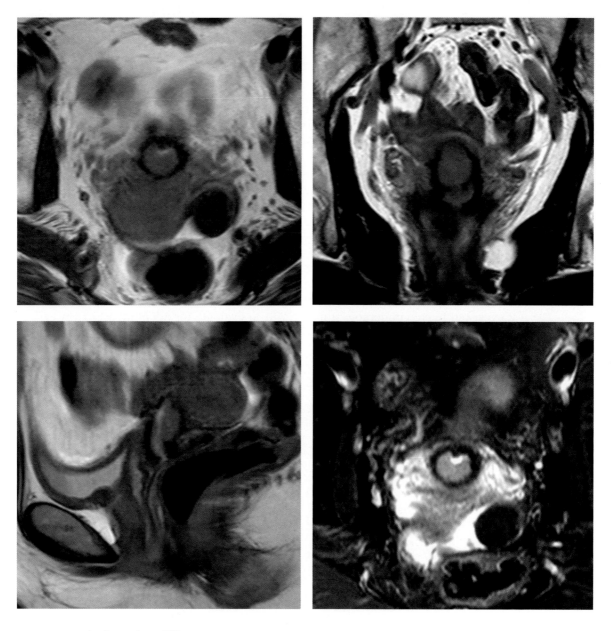

A. Less than IIB
B. IIB or greater

8   A 30-year-old female with menorrhagia undergoes a pelvic MRI. What junctional zone thickness is commonly used to indicate a high specificity for the diagnosis of adenomyosis?

A. >4 mm

B. >8 mm

C. >12 mm

D. >16 mm

9   A 56-year-old female with postmenopausal bleeding undergoes a transvaginal ultrasound. What is the most likely diagnosis for the adnexal mass?

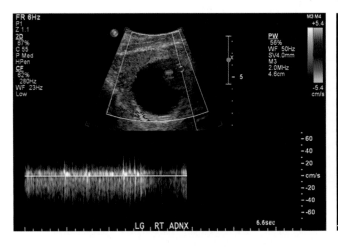 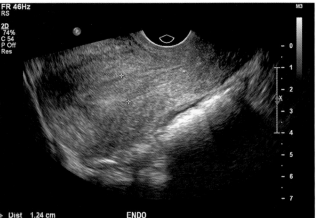

A. Cystadenocarcinoma

B. Granulosa cell tumor

C. Endometrioma

D. Immature teratoma

10   A 25-year-old female undergoes a pelvic MRI to evaluate for adenomyosis. How should the junctional zone thickness be measured?

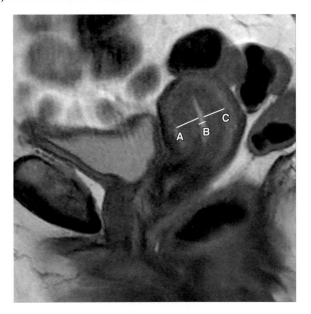

A. Line A + Line B

B. Line A + Line B + Line C

C. Line A + Line C − Line B

D. Line A or Line C

11 A 60-year-old female with cervical cancer undergoes a pelvic MRI. According to the FIGO staging system, what stage is this neoplasm?

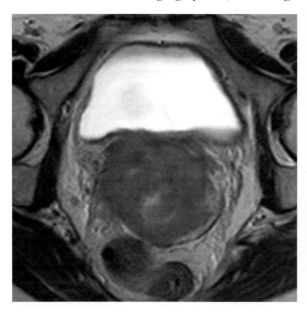 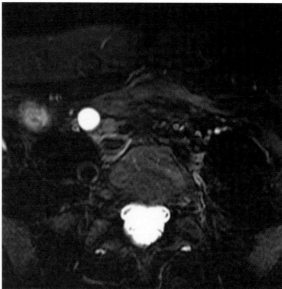

A. IIA
B. IIB
C. IIIA
D. IIIB

12 The cornerstone of cervical cancer staging with pelvic MRI is thin-section T2-weighted imaging without fat saturation angled to the short axis of the cervix. The pulse sequence commonly used for this purpose utilizes a multislice fast spin echo technique. Which of the following modifications would increase the image acquisition time required for this pulse sequence?

A. A reduction in the echo train length
B. An increase in the echo time
C. A reduction in the repetition time
D. An increase in the frequency-encoding matrix

13 A 22-year-old female with vaginal bleeding and a positive urine pregnancy test undergoes a pelvic ultrasound. A gestational sac is identified containing a yolk sac and a fetal pole. No fetal cardiac activity is detected. According to the Society of Radiologists in Ultrasound (SRU) 2012 guidelines, at what crown rump length size is absent fetal cardiac activity considered diagnostic of fetal loss?

A. ≥3 mm
B. ≥5 mm
C. ≥7 mm
D. ≥9 mm

14 A 32-year-old female with multiple uterine fibroids undergoes consultation for uterine artery embolization. She is deemed a suitable candidate. A preprocedure MRI is performed, and large bilateral corkscrew-shaped vessels are identified extending from the aorta to the uterus. Based on this finding, what is the best next step?

A. Uterine artery embolization is contraindicated.
B. Unilateral uterine artery embolization should be performed.
C. Bilateral uterine artery embolization should be performed.
D. Bilateral uterine and gonadal artery embolization should be performed.

15 A 25-year-old female with primary infertility undergoes a pelvic MRI to assess for congenital anomalies. How should the images be interpreted?

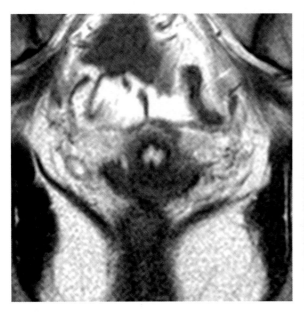 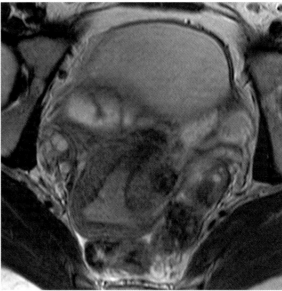

    A. Normal examination
    B. Uterus didelphys
    C. Bicornuate bicollis uterus
    D. Septate uterus

16 A 55-year-old female with postmenopausal bleeding is diagnosed with endometrial cancer. A pelvic MRI is performed for staging, and the mass is shown to involve >50% of the myometrial thickness. There is no evidence of cervical, vaginal, nodal, or metastatic disease. According to the FIGO staging system, what is the clinical stage of this neoplasm?

    A. IA
    B. IB
    C. II
    D. IIIA

17 Which of the following has a classic association with a "T-shaped uterus"?

    A. Diffuse adenomyosis
    B. Exposure to a fetal carcinogen
    C. Multifocal leiomyomata
    D. Endometrial cancer
    E. Pelvic inflammatory disease

18 A 44-year-old female with pelvic pain undergoes a pelvic MRI, and a large mass is identified. What is the most likely diagnosis?

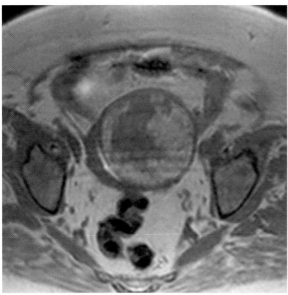

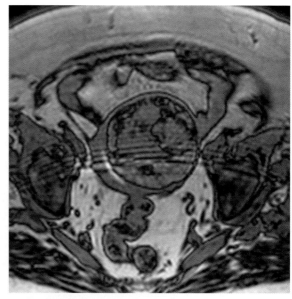

Axial T1w GRE

Axial T1w GRE

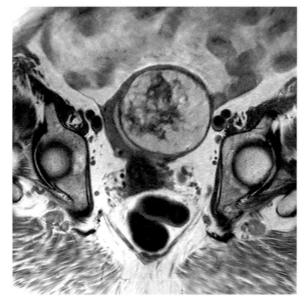

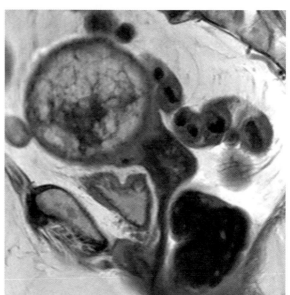

Axial T2w FSE

Sagittal T2w FSE

    A. Leiomyoma
    B. Dermoid
    C. Endometrial cancer
    D. Uterine sarcoma

19 A 30-year-old G0P0 female with vaginal bleeding and a serum hCG level of 200,000 mIU/mL undergoes a transvaginal ultrasound. What is the most likely diagnosis?

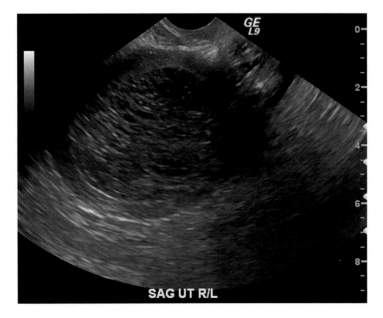

A. Retained products of conception
B. Gestational trophoblastic disease
C. Diffuse adenomyosis
D. Large intrauterine blood clots

20 A 64-year-old female with endometrial cancer presents for staging evaluation with MRI of the pelvis. What is the best pulse sequence for measuring the depth of myometrial invasion?

A. 3D T1w fat-saturated GRE postcontrast
B. 3D T1w fat-saturated GRE precontrast
C. 2D T2w FSE without fat saturation
D. 2D T2w FSE with fat saturation

21 A 30-year-old female with pelvic fullness undergoes a pelvic ultrasound. How should this fibroid be classified?

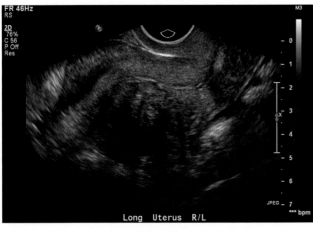
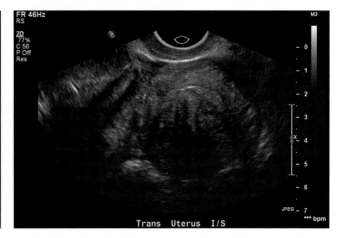

A. Intracavitary
B. Intramural
C. Pedunculated
D. Submucosal
E. Subserosal

22 A 30-year-old female with menorrhagia undergoes a transvaginal ultrasound, and a Nabothian cyst is identified. Which of the following contributes to the appearance of bright pixels deep to the cyst?

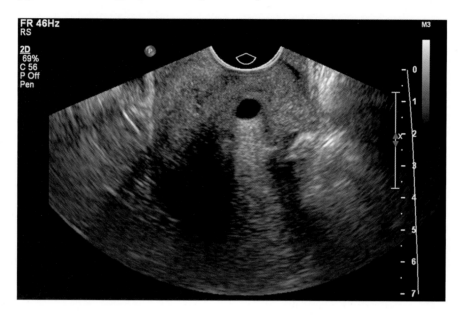

A. Attenuation correction artifact
B. Refraction artifact
C. Reverberation artifact
D. Side lobe artifact

23 A 24-year-old G4P3 female presents with secondary infertility. What is the most likely explanation for the appearance of the fundal endometrial canal?

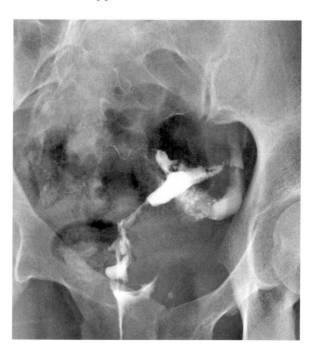

A. Endometrial cancer
B. Adhesive disease
C. Fetal diethylstilbestrol exposure
D. Uterine fibroids

24   A 32-year-old female with secondary infertility undergoes a hysterosalpingogram. How should the imaging be interpreted?

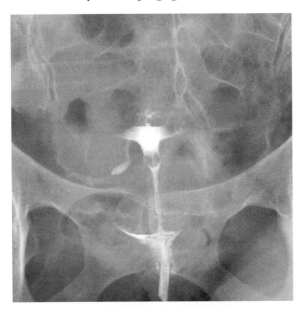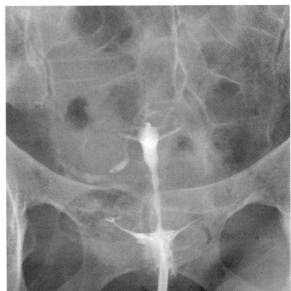

    A. Zero patent fallopian tubes
    B. One patent fallopian tube
    C. Two patent fallopian tubes

25   A 19-year-old female with pelvic pain undergoes a pelvic MRI. A unicornuate uterus with a rudimentary horn is diagnosed. How should the rudimentary horn be managed?

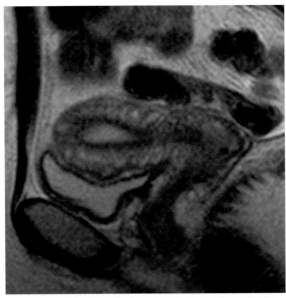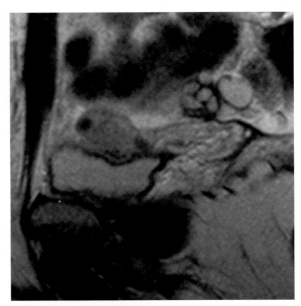

Left parasagittal T2W FSE   *Right parasagittal T2W FSE*

    A. Operative resection
    B. Hysteroscopic recanalization
    C. Oral contraceptive pills
    D. Endometrial ablation

26 A 40-year-old female with pelvic discomfort undergoes a pelvic ultrasound, and a large myometrial mass is identified. What is the most common way uterine leiomyosarcoma is differentiated from uterine leiomyoma?

A. Detecting intratumoral hemorrhage on T1-weighted images
B. Detecting rapid tumor growth over a short period of time
C. Retrospective histologic analysis after surgical removal
D. Prospective histologic analysis with percutaneous biopsy

27 A 67-year-old female with breast cancer on tamoxifen therapy undergoes a pelvic ultrasound for irregular bleeding. What endometrial thickness is considered an indication for endometrial biopsy in a postmenopausal woman receiving tamoxifen therapy?

A. ≥5 mm
B. ≥6 mm
C. ≥7 mm
D. ≥8 mm

28 A 20-year-old female undergoes a hysterosalpingogram. What is the best next step?

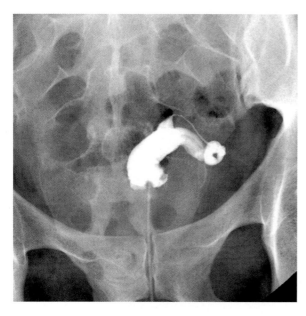 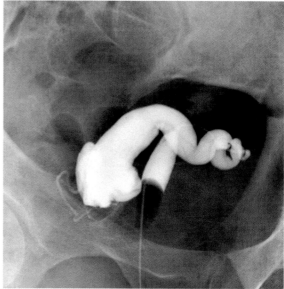

A. Advance the catheter
B. Inject more contrast material
C. Pull back the catheter
D. Drain the contrast material

29 A 25-year-old female with primary infertility undergoes a hysterosalpingogram. What is the most likely explanation for the imaging findings?

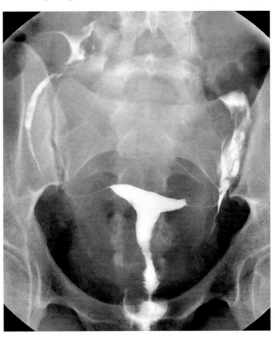

A. Normal study
B. Congenital variant
C. Pelvic inflammatory disease
D. Pelvic mass

30 A 30-year-old female desiring sterility undergoes bilateral fallopian tube microinsert placement. She returns for a hysterosalpingogram to document microinsert position and tubal occlusion. What is the best explanation for the small collections of contrast material alongside the endometrial canal?

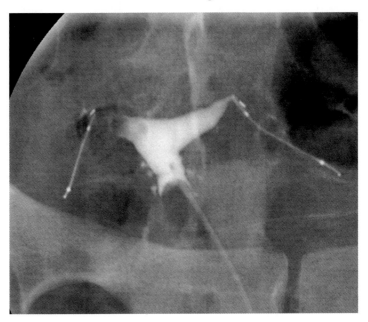

A. Normal variant
B. Fibroids
C. Venous intravasation
D. Endometrial cancer
E. Adenomyosis

ANSWERS AND EXPLANATIONS

1 Answer B. In a woman with postmenopausal bleeding, further evaluation is required with endometrial biopsy or transvaginal ultrasound to assess for malignancy using the following algorithm:

- If an endometrial biopsy is performed first and yields diagnostic tissue, transvaginal ultrasound is not required.
- If a transvaginal ultrasound is performed first and the endometrial stripe is ≥5 mm, endometrial biopsy is required.
- If a transvaginal ultrasound is performed first and the endometrial stripe is <5 mm, endometrial biopsy is not required.

An endometrial stripe measurement ≤4 mm in the setting of postmenopausal bleeding has a negative predictive value >99% for endometrial cancer. Therefore, transvaginal ultrasound can serve as a triage tool to determine which patients with postmenopausal bleeding require endometrial biopsy.

References: Karlsson B, Granberg S, Wikland M, et al. Transvaginal ultrasound of the endometrium in women with postmenopausal bleeding—a Nordic multicenter study. *Am J Obstet Gynecol* 1995;172:1488–1494.

The American Congress of Obstetricians and Gynecologists. The role of transvaginal ultrasonography in the evaluation of postmenopausal bleeding. *The American Congress of Obstetricians and Gynecologists (ACOG) Committee Opinion 440. 2009 and 2013.*

2 Answer C. The image demonstrates a diffusely thickened junctional zone compatible with adenomyosis. A junctional zone measurement >12 mm is specific for the diagnosis. A junctional zone measurement 9 to 12 mm is equivocal for adenomyosis, and a junctional zone measurement ≤8 mm is normal. The diagnosis of adenomyosis is important because adenomyosis is more resistant to catheter-directed embolic treatment compared to fibroids, the operative approach for fibroids and adenomyosis differs, and diffuse adenomyosis can be mistaken for malignancy on imaging.

The imaging findings of fibroids (Answer B) can overlap with those of adenomyosis, but fibroids are typically more well defined with circumscribed margins. Adenomyosis tends to be a diffuse process though focal adenomyomas do occur. Endometrial cancer (Answer D) is not the best choice because the endometrium is normal. A cesarean-section scar (Answer E) would be inferiorly located along the anterior lower uterine segment and would manifest as a thin signal abnormality associated with myometrial volume loss.

References: Popovic M, Puchner S, Berzaczy D, et al. Uterine artery embolization for the treatment of adenomyosis: a review. *J Vasc Interv Radiol* 2011;22:901–909.

Shwayder J, Sakhel K. Imaging for uterine myomas and adenomyosis. *J Minim Invasive Gynecol* 2013;21(3):362–376.

Stamatopoulos CP, Mikos T, Grimbizis GF, et al. Value of magnetic resonance imaging in diagnosis of adenomyosis and myomas of the uterus. *J Minim Invasive Gynecol* 2012;19:620–626.

3   **Answer A.**   The endometrial stripe should be measured in the long-axis view of the uterus during transvaginal scanning. It should encompass the maximum anteroposterior thickness of the endometrium including the anterior and posterior layers and excluding any endometrial fluid. Inaccurate measurement technique can result in an over- or underestimation of the true endometrial thickness and lead to inappropriate management.

References: Davidson KG, Dubinsky TJ. Ultrasonographic evaluation of the endometrium in postmenopausal vaginal bleeding. *Radiol Clin North Am* 2003;41:769–780.
The American Congress of Obstetricians and Gynecologists. The role of transvaginal ultrasonography in the evaluation of postmenopausal bleeding. *The American Congress of Obstetricians and Gynecologists (ACOG) Committee Opinion 440.* 2009 and 2013.

4   **Answer C.**   An endometrial stripe measurement ≥5 mm in the setting of postmenopausal bleeding is an indication for endometrial biopsy. An endometrial stripe measurement ≤4 mm in this setting has a negative predictive value for endometrial cancer >99%, and therefore can be used to select patients who may not benefit from endometrial biopsy.

There is not an established endometrial stripe measurement threshold for triggering endometrial biopsy in asymptomatic postmenopausal women. This is because asymptomatic women (i.e., those without postmenopausal bleeding) have a very low likelihood of endometrial cancer. Thus, the positive predictive value of any stripe measurement in this setting is low (2.4% for stripe measurements >6 mm in one study of 1,750 asymptomatic women [Fleischer, 2001]).

References: Fleischer AC, Wheeler JE, Lindsay I, et al. An assessment of the value of ultrasonographic screening for endometrial disease in postmenopausal women without symptoms. *Am J Obstet Gynecol* 2001;184:70–75.
Karlsson B, Granberg S, Wikland M, et al. Transvaginal ultrasound of the endometrium in women with postmenopausal bleeding—a Nordic multicenter study. *Am J Obstet Gynecol* 1995;172:1488–1494.
The American Congress of Obstetricians and Gynecologists. The role of transvaginal ultrasonography in the evaluation of postmenopausal bleeding. *The American Congress of Obstetricians and Gynecologists (ACOG) Committee Opinion 440.* 2009 and 2013.

5   **Answer C.**   The images demonstrate a small nonspecific fluid collection within the endometrial canal without specific signs of an early intrauterine pregnancy. Specifically, there is no yolk sac and no fetal parts. Therefore, the differential diagnosis includes:

a. A normal early intrauterine pregnancy (most likely)
b. An abnormal intrauterine pregnancy
c. A pseudogestational sac or decidual cyst of ectopic pregnancy (rare)

In a patient with a positive pregnancy test, a small endometrial fluid collection is much more likely to be an immature gestational sac than a cyst of ectopic pregnancy because ectopic pregnancy is rare. However, if no specific sign of intrauterine pregnancy is identified, then follow-up is suggested to confirm viability and exclude ectopic pregnancy. If a specific sign of intrauterine pregnancy is identified (e.g., yolk sac, fetal parts), then ectopic pregnancy is virtually excluded with the exception of a heterotopic pregnancy (i.e., combined intrauterine and ectopic pregnancy). A heterotopic pregnancy is rare in the general population (~1:30,000 pregnancies) but is more frequent in patients undergoing fertility treatment.

References: Doubilet PM, Benson CB. First, do no harm…to early pregnancies. *JUM* 2010;29:685–689.
Doubilet PM, Benson CB, Bourne T, et al. Diagnostic criteria for nonviable pregnancy early in the first trimester. *N Engl J Med* 2013;369:1443–1451.
Levine D. Ectopic pregnancy. *Radiology* 2007;245:385–397.

6 **Answer A.**   Reducing the number of radiation pulses per second will decrease the radiation dose to the patient and the operator. Placing a lead apron on the operator (Answer B) is extremely effective for reducing the radiation dose to the operator, but will do nothing to reduce the radiation dose to the patient. Both moving the image intensifier away from the patient (Answer C) and opening the collimation (Answer D) will increase the radiation dose to the patient and operator. As the image intensifier moves away from the patient, the ABC (**A**utomatic **B**rightness **C**ontrol) will detect that the image is less bright and will increase the radiation output to maintain a similar level of image brightness throughout the study. Use of collimation decreases the radiation exposure by blocking x-rays at the periphery of the image; therefore, opening the collimation will allow these x-rays through, increasing the radiation exposure.

References: Geise RA. The AAPM/RSNA physics tutorial for residents. Fluoroscopy: recording of fluoroscopic images and automatic exposure control. *Radiographics* 2001;21:227–236.
Mahesh M. The AAPM/RSNA physics tutorial for residents. Fluoroscopy: patient radiation exposure issues. *Radiographics* 2001;21:1033–1045.
Wang J, Blackburn FJ. The AAPM/RSNA physics tutorial for residents. X-ray image intensifiers for fluoroscopy. *Radiographics* 2000;20:1471–1477.

7 **Answer A.**   There is no evidence of invasion through the endocervical stroma into the parametrium. Note the intact low-signal intensity ring bounding the mass on the short axis T2-weighted images. The soft tissue structure posterior to the cervix is a diminutive retroverted uterus.

Detection of parametrial invasion on MRI (i.e., invasion into the tissues lateral to the cervix) is clinically important because it determines surgical candidacy. Cervical cancer invading the parametrium is consistent with FIGO (**I**nternational **F**ederation of **G**ynecology and **O**bstetrics) stage IIB disease. Patients who traditionally are treated with radiation and chemotherapy (instead of surgery) include those with: (1) invasive disease (IIB or higher FIGO stage) and/or (2) large tumors (>4 cm in diameter). The critical features on MRI are therefore detection of parametrial invasion and an accurate diameter measurement.

An abbreviated version of the FIGO staging of cervical cancer is shown in the table. The most important management points for the radiologist is discriminating IIB and higher disease from IIA and lower disease, and providing an accurate size measurement.

FIGO Stage	Description
I	Confined to the cervix. Stage I disease is further stratified by mass visibility, mass size (>4 cm or ≤4 cm), and depth of stromal invasion.
IIA	Invasion of the upper two-thirds of the vagina. Stage IIA disease is further substratified by mass size (>4 cm or ≤4 cm).
IIB	Parametrial invasion.
IIIA	Invasion of the lower third of the vagina.
IIIB	Invasion of the pelvic sidewall and/or hydronephrosis.
IVA	Invasion of adjacent organs other than the ureter or vagina.
IVB	Metastatic disease.

References: Cervix uteri. In: Edge SB, Byrd DR, Compton CC, et al., (eds). *AJCC cancer staging manual*, 7th ed. New York, NY: Springer, 2010:395–402.

Sala E, Wakely S, Senior E, et al. MRI of malignant neoplasms of the uterine corpus and cervix. *AJR Am J Roentgenol* 2007;188:1577–1587.

8 **Answer C.** The most widely validated criterion for the noninvasive diagnosis of adenomyosis is a junctional zone thickness measurement >12 mm. This has a reported specificity >95% and a reported sensitivity of 60% to 65%. Junctional zone thickness measurements 9 to 12 mm are considered indeterminate for adenomyosis and junctional zone thickness measurements ≤8 mm are considered normal. Approximately 20% of patients have a nonmeasurable junctional zone on MRI, and therefore, this criterion cannot be used for all patients.

Other signs of adenomyosis unrelated to the junctional zone thickness measurement include: (1) focal adenomyoma (T2-hypointense mass similar to a fibroid but lacking peripheral hypervascularity and containing small microcysts; the imaging findings of fibroids and adenomyomas overlap) and (2) subcentimeter submucosal microcysts (cysts of ectopic endometrial tissue) embedded within the junctional zone or outer myometrium.

References: Hauth EA, Jaeger JH, Libera H, et al. MR imaging of the uterus and cervix in healthy women: determination of normal values. *Eur Radiol* 2007;17:734–742.

Novellas S, Chassang M, Delotte J, et al. MRI characteristics of the uterine junctional zone: from normal to the diagnosis of adenomyosis. *AJR Am J Roentgenol* 2011;196:1206–1213.

Reinhold C, Tafazoli F, Mehio A, et al. Uterine adenomyosis: endovaginal US and MR imaging features with histopathologic correlation. *Radiographics* 1999;19:S147–S160.

9 **Answer B.** The left image demonstrates a complex adnexal mass with a vascularized mural nodule, and the right image labeled "endo" shows abnormal thickening of the endometrial stripe. The presence of a complex ovarian mass and concomitant endometrial thickening in a postmenopausal woman is suggestive of a granulosa cell tumor. Granulosa cell tumor is a sex cord–stromal neoplasm of the ovary that characteristically expresses sex steroids such as estrogen. As a result, granulosa cell tumors of the ovary are commonly associated with endometrial hyperplasia (two-thirds of patients). Unopposed estrogen expression can occasionally result in endometrial carcinoma. Treatment of granulosa cell tumor is usually surgical. Most are detected at an early stage and are not associated with endometrial cancer; therefore, the prognosis is generally excellent.

References: Colombo N, Parma G, Zanagnolo V, et al. Management of ovarian stromal cell tumors. *J Clin Oncol* 2007;25:2944–2951.

Schumer ST, Cannistra SA. Granulosa cell tumor of the ovary. *J Clin Oncol* 2003;21:1180–1189.

10 **Answer D.** Unlike the endometrial stripe measurement, the junctional zone measurement is only measured on a single wall of the uterus (i.e., anterior and posterior measurements are not summed). Junctional zone measurements should be made on the midsagittal image along the uterine long axis, and at multiple locations along the anterior and posterior wall. Adenomyosis can be focal or diffuse and therefore can occur at any location. A junctional zone measurement >12 mm on the midsagittal image is specific (>95%) for the diagnosis; measurements 9 to 12 mm are equivocal and measurements ≤8 mm are normal.

References: Hauth EA, Jaeger JH, Libera H, et al. MR imaging of the uterus and cervix in healthy women: determination of normal values. *Eur Radiol* 2007;17:734–742.

Novellas S, Chassang M, Delotte J, et al. MRI characteristics of the uterine junctional zone: from normal to the diagnosis of adenomyosis. *AJR Am J Roentgenol* 2011;196:1206–1213.

Reinhold C, Tafazoli F, Mehio A, et al. Uterine adenomyosis: endovaginal US and MR imaging features with histopathologic correlation. *Radiographics* 1999;19:S147–S160.

11 Answer D. The images demonstrate a bulky cervical cancer obstructing the right ureter resulting in hydronephrosis. Note the dilated ureter on the axial T2-weighted fat-suppressed image. These findings are compatible with FIGO stage IIIB disease. In this case, the tumor is so large that no normal cervical tissue can be identified. Management of IIIB disease consists of radiation and chemotherapy. Hydronephrosis is a typical complication of advanced invasive cervical cancer because the distal ureter courses near the parametrial tissues lateral to the cervix.

References: Cervix uteri. In: Edge SB, Byrd DR, Compton CC, et al., (eds). *AJCC cancer staging manual*, 7th ed. New York, NY: Springer, 2010:395–402.
Sala E, Wakely S, Senior E, et al. MRI of malignant neoplasms of the uterine corpus and cervix. *AJR Am J Roentgenol* 2007;188:1577–1587.

12 Answer A. Reducing the echo train length will increase the image acquisition time for a multislice fast spin echo pulse sequence. The image acquisition time for a 2D fast spin echo sequence can be estimated using the following formula, which can also be used to predict the effect of parameter modifications on sequence length:

$$\text{Time is proportional to} : \left(TR \times N_p \times NSA \right) / ETL$$

Where TR is repetition time, N_p is the number of phase-encoding steps, NSA is the number of signal averages, and ETL is the echo train length. ETL is the major advantage of fast spin echo imaging over traditional spin echo imaging—it dramatically reduces the length of time required for image acquisition. The formula for a traditional 2D spin echo sequence is the same as listed above without the ETL factor.

If a 3D sequence is acquired instead of a 2D sequence, an additional variable will be multiplied with the numerator: the number of phase-encoding steps in the z-axis direction.

Changes to the echo time (TE, Answer B) and/or changes to the frequency-encoding matrix (N_p, Answer D) will not have a significant effect on the image acquisition time. Reducing the repetition time (TR, Answer C) will tend to decrease the image acquisition time, not increase it.

References: Mamourian AC. *Practical MR physics*, 1st ed. New York: Oxford University Press, 2010.
McRobbie DW, Moore EA, Graves MJ, et al. *MRI: from picture to proton*, 2nd ed. New York: Cambridge University Press, 2007.

13 Answer C. A crown rump length (CRL) ≥7 mm with no fetal cardiac activity is diagnostic of fetal loss. The guidelines for the diagnosis of early pregnancy failure were revised in 2012–2013. The following represent the current criteria considered diagnostic of pregnancy failure:

1. Crown rump length ≥7 mm and no fetal cardiac activity
2. Mean sac diameter ≥25 mm and no fetal pole
3. No embryo with cardiac activity ≥2 weeks after a scan showing a gestational sac but no yolk sac
4. No embryo with cardiac activity ≥11 days after a scan showing a gestational sac and a yolk sac

Older guidelines used a 5-mm CRL threshold for the detection of fetal cardiac activity, but this was based on small series with wide confidence intervals. Newer guidelines utilize a ≥7-mm cutoff to ensure that the threshold has 100% specificity and 100% positive predictive value for fetal demise.

References: American Institute of Ultrasound in Medicine. AIUM practice guideline for the performance of obstetric ultrasound examinations. 2013. http://www.aium.org/resources/guidelines/obstetric.pdf
Doublet PM, Benson CB, Bourne T, et al. Diagnostic criteria for nonviable pregnancy early in the first trimester. *N Engl J Med* 2013;369:1443–1451.

14   **Answer D.**   Large fibroids may receive collateral flow from enlarged, corkscrew-shaped ovarian (i.e., gonadal) arteries. When this finding is identified, if superselective embolization of the ovarian arteries is not performed in addition to embolization of the uterine arteries, the procedure will have a higher likelihood of treatment failure.

Dilated ovarian arteries can be identified by their corkscrew-shaped appearance in the coronal plane. Both the right and left ovarian arteries typically arise from the abdominal aorta below the level of the renal arteries. Occasionally, one or more will arise from the renal arteries.

Intrauterine anastomoses (flow from the right uterine artery supplying the left uterus and vice versa) preclude unilateral uterine artery embolization as an effective treatment of fibroids (Answer B). In general, bilateral uterine artery embolization is required, regardless of whether there are utero-ovarian anastomoses.

References: Kim HS, Paxton BE, Lee JM. Long-term efficacy and safety of uterine artery embolization in young patients with and without uteroovarian anastomoses. *J Vasc Interv Radiol* 2008;19:195–200.

Kirby JM, Burrows D, Haider E, et al. Utility of MRI before and after uterine fibroid embolization: why to do it and what to look for. *Cardiovasc Intervent Radiol* 2011;34:705–716.

Pelage JP, Walker WJ, Le Dref O, et al. Ovarian artery: angiographic appearance, embolization and relevance to uterine fibroid embolization. *Cardiovasc Intervent Radiol* 2003;26:227–233.

15   **Answer A.**   The image at the level of the cervix demonstrates normal folds indenting the endocervical canal. Endocervical folds can be mistaken for a fibrous septum, and therefore, it is important to recognize them as a normal finding. The differentiating feature between normal endocervical folds and a congenital septum is connectivity to the uterine fundus. A septum will generally always begin at the fundus and extend inferiorly. If an apparent septum is identified only at the level of the cervix, it is much more likely to be a normal fold than a true septum.

Uterus didelphys (Answer B) is a Müllerian duct fusion anomaly resulting in two separate uterine horns and two separate cervices. The two uterine horns and two cervices are completely separate in this condition. Uterus didelphys generally does not require specific treatment.

Bicornuate bicollis uterus (Answer C) is a Müllerian duct fusion anomaly resulting in two separate uterine horns and two endocervical canals; it differs from a uterus didelphys because the cervical tissue surrounding the two endocervical canals is fused. This condition generally does not require specific treatment.

Septate uterus (Answer D) is a congenital resorption anomaly that results in separation of the endometrial and sometimes endocervical canal into two halves by an internal septum. It is caused by a failure of the fused uterus to resorb the fused internal tissue in utero. A uterine septum can be partial or complete, and can be composed of muscle and/or fibrous tissue. In patients with infertility, it is treated with hysteroscopic resection.

References: Dykes TM, Siegel C, Dodson W. Imaging of congenital uterine anomalies: review and self-assessment module. *AJR Am J Roentgenol* 2007;189:S1–S10.

El Jack AK, Siegelman ES. "Pseudoseptum" of the uterine cervix on MRI. *J Magn Reson Imaging* 2007;26:963–965.

Mueller GC, Hussain HK, Smith YR, et al. Müllerian duct anomalies: comparison of MRI diagnosis and clinical diagnosis. *AJR Am J Roentgenol* 2007;189:1294–1302.

Troiano RN, McCarthy SM. Müllerian duct anomalies: imaging and clinical issues. *Radiology* 2004;233:19–34.

16 **Answer B.**   Endometrial cancer invading more than 50% of the myometrial thickness is considered FIGO (**I**nternational **F**ederation of **G**ynecology and **O**bstetrics) stage IB disease. Because the majority (~80%) of patients with endometrial cancer present with clinical stage I disease (IA or IB), the primary role of MR imaging is to determine the depth of myometrial invasion—in particular, discriminating clinical stage IA disease (<50% myometrial invasion) from clinical stage IB disease (>50% myometrial invasion). This is important because patients with clinical stage IA disease have a much lower likelihood of having nodal metastases than patients diagnosed with clinical stage IB disease. In patients with clinical stage IA disease and small (<2 to 3 cm) low-grade tumors, lymph node dissection should not be routinely performed. In patients with clinical stage IB disease, lymph node dissection should be routinely performed.

An abbreviated version of the FIGO staging of endometrial cancer is shown below. The most important decision point for the radiologist is discriminating clinical stage IA from IB disease.

FIGO Stage	Description
IA	<50% myometrial invasion
IB	>50% myometrial invasion
II	Cervical stromal invasion
IIIA	Serosal, fallopian tube, or ovary invasion
IIIB	Vaginal or parametrial invasion
IIIC	Nodal metastases (regional or periaortic)
IV	Rectal invasion, bladder invasion, distant metastases

References: American Joint Committee on Cancer. Uterine cancer. In: *AJCC cancer staging manual*, 7th ed. New York, NY: Springer, 2010:403–409.

Frei KA, Kinkel K, Bonel HM, et al. Prediction of deep myometrial invasion in patients with endometrial cancer: clinical utility of contrast-enhanced MR imaging—a meta-analysis and Bayesian analysis. *Radiology* 2000;216:444–449.

Sala E, Wakely S, Senior E, et al. MRI of malignant neoplasms of the uterine corpus and cervix. *AJR Am J Roentgenol* 2007;188:1577–1587.

Vargas R, Rauh-Hain JA, Clemmer J, et al. Tumor size, depth of invasion, and histologic grade as prognostic factors of lymph node involvement in endometrial cancer: a SEER analysis. *Gynecol Oncol* 2014;133(2):216–220.

17 **Answer B.**   Diethylstilbestrol (DES) is a fetal teratogen that was used in the mid-20th century for the prevention of pregnancy-related side effects. Maternal use of DES resulted in multiple fetal anomalies. Among them, the "T-shaped" uterus is classic, with longitudinal constriction and hypoplasia of the endometrial cavity, and an irregular appearance of the endometrial cavity walls. Hydrosalpinges are also common. Other associations include ectopic pregnancy, spontaneous abortion, vaginal clear cell adenocarcinoma, and cervical clear cell adenocarcinoma. DES use was discontinued many years ago and therefore the number of patients with this history is shrinking.

References: Kaufman RH, Adam E, Binder GL, et al. Upper genital tract changes and pregnancy outcome in offspring exposed in utero to diethylstilbestrol. *Am J Obstet Gynecol* 1980;137:299–308.

Rennell CL. T-shaped uterus in diethylstilbestrol (DES) exposure. *AJR Am J Roentgenol* 1979;132:979–980.

van Gills AP, Tham RT, Falke TH, et al. Abnormalities of the uterus and cervix after diethylstilbestrol exposure: correlation of findings on MR and hysterosalpingography. *AJR Am J Roentgenol* 1989;153:1235–1238.

18   **Answer A.**   The images demonstrate a large fat-containing mass arising from the uterus and splaying the endometrial canal consistent with a lipoleiomyoma (i.e., a fat-containing fibroid). Note the India ink artifact on the opposed-phase T1-weighted GRE sequence indicating macroscopic fat. Fibroids have a diverse appearance with variable degrees of necrosis, enhancement, vascularity, fat, lipid, myxoid tissue, hemorrhage (i.e., "red" degeneration), etc. In general, regardless of the imaging appearance, a circumscribed mass within the myometrium is more likely to be a fibroid than any other entity.

A dermoid (Answer B) can also contain fat, but this mass is in the uterus and does not arise from the ovary. Endometrial cancer (Answer C) and uterine sarcoma (Answer D) do not typically contain fat. Endometrial cancer (Answer C) arises from the endometrium and may infiltrate the myometrium, but a rounded myometrial mass would be a strange presentation for endometrial cancer.

References: Murase E, Siegelman ES, Outwater EK, et al. Uterine leiomyomas: histopathologic features, MR imaging findings, differential diagnosis, and treatment. *Radiographics* 1999;19:1179–1197.

Ueda H, Togashi K, Konishi I, et al. Unusual appearances of uterine leiomyomas: MR imaging findings and their histopathologic backgrounds. *Radiographics* 1999;19:S131–S145.

19   **Answer B.**   The images demonstrate a large central uterine mass with numerous small cystic spaces that in the context of a markedly elevated serum hCG level is consistent with gestational trophoblastic disease (e.g., hydatidiform mole). Gestational trophoblastic disease is a complication with malignant potential resulting from abnormal trophoblastic tissue. It includes hydatidiform mole (partial vs. complete), invasive mole (a locally invasive mole that rarely metastasizes), and choriocarcinoma (a malignant mass associated with hemorrhagic metastases [e.g., lung and brain]). Gestational trophoblastic disease is usually detected by imaging or by an abnormally elevated hCG level in a pregnant or recently pregnant patient. Treatment consists of surgical evacuation, with or without systemic chemotherapy.

Retained products of conception (Answer A) can appear morphologically identical to gestational trophoblastic disease; differentiation is based on the hCG level. In this case, not only is the serum hCG level markedly elevated, but the patient has not been previously pregnant (G0P0). Although adenomyosis (Answer C) can be mass-like and exhibit small cystic spaces (i.e., ectopic endometrial glands), it is not the best answer in the setting of a markedly elevated serum hCG level. Similarly, large blood clots (Answer D) would not explain the serum hCG level.

References: Green CL, Angtuaco TL, Shah HR, et al. Gestational trophoblastic disease: a spectrum of radiologic diagnosis. *Radiographics* 1996;16:371–384.

Seckl MJ, Sebire NJ, Berkowitz RS. Gestational trophoblastic disease. *Lancet* 2010;376:717–729.

Wagner BJ, Woodward PJ, Dickey GE. From the archives of the AFIP: gestational trophoblastic disease: radiologic-pathologic correlation. *Radiographics* 1996;16:131–148.

20 Answer A.   The ideal sequence for measuring the depth of myometrial invasion is a dynamic contrast-enhanced 3D T1w GRE with fat saturation. This has improved diagnostic ability over anatomic T2w FSE imaging. Early time-point imaging (≤1 minute) is ideal for early myometrial invasion, equilibrium timepoint imaging (2 to 3 minutes) is ideal for deep myometrial invasion, and delayed timepoint imaging (4 to 5 minutes) is ideal for cervical stromal invasion. 3D imaging is important because the depth of invasion should be assessed in multiple planes. A 2D sequence would not allow easy postprocessing into off-axis orientations (due to nonisotropic voxels and stair-stepping artifact).

Although 2D T2w FSE (Answers C and D) is a routine part of endometrial cancer staging protocols, it is less accurate than dynamic post–contrast imaging for determining the depth of myometrial invasion. When performed, it should be done without fat saturation to improve visualization of the relationship between the primary tumor and the surrounding fat.

References: Frei KA, Kinkel K, Bonel HM, et al. Prediction of deep myometrial invasion in patients with endometrial cancer: clinical utility of contrast-enhanced MR imaging—a meta-analysis and Bayesian analysis. *Radiology* 2000;216:444–449.

Sala E, Wakely S, Senior E, et al. MRI of malignant neoplasms of the uterine corpus and cervix. *AJR Am J Roentgenol* 2007;188:1577–1587.

21 Answer D.   The images demonstrate a large heterogeneous fibroid within the posterior uterine fundus exerting broad mass effect upon the endometrial stripe consistent with a submucosal fibroid. Submucosal fibroids are associated with uterine bleeding and infertility. Removal or embolization of submucosal fibroids can reduce bleeding and improve fertility.

There are seven major categories of uterine fibroids:

Fibroid Type	Comment
Intracavitary	Within the endometrial cavity, connected to the myometrium by a stalk
Submucosal	Within the myometrium immediately beneath the endometrial lining
Intramural	Within the myometrium
Subserosal	Within the myometrium immediately beneath the uterine serosa
Pedunculated	External to the uterus, connected to the myometrium by a stalk
Cervical	Within the cervix
Broad ligament	Separate from the uterus within the adnexa

No fibroid type is an absolute contraindication to uterine artery embolization, but there are two caveats: Embolization of an intracavitary fibroid can lead to "birthing" of the fibroid, and embolization of a pedunculated fibroid can lead to hypothetical separation of the fibroid from the uterus.

References: Bulman BA, Ascher SM, Spies JB. Current concepts in uterine fibroid embolization. *Radiographics* 2012;32:1735–1750.

Parker WH. Etiology, symptomatology, and diagnosis of uterine myomas. *Fertil Steril* 2007;87:725–736.

22 **Answer A.** "Posterior acoustic enhancement" (i.e., "increased through transmission") is caused by two things: (1) lack of amplitude attenuation of the ultrasound beam as it passes through the cyst and (2) attenuation correction artifact.

The ultrasound machine makes several assumptions. It assumes that (1) the speed of sound is constant, (2) the true distance of an object from the transducer is only related to the travel time of the returning echo, (3) the path of the ultrasound beam is always straight, (4) each echo it receives only encountered a single reflection, and (5) tissues at a similar depth always will be attenuated to a similar degree. These assumptions can lead to imaging artifacts.

To compensate for the last of these, the ultrasound machine uses "time gain compensation" to increase the gain on echoes returning from deeper structures (i.e., echoes that take a longer time to return to the transducer). If it did not do this, there would be a progressive loss of signal moving from the superficial field to the deep field. The gain at each depth is constant; all pixels at the same depth are affected equally. Therefore, when the ultrasound beam passes through a structure that causes minimal sound attenuation compared to the adjacent tissues (e.g., through a cyst), the beam will lose less strength (i.e., amplitude) at that location than is expected. When the "time gain compensation" is applied to the tissues deep to the cyst, the tissues immediately below the cyst will be brightened more than other structures at the same depth, resulting in greater pixel brightness and a hyperechoic artifact.

References: Feldman MK, Katyal S, Blackwood MS. US artifacts. *Radiographics* 2009;29:1179–1189.
Pozniak MA, Zagzebski JA, Scanlan KA. Spectral and color Doppler artifacts. *Radiographics* 1992;12:35–44.

23 **Answer B.** The imaging demonstrates an irregular filling defect of the fundal endometrial canal associated with bilateral fallopian tube occlusion and venous intravasation. The irregularity of the filling defect and associated fallopian tube occlusions are suggestive of scar tissue formation. Endometrial scarring is commonly the result of prior pregnancy or intervention (e.g., dilatation and curettage [D&C]) and is associated with infertility, pregnancy loss, irregular menses, and pelvic pain. When diffuse, the entire cavity can become occluded (i.e., Asherman syndrome).

Endometrial cancer (Answer A) would be unusual in a patient of this age—it typically manifests in the fifth or sixth decade of life—and would present as a filling defect in the endometrial canal when seen at hysterosalpingography. Fetal diethylstilbestrol (DES) exposure (Answer C) would be extremely unlikely in a patient of this age; DES use was discontinued before this 24-year-old patient would have been conceived. The imaging findings are not consistent with uterine fibroids (Answer D). Fibroids stretch the endometrial cavity and/or produce smooth rounded filling defects.

References: Ahmadi F, Siahbazi S, Akhbari F, et al. Hysterosalpingography finding in intra uterine adhesion (Asherman's syndrome): a pictorial essay. *Int J Fertil Steril* 2013;7:155–160.
Simpson WL, Beitia LG, Mester J. Hysterosalpingography: a reemerging study. *Radiographics* 2006;26:419–431.
Steinkeler JA, Woodfield CA, Lazarus E, et al. Female infertility: a systematic approach to radiologic imaging and diagnosis. *Radiographics* 2009;29:1353–1370.

24 **Answer A.** The images demonstrate nonvisualization of the fallopian tubes, deformity of the fundal endometrium related to inadvertent catheter puncture, intravasation into small fundal myometrial vessels, and filling of a right pelvic vein, consistent with venous intravasation. Note that the tubular contrast material-filled structure in the right adnexa arises from the site of fundal intravasation, and not the uterine cornua as would be expected for a fallopian tube. The crescent-shaped contrast material at the base of the image is within the vagina and not the intraperitoneal cavity.

Intravasation into pelvic veins and/or lymphatics can occur with a pressurized endometrial cavity (i.e., a high-pressure HSG injection) or inadvertent catheter puncture of the myometrium (as in this case). Other than potentially confusing intravasation for fallopian tube patency, it is a clinically insignificant finding. No adjuvant antibiotic prophylaxis is necessary. Rarely, allergic-like reactions to the intravasated contrast material can occur.

References: Bateman BG, Nunley WC, Kitchin JD. Intravasation during hysterosalpingography using oil-base contrast media. *Fertil Steril* 1980;34:439–443.

Simpson WL, Beitia LG, Mester J. Hysterosalpingography: a reemerging study. *Radiographics* 2006;26:419–431.

25   Answer A.   Rudimentary horns associated with unicornuate uteri are usually surgically removed because of their association with cyclic pelvic pain, endometriosis, ectopic pregnancy, and pregnancy-associated uterine rupture. Rudimentary horns often have functioning endometrial tissue but may not communicate with the primary endometrial canal. When pregnancies occur within a rudimentary horn, it can lead to uterine rupture. Therefore, it is important to look for a rudimentary horn when a unicornuate uterus is identified. In an asymptomatic woman who is unable to become pregnant, the rudimentary horn can be left in situ. Pelvic MRI is the best noninvasive tool for the detection of rudimentary horns and the characterization of Müllerian duct anomalies.

References: Brucker SY, Rall K, Campo R, et al. Treatment of congenital malformations. *Semin Reprod Med* 2011;29:101–112.

Jayasinghe Y, Rane A, Stalewski H, et al. The presentation and early diagnosis of the rudimentary horn. *Obstet Gynecol* 2005;105:1456–1467.

Khati NJ, Frazier AA, Brindle KA. The unicornuate uterus and its variants: clinical presentation, imaging findings, and associated complications. *J Ultrasound Med* 2012;31:319–331.

26   Answer C.   Unfortunately, there are no validated reliable imaging-based methods to distinguish the rare leiomyosarcoma from the common leiomyoma (i.e., fibroid). Therefore, the diagnosis is usually made retrospectively after a presumed fibroid has been surgically removed. Some features that have been suggested for discriminatory purposes include large size, rapid growth, hemorrhage, necrosis, irregular margins, heterogeneous enhancement, and hyperintensity on T2-weighted images. However, each of these findings can also be seen with benign uterine fibroids, and fibroids are much more common than leiomyosarcoma. As a result, the positive predictive value of these characteristics is very low. Many leiomyosarcomas of the uterus are only diagnosed histologically after removal of a presumed fibroid. Recently, diffusion-weighted imaging has been explored as a way to improve imaging-based differentiation, but at the current time, this approach has not been validated. Because fibroids are so much more common than leiomyosarcoma, and the positive predictive value of any imaging discriminatory marker is poor, percutaneous biopsy (Answer D) is typically not a feasible option for establishing the diagnosis (i.e., it is unclear which masses would benefit from biopsy).

References: Parker WH, Fu YS, Berek JS. Uterine sarcoma in patients operated on for presumed leiomyoma and rapidly growing leiomyoma. *Obstet Gynecol* 1994;84:414–418.

Thomassin-Naggara I, Dechoux S, Bonneau C, et al. How to differentiate benign from malignant myometrial tumours using MR imaging. *Eur Radiol* 2013;23:2306–2314.

27 Answer A.   Although tamoxifen use is associated with endometrial hyperplasia, there is no allowance made for symptomatic postmenopausal women receiving tamoxifen therapy relative to their need for endometrial biopsy. Therefore, the endometrial stripe thickness threshold for symptomatic postmenopausal women on tamoxifen therapy is the same as the threshold used for the general symptomatic postmenopausal population: ≥5 mm.

References: Bezircioglu I, Baloglu A, Tarhan MO, et al. Evaluation of endometrium by transvaginal ultrasonography and Doppler in tamoxifen-treated women with breast cancer. *Eur J Gynaecol Oncol* 2012;33:295–299.

The American Congress of Obstetricians and Gynecologists. The role of transvaginal ultrasonography in the evaluation of postmenopausal bleeding. *The American Congress of Obstetricians and Gynecologists (ACOG) Committee Opinion 440*. 2009 and 2013.

28 Answer C.   The images demonstrate a hypoplastic leftward-deviated endometrial canal communicating with a hydrosalpinx. The differential diagnosis includes the following: (1) unicornuate uterus with or without a rudimentary horn, (2) bicornuate unicollis uterus in which the balloon is too deep and effectively cannulated only one of the uterine horns, (3) bicornuate bicollis uterus in which only one of the cervices was cannulated, (4) complete septate uterus in which only one side of the septum was cannulated (unlikely given the banana-shaped appearance), and (5) uterus didelphys in which only one of the cervices was cannulated. The best next step is to pull back the catheter to determine if there is another communicating uterine horn. Once the catheter has been pulled back, additional contrast material should be injected. If the differential diagnosis remains in doubt, or if a unicornuate uterus with no communicating rudimentary horn is demonstrated, a pelvic MRI should be considered for further evaluation of the pelvic anatomy.

References: Behr SC, Courtier JL, Qayyum A. Imaging of Müllerian duct anomalies. *Radiographics* 2012;32:E233–E250.

Simpson WL, Beitia LG, Mester J. Hysterosalpingography: a reemerging study. *Radiographics* 2006;26:419–431.

29 Answer D.   The images demonstrate marked displacement of otherwise normal-appearing fallopian tubes consistent with local mass effect. There is also subtle elongation of and indentation upon the right endometrial canal. These findings are consistent with pelvic masses. In a young patient, large parauterine masses are most likely to represent fibroids. The following pelvic MR images were obtained in the same patient, confirming the suspected diagnosis. Compare the shape of the uterus on the MR images to the mass effect on the HSG.

The HSG findings are not normal (Answer A) because the fallopian tubes are not in a normal position. Pelvic inflammatory disease (Answer C) can result in a variety of findings including hydrosalpinges, salpingitis isthmica nodosa, pelvic inclusion cysts, and scarring, but none of those findings are present in this case. The images are not typical for a congenital variant (Answer B).

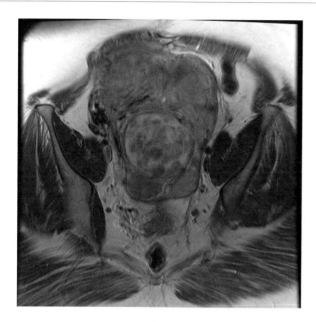
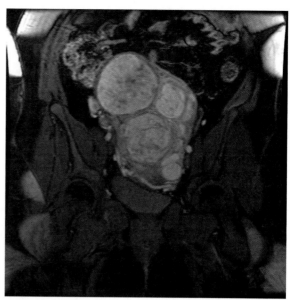

References: Dunnick NR, Sandler CM, Newhouse JH. *Textbook of uroradiology*, 5th ed. Philadelphia, PA: Lippincott Williams & Wilkins, 2012.
Simpson WL, Beitia LG, Mester J. Hysterosalpingography: a reemerging study. *Radiographics* 2006;26:419–431.

30 Answer E.   Small flask-shaped projections of contrast material external to the endometrial canal is consistent with adenomyosis. Adenomyosis is characterized by ectopic in-growth of endometrial glands into the myometrium. The condition is associated with endometriosis. On pelvic MRI, typical adenomyosis appears as focal or diffuse thickening of the junctional zone with or without internal subcentimeter myometrial cysts. Occasionally, adenomyosis can present as a focal mass that resembles a fibroid (i.e., adenomyoma).

References: Reinhold C, Tafazoli F, Mehio A, et al. Uterine adenomyosis: endovaginal US and MR imaging features with histopathologic correlation. *Radiographics* 1999;19:S147–S160.
Simpson WL, Beitia LG, Mester J. Hysterosalpingography: a reemerging study. *Radiographics* 2006;26:419–431.

QUESTIONS

1 A 50-year-old female with pelvic pain undergoes a pelvic MRI that demonstrates a 4.5-cm left ovarian cyst (depicted in the center of the image). Along what direction is the frequency-encoding gradient increasing in this sagittal T2-weighted image?

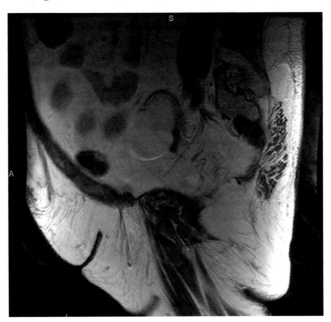

   A. Superior-to-inferior
   B. Inferior-to-superior
   C. Right-to-left
   D. Left-to-right

2 A 50-year-old female undergoes a pelvic MRI, and chemical shift artifact of the first kind is identified along the margins of an ovarian cyst. Assuming a receiver bandwidth of ±64 kHz (128 kHz) and a frequency matrix size of 128, what is the expected size of the pixel shift at 1.5 Tesla?

   A. 0.2 pixels
   B. 0.4 pixels
   C. 2.0 pixels
   D. 4.0 pixels

3 A 22-year-old female with right lower quadrant pain undergoes a contrast-enhanced CT of the abdomen and pelvis. What is the most likely cause of the dominant abnormality?

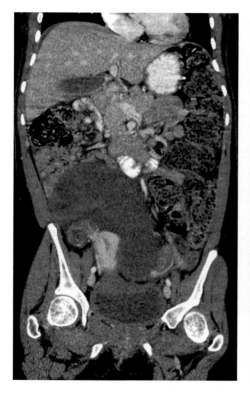 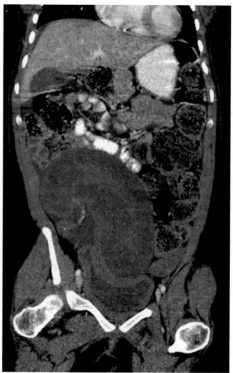

A. Infection
B. Ischemia
C. Inflammation
D. Malignancy

4 A 32-year-old G1P1 female presents with secondary infertility. Which of the following best characterizes the role of ultrasound in the diagnosis of polycystic ovary syndrome (PCOS)?

A. Numerous bilateral ovarian cysts are a highly sensitive marker of PCOS.
B. Numerous bilateral ovarian cysts are a highly specific marker of PCOS.
C. Ultrasound has only a supportive role in the diagnosis of PCOS.
D. Ultrasound has no role in the diagnosis of PCOS.

5 Why is STIR never used for fat suppression in T1-weighted contrast-enhanced pulse sequences?

A. Gadolinium variably shortens T1, resulting in unpredictable tissue suppression.
B. Gadolinium variably shortens T2, resulting in unpredictable tissue suppression.
C. Fat protons are not affected by the 180-degree inversion pulse.
D. Fat protons are not affected by the 90-degree inversion pulse.

6   A 38-year-old female with a negative urine pregnancy test and recurrent left lower quadrant pain undergoes a pelvic ultrasound with color Doppler imaging. A 3.5-cm abnormality is identified in the left ovary. Her symptoms persist, and follow-up ultrasound performed 2 months later is unchanged. What is the best next step?

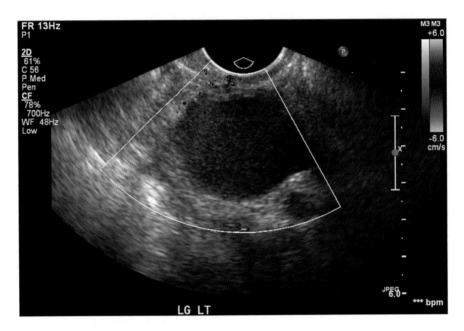

A. Further imaging: follow-up ultrasound in 2 months
B. Further imaging: contrast-enhanced pelvic MRI now
C. Percutaneous biopsy
D. Cystectomy performed by a gynecologist
E. Cystectomy performed by a gynecology oncologist

7   A 28-year-old female with fever, leukocytosis, and adnexal pain undergoes a pelvic ultrasound. The serum bHCG level is 0 mIU/mL. What is the best next step?

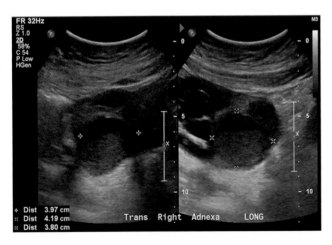 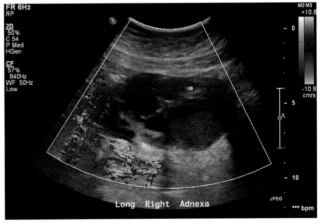

A. Ignore (benign finding)
B. Imaging follow-up
C. Intravenous antibiotic therapy
D. Intravenous antibiotic therapy and drainage
E. Surgical resection

8   The management of asymptomatic ovarian and adnexal cysts is in part dependent on whether a cyst is detected in a premenopausal or a postmenopausal patient. What is the definition of postmenopause in patients who have not had a hysterectomy?

A. Two cycles of amenorrhea after the age of 50 years
B. Six cycles of amenorrhea from the last menstrual period
C. One year of amenorrhea from the last menstrual period
D. One year of amenorrhea after the age of 50 years

9   A 32-year-old female with no past medical history undergoes a transvaginal pelvic ultrasound for menorrhagia. A 3.5-cm left adnexal cyst is identified. The patient has no pelvic pain. How should this finding be dictated in the radiologist's report?

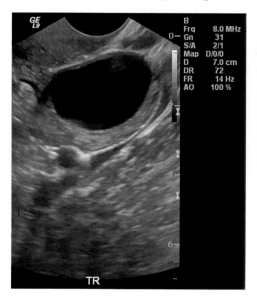 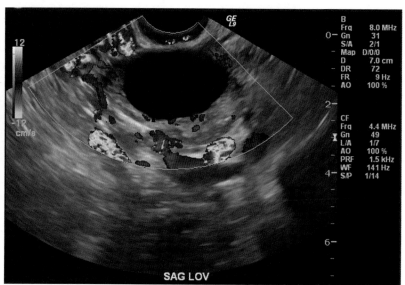

A. The finding should not be mentioned.
B. The finding is likely benign with no follow-up recommended.
C. The finding is likely benign with 1-year follow-up recommended.
D. The finding is possibly malignant with 1-year follow-up recommended.
E. The finding is possibly malignant with surgical consultation recommended.

10   A 72-year-old female with no past medical history undergoes a transvaginal pelvic ultrasound for postmenopausal bleeding. A 3.5-cm simple left adnexal cyst is identified. The patient has no pelvic pain. How should this finding be dictated in the radiologist's report?

A. The finding should not be mentioned.
B. The finding is likely benign with no follow-up recommended.
C. The finding is likely benign with 1-year follow-up recommended.
D. The finding is possibly malignant with 1-year follow-up recommended.
E. The finding is possibly malignant with surgical consultation recommended.

11   A 40-year-old female undergoes a transvaginal ultrasound, and a cystic adnexal mass is identified. A repeat study performed 2 months later shows no interval change. Which of the following imaging findings most strongly suggests a malignant etiology?

A. Two 4-mm-thick septations
B. Diffuse low-level internal echoes
C. Tubular configuration with a "waist sign"
D. Solid-appearing area with concave margins and no internal flow

12   A 35-year-old female with lower abdominal pain undergoes a contrast-enhanced CT of the abdomen and pelvis. A 6-cm mass is identified in the left pelvis. What is the most likely diagnosis?

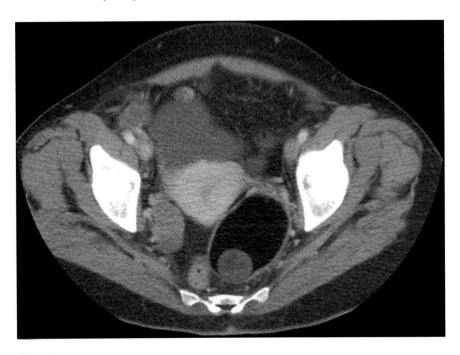

A. Mature cystic teratoma
B. Immature teratoma
C. Liposarcoma
D. Lipoma

13   A 22-year-old female with pelvic inflammatory disease complicated by infected peritoneal fluid presents for transgluteal catheter drainage. Of the following routes of access, which is most likely to result in successful drainage with the least risk of complication?

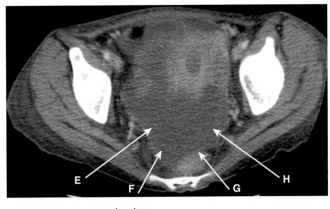
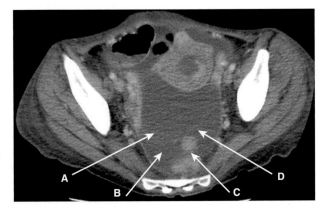

A. A
B. B
C. C
D. D
E. E
F. F
G. G
H. H

14 In utero diethylstilbestrol exposure has a strong association with which of the following malignancies?

   A. Uterine sarcoma

   B. Endometrial adenocarcinoma

   C. Vaginal clear cell adenocarcinoma

   D. Ovarian carcinosarcoma

15 Which of the following is a risk factor for *Actinomyces israelii* infection of the fallopian tubes?

   A. Unprotected sexual intercourse

   B. Intrauterine device placement

   C. Oral contraceptive use

   D. Uterus didelphys

16 A 32-year-old G2P2 female undergoes hysteroscopic placement of bilateral fallopian tube occlusion devices. Three months later, a hysterosalpingogram is performed. How should the resulting imaging be interpreted?

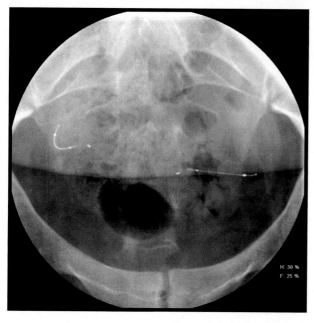 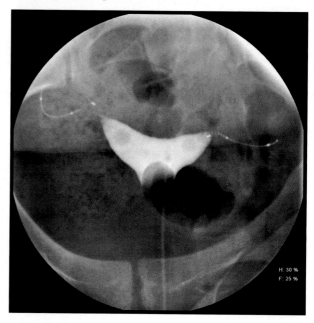

   A. Normal device position, bilateral tubal occlusion

   B. Normal device position, insufficient tubal occlusion

   C. Abnormal device position, bilateral tubal occlusion

   D. Abnormal device position, insufficient tubal occlusion

17 A 40-year-old G1P1 female who recently immigrated to the United States from a third-world country presents with incontinence. She has no known surgical or cancer history, and a pelvic examination is normal. A cystogram is performed, and a vesicovaginal fistula is identified. Which of the following risk factors best explains the imaging findings?

   A. Multistrain human papillomavirus infection

   B. Recurrent *Clonorchis sinensis* infection

   C. Childbirth complicated by prolonged labor

   D. Low-fiber, high-carbohydrate diet

18 A 57-year-old female presents with vaginal cancer. What is the most common cell type and risk factor for vaginal cancer in the United States?

   A. Squamous cell carcinoma; pelvic radiation therapy

   B. Squamous cell carcinoma; human papillomavirus infection

   C. Adenocarcinoma; in utero diethylstilbestrol exposure

   D. Adenocarcinoma; *Chlamydia trachomatis* infection

19 A 50-year-old female with pelvic discomfort undergoes a pelvic MRI, and a left ovarian mass is identified. Other images (not shown) reveal bilateral pleural effusions and ascites. Her serum CA-125 level is elevated. The following images are representative of the entire ovarian mass. Which of the following best characterizes this patient's prognosis and expected treatment course?

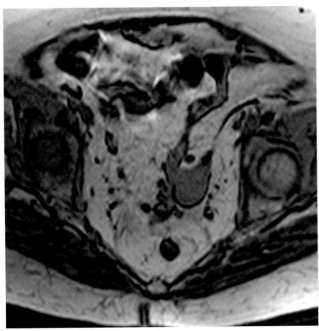

Axial T1w GRE with fat saturation

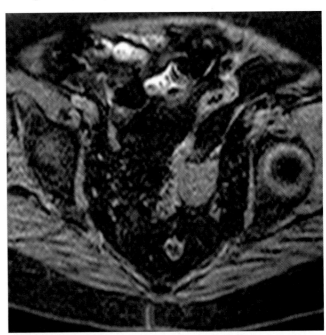

Axial T1w GRE with fat saturation postcontrast

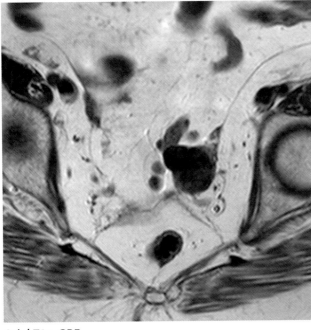

Axial T1w GRE

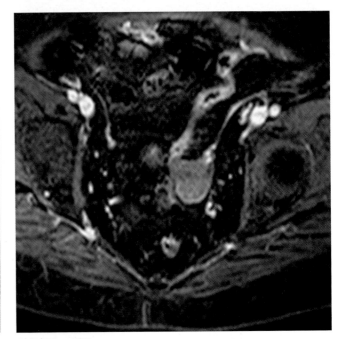

Axial T2w FSE

A. Excellent prognosis following systemic chemotherapy
B. Excellent prognosis following ipsilateral oophorectomy
C. Dismal prognosis despite systemic chemotherapy
D. Dismal prognosis despite ipsilateral oophorectomy

20   A 55-year-old female requests information about the combined use of serum
     CA-125 and transvaginal ultrasound for ovarian cancer screening. Which of the
     following statements best summarizes the current consensus on ovarian cancer
     screening in average-risk patients?

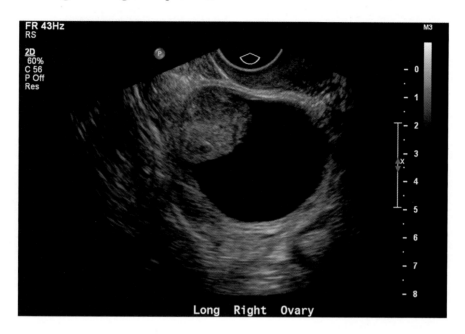

A. Neither CA-125 nor pelvic ultrasound is effective for screening average-risk
   patients.
B. CA-125 is effective for screening average-risk patients, but pelvic ultrasound
   is not.
C. Pelvic ultrasound is effective for screening average-risk patients, but CA-125
   is not.
D. CA-125 and pelvic ultrasound are effective for screening average-risk
   patients but only in combination.

21   A senior investigator at a major academic institution is interested in
     detecting new treatments for ovarian carcinomatosis. He plans to make
     thickness measurements of the omental cake by CT in affected patients
     1, 3, 6, and 12 months after the initial laparoscopic diagnosis in the absence
     of intercurrent systemic therapy. He plans to use this information as a
     control against which he can compare the effect of novel therapeutic agents.
     However, most patients with ovarian carcinomatosis at his institution receive
     standard-of-care systemic therapy, so he is having difficulty identifying a
     control group for his study. Which of the following approaches is most
     appropriate?

A. He should ask his gynecology colleagues to delay systemic chemotherapy
   for at least 12 months in patients newly diagnosed with ovarian cancer, and
   then use this group as his control.
B. He should randomize patients newly diagnosed with ovarian cancer to
   receive either standard-of-care systemic therapy or no therapy for
   12 months, and then use the "no therapy" group as his control.
C. He should instead contrast the growth rate of ovarian carcinomatosis in the
   setting of one IND- and IRB-approved novel therapeutic agent against that
   of another IND- and IRB-approved novel therapeutic agent.
D. He should instead contrast the growth rate of ovarian carcinomatosis in the
   setting of standard-of-care systemic therapy against that of an IND- and IRB-
   approved novel therapeutic agent.

22   A 24-year-old female presents for MR imaging of the pelvis after her primary care physician discovered an ovoid soft palpable mass. What is the most likely diagnosis?

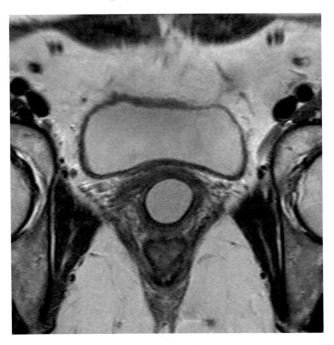 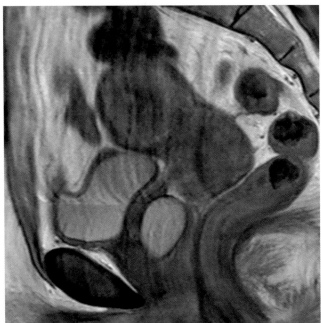

A. Bartholin gland cyst
B. Gartner duct cyst
C. Urethral diverticulum
D. Skene gland cyst

23   A 25-year-old female with right lower quadrant pain undergoes a transvaginal ultrasound to "rule out torsion." Her right ovary measures 2 × 3 × 2 cm, and her left ovary measures 2 × 3 × 2 cm. How should the images be interpreted?

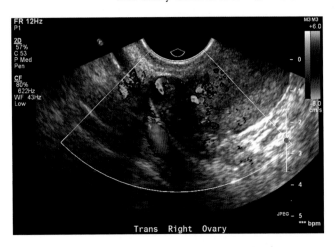 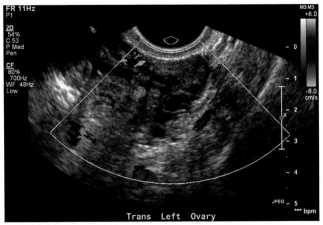

A. Normal ovaries; the apparent diminished flow in the left ovary is likely technical.
B. There is diminished flow in the left ovary that is equivocal for ovarian torsion.
C. There is diminished flow in the left ovary consistent with acute ovarian torsion.
D. There is diminished flow in the left ovary consistent with chronic ovarian torsion.

24 A 22-year-old female with right lower quadrant pain and a positive pregnancy test undergoes a transvaginal ultrasound. Which of the following is a risk factor for tubal ectopic pregnancy?

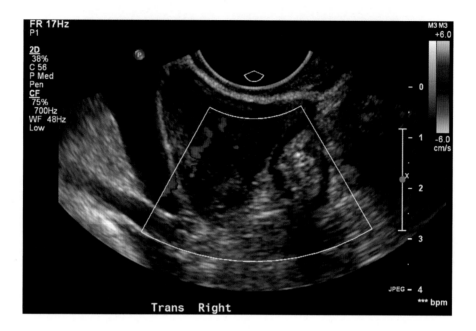

A. Human papillomavirus infection
B. *Neisseria gonorrhoeae* infection
C. Prior uncomplicated vaginal delivery
D. Prior uncomplicated cesarean section

25 A young investigator is designing a clinical trial comparing two imaging modalities for cervical cancer staging. Prior to Institutional Review Board submission, she is required to attest that she will conduct her research in an ethical fashion. Match the following research practices (lettered) with the appropriate guiding ethical principle (numbered) as outlined in the Belmont Report.

A. Informed consent process	1. Justice
B. Risk/benefit assessment	2. Respect for persons
C. Protection of vulnerable subjects	3. Beneficence

26 A 28-year-old female with hypotension and severe pelvic pain presents for pelvic ultrasound. A urine beta-HCG is positive, and no normal pregnancy is identified. If this patient has an ectopic pregnancy, where is it most likely to be located?

A. Uterus
B. Fallopian tube
C. Ovary
D. Cul-de-sac
E. Cervix

27 A 24-year-old female presents for MR imaging of the pelvis after her primary care physician discovered an ovoid soft palpable mass. What is the most likely diagnosis?

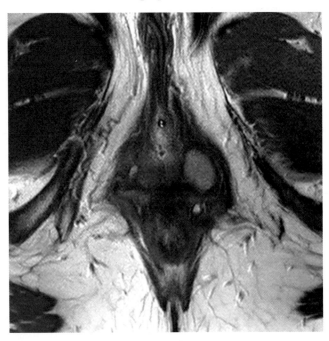

A. Bartholin gland cyst
B. Gartner duct cyst
C. Urethral diverticulum
D. Skene gland cyst

28 A 24-year-old female with primary infertility undergoes a hysterosalpingogram for tubal evaluation. Which of the following best explains the imaging findings?

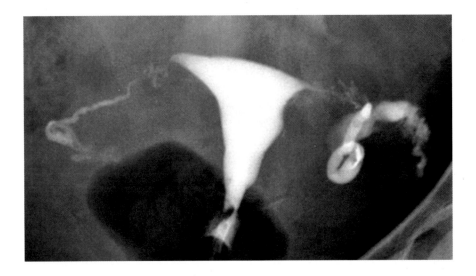

A. Normal study
B. Prior *Chlamydia trachomatis* infection
C. Congenital mesonephric duct abnormality
D. Fetal diethylstilbestrol exposure

29 A 40-year-old female with chronic pelvic pain undergoes a transvaginal pelvic ultrasound. A repeat study performed 2 months later shows persistent findings. What is the most likely diagnosis?

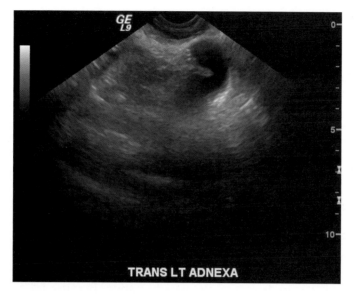

A. Ovarian serous cystadenoma
B. Ovarian mucinous adenocarcinoma
C. Hydrosalpinx
D. Endometrioma

30 The fallopian tube is composed of four major segments. Match the segments of the fallopian tube (lettered) with the labels shown in the figure (numbered).

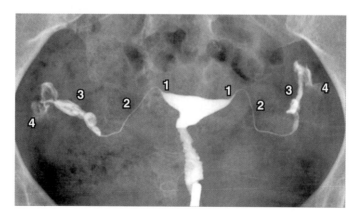

A. Ampullary	1. Segment 1
B. Interstitial	2. Segment 2
C. Infundibular	3. Segment 3
D. Isthmic	4. Segment 4

ANSWERS AND EXPLANATIONS

1 **Answer A.** The frequency-encoding gradient in this image increases from superior to inferior. This cyst in the center of the image demonstrates chemical shift artifact of the first kind along the superior and inferior margins; with this artifact, the spatial mapping of fat is erroneously shifted relative to water. Chemical shift artifact only occurs along the frequency-encoding axis. Therefore, Answer C and Answer D are incorrect. The black line where fat pixels were shifted away from the wall of the cyst is along the superior margin, and the white line into which pixels were shifted from fat into the cyst is along the inferior margin. This indicates that the frequency-encoding gradient increases from superior to inferior (from the black line toward the white line). An explanation of this is provided below. Chemical shift artifact of the first kind occurs along fat–fluid and fat–tissue interfaces. The width of the artifact increases with increasing field strength and lower receiver bandwidth.

Spatial location along the frequency-encoding axis is determined by precessional frequency. The frequency-encoding gradient assigns protons along each line of the frequency-encoding axis a unique precessional frequency that can be used later to determine its spatial location. Because fat protons do not precess at the same frequency as do water protons, the mapping is erroneous, with the slower fat protons being erroneously shifted downward along the frequency-encoding gradient (slower precession frequency than expected). Look at the graph below and imagine that the x-axis voxels labeled "water" represent the cyst from the image, and the x-axis voxels labeled "fat" represent the adjacent fat from the image. The y-axis is gradient frequency; two different frequency-encoding gradients are shown as red and blue lines. These lines show the frequencies assigned (by position) to the different voxels.

The graph shows that the steepness of the frequency-encoding gradient is a reflection of the width of the receiver bandwidth. The receiver bandwidth is basically the range of frequencies encoded by the frequency-encoding gradient for a given matrix size. Therefore, a higher receiver bandwidth (e.g., the red line, steep slope) will be less affected by a small frequency shift (e.g., 220 Hz at 1.5 Tesla) because the shift may occur entirely within a single voxel. Choose a spot on the red line and trace backward 220 Hz using the y-axis. Notice that this new position may remain within the same voxel. As the receiver bandwidth decreases (e.g., blue line), the shift will cross voxels, moving signal intensity contributed by fat from one voxel into another. Choose a spot on the blue line and trace backward 220 Hz using the y-axis. Notice that this new position will be within a different voxel.

The direction of the chemical shift of the fat protons will be from high to low frequency because fat protons precess slower than do water protons. Therefore, the fat–water interface at the high end of the gradient will experience a shift of fat protons into the cyst (creating a bright band of added signal), and the fat–water interface at the low end of the gradient will experience a shift of fat protons away from the cyst (creating a black band of absent signal). Why not always maximize the receiver bandwidth? High receiver bandwidths have more noise per pixel. Therefore, high receiver bandwidths come at the cost of reduced SNR (signal-to-noise ratio).

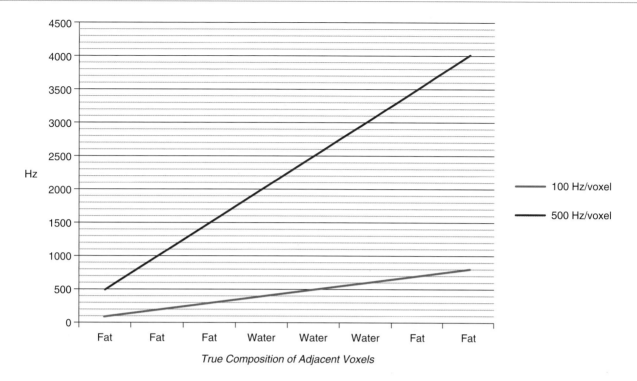

True Composition of Adjacent Voxels

References: Kamel IR, Merkle EM. *Body MR Imaging at 3 Tesla*, 1st ed. New York: Cambridge University Press, 2011.
Mamourian AC. *Practical MR physics*, 1st ed. New York: Oxford University Press, 2010.
McRobbie DW, Moore EA, Graves MJ, et al. *MRI: from picture to proton*, 2nd ed. New York: Cambridge University Press, 2007.

2   **Answer A.**   Fat protons precess slower than do water protons by 3.5 ppm when exposed to the same magnetic field. This results in a difference in Larmor frequency by approximately 220 Hz at 1.5 Tesla and approximately 440 Hz at 3.0 Tesla. This information can be used with the receiver bandwidth and frequency matrix size to calculate the width of the chemical shift artifact using the following equation:

$$\text{Chemical shift} \left(220\,\text{Hz at 1.5 Tesla or } 440\,\text{Hz at 3.0 Tesla}\right) / \\ \left(\text{receiver bandwidth}/\text{frequency matrix}\right)$$

Therefore, at 1.5 Tesla with a receiver bandwidth of 128 kHz (128,000 Hz) and a frequency matrix of 128, the pixel shift is

$$220\,\text{Hz}/\left(128{,}000\,\text{Hz}/128\,\text{pixels}\right) = 220\,\text{Hz}/\left(1{,}000\,\text{Hz}/\text{pixel}\right) = 0.2\,\text{pixels}$$

If a 3-Tesla system is used instead, notice that the size of the shift would double:

$$440\,\text{Hz}/\left(128{,}000\,\text{Hz}/128\,\text{pixels}\right) = 440\,\text{Hz}/\left(1{,}000\,\text{Hz}/\text{pixel}\right) = 0.4\,\text{pixels}$$

If a smaller bandwidth is used (e.g., 64 kHz, 3.0 Tesla), the size of the shift would increase again:

$$440\,\text{Hz}/\left(64{,}000\,\text{Hz}/128\,\text{pixels}\right) = 440\,\text{Hz}/\left(500\,\text{Hz}/\text{pixel}\right) = 0.9\,\text{pixels}$$

References: Kamel IR, Merkle EM. *Body MR Imaging at 3 Tesla*, 1st ed. New York: Cambridge University Press, 2011.
Mamourian AC. *Practical MR physics*, 1st ed. New York: Oxford University Press, 2010.
McRobbie DW, Moore EA, Graves MJ, et al. *MRI: from picture to proton*, 2nd ed. New York: Cambridge University Press, 2007.

3 **Answer B.** The images demonstrate swirling of the vasculature in the right adnexa, tethering of the urinary bladder and uterus to the right, and a large low-attenuation right adnexal mass consistent with an edematous and ischemic ovary in the setting of ovarian torsion. The twisted vascular pedicle is pathognomonic, while ipsilateral deviation of the uterus and bladder is supportive of the diagnosis. The ovary is massively enlarged secondary to vascular volvulus, necrosis, and edema. Malignancy would be unusual in a patient of this age (Answer D). By the time the ovary is this enlarged, it is likely no longer viable, but the best next step remains operative evaluation.

References: Duigenan S, Oliva E, Lee SI. Ovarian torsion: diagnostic features on CT and MRI with pathologic correlation. *AJR Am J Roentgenol* 2012;198:W122–W131.

Chang HC, Bhatt S, Dogra VS. Pearls and pitfalls in diagnosis of ovarian torsion. *Radiographics* 2008;28:1355–1368.

4 **Answer C.** Polycystic ovary syndrome (PCOS) is a heterogeneous disorder characterized by androgen excess, oligo- or anovulation, and polycystic ovaries. However, PCOS can manifest in a variety of ways, and the diagnosis is not always clear-cut. Patients may have only two of the three typical criteria, and no one criterion is sufficient for the diagnosis. Therefore, ultrasound provides a supportive role. Many patients who do not have PCOS have "polycystic ovaries," and many patients with the clinical findings of PCOS do not have typical imaging findings.

Ultrasound criteria that are supportive for the diagnosis of PCOS (representing one of the three key criteria) as established by the ESHRE/ASRM Consensus Workshop Group include one or both ovaries with:

12 or more follicles 2 to 9 mm in diameter and/or ovarian volume >10 mL

Ovarian volume is calculated by the following formula: length × width × height × 0.5. The distribution of the follicles, the stromal echotexture, and the stromal volume are not considered relevant. The definition does not apply in women taking oral contraceptive pills because oral contraceptives can alter the appearance of the ovaries.

References: Balen A, Michelmore K. What is polycystic ovary syndrome? Are national views important? *Hum Reprod* 2002;17:2219–2227.

Lujan ME, Chizen DR, Pierson RA, et al. Diagnostic criteria for polycystic ovary syndrome: pitfalls and controversies. *J Obstet Gynaecol Can* 2008;30:671–679.

Norman RJ, Dewailly D, Legro RS, et al. Polycystic ovary syndrome. *Lancet* 2007;370:685–697.

Rotterdam ESHRE/ASRM-Sponsored PCOS Consensus Workshop Group. Revised 2003 consensus on diagnostic criteria and long-term health risks related to polycystic ovary syndrome. *Fertil Steril* 2004;81:19–25.

5 **Answer A.** Gadolinium-containing contrast material primarily functions by indirectly shortening the T1 times of nearby tissue. The precise effect on T1 is unpredictable and based partially on the concentration of contrast material in a given voxel. Therefore, the T1 time of some tissues could be inadvertently matched to the T1 time of fat and inappropriately suppressed following an STIR inversion recovery pulse.

STIR is an inversion recovery technique. All tissues in the slice are subjected to a 180-degree inversion recovery RF pulse prior to the excitation RF pulse, with the timing of the 180-degree RF pulse being determined by the T1 time of fat. The length of time between the 180-degree inversion RF pulse and the excitation RF pulse is known as the inversion time (TI).

The excitation RF pulse is performed when the longitudinal recovery of fat protons subjected to the 180-degree inversion RF pulse crosses the zero or "null" point of magnetization. This timing is determined by a predetermined calculation. If the magnetization of fat is at the zero point, it will not generate any signal when exposed to the excitation RF pulse. Any other tissues that have a similar or identical

T1 time to fat (e.g., soft tissue with a shortened T1 time due to gadolinium-containing contrast material) will also be suppressed in a similar fashion.

The principal mechanism of the STIR inversion RF pulse is based on T1 relaxation, not T2 relaxation (Answer B). STIR results in more homogeneous fat suppression compared to frequency-selective techniques because it is less affected by magnetic field inhomogeneity (i.e., T1 times are fixed characteristics of tissue while resonance frequencies are affected by magnetic field strength; magnetic field strength varies locally due to B_0 inhomogeneity, varying local magnetic moments, and susceptibility effects).

References: Delfaut EM, Beltran J, Johnson G, et al. Fat suppression in MR imaging: techniques and pitfalls. *Radiographics* 1999;19:373–382.
McRobbie DW, Moore EA, Graves MJ, et al. 2007. *MRI: from picture to proton*, 2nd ed. New York: Cambridge University Press.

6 **Answer D.** The image demonstrates a cystic mass in the left ovary that contains numerous low-level echoes compatible with a benign endometrioma. No solid nodule is identified. Further imaging (Answers A and B) is unlikely to add value, and the patient is symptomatic. Definitive management is surgical. In many cases, endometriomas can be excised without removing the ipsilateral ovary.

The mass has no features of malignancy, and therefore a cancer surgery (Answer E) is not necessary. Percutaneous biopsy (Answer C) is in general contraindicated for the evaluation of a cystic ovarian mass due to the risk of perforation and spillage.

References: Abbott JA, Hawe J, Clayton RD, et al. The effects and effectiveness of laparoscopic excision of endometriosis: a prospective study with 2–5 year follow-up. *Hum Reprod* 2003;18:1922–1927.
Hart RJ, Hickey M, Maouris P, et al. Excisional surgery versus ablative surgery for ovarian endometrioma. *Cochrane Database Syst Rev* 2005;20:CD004992.
Seracchioli R, Mabrouk M, Frasca C, et al. Long-term cyclic and continuous oral contraceptive therapy and endometrioma recurrence: a randomized controlled trial. *Fertil Steril* 2010;93:52–56.

7 **Answer C.** The clinical history and imaging findings are consistent with a hydro/pyosalpinx and a small tuboovarian abscess in the setting of pelvic inflammatory disease. The best next step is intravenous antibiotic therapy. Percutaneous drainage is likely not needed. The majority of small tuboovarian abscesses <8 cm will respond to antibiotic therapy alone. Large abscesses (>8 cm) and those that fail antibiotic therapy can be drained safely percutaneously. Common routes of access include transvaginal, transrectal, transabdominal, and transgluteal.

References: Dewitt J, Reining A, Allsworth JE, et al. Tuboovarian abscesses: is size associated with duration of hospitalization and complications? *Obstet Gynecol Int* 2010; doi: 10.1155/2010/847041.
Goharkhay N, Verma U, Maggiorotto F. Comparison of CT- or ultrasound-guided drainage with concomitant intravenous antibiotics vs. intravenous antibiotics alone in the management of tubo-ovarian abscesses. *Ultrasound Obstet Gynecol* 2007;29:65–69.
Perez-Medina T, Huertas MA, Baho JM. Early ultrasound-guided transvaginal drainage of tubo-ovarian abscesses: a randomized study. *Ultrasound Obstet Gynecol* 1996;7:435–438.

8 **Answer C.** Postmenopause is a retrospective diagnosis defined as the state following 1 year of amenorrhea from the last menstrual period. Although the average age of menopause is 51 to 53 years in Western countries, the age it occurs varies widely (i.e., 40 to 60 years of age). Therefore, there is no age threshold for the diagnosis in patients without a prior hysterectomy (Answers A and D). In patients who have had a hysterectomy but retain their ovaries (precluding assessment of menstrual status), menopause is defined as age 50.

References: Levine D, Brown DL, Andreotti RF, et al. Management of asymptomatic ovarian and other adnexal cysts imaged at US: Society of Radiologists in Ultrasound Consensus Conference Statement. *Radiology* 2010;256:943–954.

Soules MR, Sherman S, Parrott E, et al. Executive summary: Stages of Reproductive Aging Workshop (STRAW). *Fertil Steril* 2001;76:874–878.

te Velde ER, Pearson PL. The variability of female reproductive ageing. *Hum Reprod* 2002;8:141–154.

9   **Answer B.**   According to the Society of Radiologists in Ultrasound Consensus Conference Statement (2010), asymptomatic simple adnexal cysts in premenopausal women >3 and ≤5 cm should be described as likely benign with no follow-up recommended. The rationale for this management is that such cysts are almost always benign, and excessive imaging follow-up creates unnecessary anxiety for minimal clinical gain.

A summary of the recommendations for the management of asymptomatic cysts in premenopausal women established by the Society of Radiologists in Ultrasound Consensus Conference Statement (2010) is provided in the following table.

Management of Asymptomatic Simple Adnexal Cysts in Premenopausal Women	
≤3 cm	The finding can be ignored or mentioned, with no follow-up recommended.
>3 and ≤5 cm	The finding should be described as almost certainly benign, with no follow-up recommended.
>5 and ≤7 cm	The finding should be described as almost certainly benign, with annual ultrasound follow-up recommended.
>7 cm	The finding should be described as too large to be definitively assessed by ultrasound, with pelvic MRI and/or surgical consultation recommended.

Reference: Levine D, Brown DL, Andreotti RF, et al. Management of asymptomatic ovarian and other adnexal cysts imaged at US: Society of Radiologists in Ultrasound Consensus Conference Statement. *Radiology* 2010;256:943–954.

10   **Answer C.**   Although postmenopausal women have a higher risk of ovarian cancer than do premenopausal women, simple cysts in this population are still extremely likely to be benign. Therefore, an asymptomatic simple adnexal cyst in a postmenopausal woman >1 and ≤7 cm should be described as likely benign with annual ultrasound follow-up recommended.

The recommendations for the management of asymptomatic simple adnexal cysts in postmenopausal women as established by the Society of Radiologists in Ultrasound Consensus Conference Statement (2010) are provided in the following table. Note the differences in recommendations for postmenopausal women (current question) and premenopausal women (previous question).

Management of Asymptomatic Simple Adnexal Cysts in Postmenopausal Women	
≤1 cm	The finding can be ignored or mentioned, with no follow-up recommended.
>1 and ≤7 cm	The finding should be described as almost certainly benign, with annual ultrasound follow-up recommended.
>7 cm	The finding should be described as too large to be definitively assessed by ultrasound, with pelvic MRI and/or surgical consultation recommended.

Reference: Levine D, Brown DL, Andreotti RF, et al. Management of asymptomatic ovarian and other adnexal cysts imaged at US: Society of Radiologists in Ultrasound Consensus Conference Statement. *Radiology* 2010;256:943–954.

11 Answer A.   Malignancy should be suspected in a cystic adnexal mass containing one or more thickened septation(s) or one or more solid vascularized nodule(s). Presence of either imaging finding is an indication for surgical evaluation, regardless of the patient's age. According to the Society of Radiologists in Ultrasound Consensus Conference Statement (2010), a "thickened" septation is defined as a septation ≥3 mm in width.

Borderline indications for surgical evaluation include multiple thin septations (≤2 mm), a nonhyperechoic nodule without internal flow, or an otherwise complex cyst of any appearance in a postmenopausal female.

Diffuse low-level internal echoes (Answer B) are a characteristic of endometriomas (due to chronic internal blood products of varying ages). A cystic structure with a tubular configuration and a "waist sign" (Answer C) is characteristic of a hydrosalpinx ("waist sign": soft tissue indentations on infolded walls of the fallopian tube). A solid-appearing avascular area with concave margins (Answer D) is characteristic of a hemorrhagic cyst (the concave margins are due to clot retraction).

References: Brown DL, Doubilet PM, Miller FH, et al. Benign and malignant ovarian masses: selection of the most discriminating grayscale and Doppler sonographic features. *Radiology* 1998;208:103–110.

Levine D, Brown DL, Andreotti RF, et al. Management of asymptomatic ovarian and other adnexal cysts imaged at US: Society of Radiologists in Ultrasound Consensus Conference Statement. *Radiology* 2010;256:943–954.

12 Answer A.   The images demonstrate a 6-cm mass in the left adnexa predominantly composed of macroscopic fat with a single nondominant solid nodule. The most likely diagnosis is mature cystic teratoma. Mature cystic teratoma of the ovary is a benign mass that is usually removed surgically due to the risk of ovarian torsion, the small risk of perforation (which can cause granulomatous peritonitis), and the small risk of malignant degeneration (e.g., squamous cell carcinoma arising from the squamous lining; this does not refer to reversion into an immature teratoma). Malignant transformation typically does not occur until the sixth or seventh decade of life.

Mature cystic teratoma is much more common than is immature teratoma. There are several notable differences between these two entities (see Table).

Mature Cystic Teratoma	Immature Teratoma
A commonly excised ovarian neoplasm	A rare ovarian neoplasm
Can be seen at all ages	Occurs in the first and second decades of life
Benign behavior	Malignant behavior
Smaller (usually 1–10 cm)	Larger (usually >15 cm)
Capsule intact	Capsular perforation
Cystic and fatty elements dominate	Large soft tissue mass
Hemorrhage is rare	Hemorrhage is common

Liposarcoma (Answer C) and lipoma (Answer D) are not the best choices. There is a claw of ovarian tissue along the anterior margin of the mass consistent with an ovarian origin.

References: Outwater EK, Siegelman ES, Hunt JL. Ovarian teratomas: tumor types and imaging characteristics. *Radiographics* 2001;21:475–490.

Saba L, Guerriero S, Sulcis R, et al. Mature and immature teratomas: CT, US, and MR imaging characteristics. *Eur J Radiol* 2009;72:454–463.

13 **Answer F.** The transgluteal approach is a safe and effective route for access to deep pelvic structures. The following is a commentary on the labeled access arrows from the question:

Arrow	Comment(s)
A	This approach is too lateral, traverses the piriformis muscle, and penetrates large vessels along the right pelvic sidewall.
B	This approach is appropriately medial but traverses the piriformis muscle. If approach F was not an option, this would be a reasonable alternative. In general, the piriformis muscle should be avoided because transpiriformis approaches often result in sciatic nerve irritation.
C	This approach is appropriately medial but penetrates the rectum.
D	This approach is too lateral, traverses the piriformis muscle, and penetrates large vessels along the left pelvic sidewall.
E	This approach is too lateral, traverses the piriformis muscle, and penetrates large vessels along the right pelvic sidewall.
F	This approach is ideal. It is appropriately medial and inferior to the piriformis muscle, thereby minimizing risk of sciatic nerve injury or irritation. It does not traverse any major vasculature and is distant from the rectum.
G	This approach is appropriately medial but penetrates the rectum.
H	This approach is too lateral, traverses the piriformis muscle, and penetrates large vessels along the left pelvic sidewall.

In general, one should maintain an approach inferior to the piriformis and close to the sacrum, as this minimizes sciatic nerve injury/irritation. The sciatic nerve runs along the inferior margin of the piriformis and courses inferolaterally. Ideal catheter placement is through the sacrospinous ligament, which attaches the sacrum to the ischial spine. This ligament seats the catheter in place and avoids damage to nearby nerves and vessels. In some cases, a transpiriformis approach must be used, but this is not ideal.

Superior to the sacrospinous ligament is the greater sciatic foramen. The transgluteal approach often enters the deep pelvis through the greater sciatic foramen, which can be divided into two general compartments: the infrapiriformis space and the suprapiriformis space. The infrapiriformis space contains the sciatic nerve (along the undersurface of the piriformis), the inferior gluteal vessels and nerve, the internal pudendal vessels and nerve, and a series of other nerves. The suprapiriformis space contains the superior gluteal vessels and nerve.

References: Harisinghani MG, Gervais DA, Hahn PF, et al. CT-guided transgluteal drainage of deep pelvic abscesses: indications, technique, procedure-related complications, and clinical outcome. *Radiographics* 2002;22:1353–1367.

Harisinghani MG, Gervais DA, Maher MM, et al. Transgluteal approach for percutaneous drainage of deep pelvic abscesses: 154 cases. *Radiology* 2003;228:701–705.

14 **Answer C.** Diethylstilbestrol (DES) is a synthetic estrogen that was administered to pregnant women in the 1940s and 1950s as a treatment for pregnancy-related complications. However, due to lack of efficacy and significant side effects (e.g., clear cell adenocarcinoma of the vagina and cervix in daughters resulting from the pregnancy), its use was eventually abandoned.

Women who were exposed to DES in utero have a significantly increased risk of clear cell adenocarcinoma of the vagina and cervix, infertility, spontaneous abortion, preterm delivery, loss of second-trimester pregnancy, ectopic pregnancy, preeclampsia, stillbirth, early menopause, cervical intraepithelial neoplasia, and breast cancer.

Imaging findings in women who were exposed to DES in utero include a "T-shaped" uterus, uterine hypoplasia, irregular uterine margins, uterine constriction, and hydrosalpinges.

References: Hoover RN, Hyer M, Pfeiffer RM, et al. Adverse health outcomes in women exposed in utero to diethylstilbestrol. *N Engl J Med* 2011;365:1304–1314.
van Gils AP, Tham RT, Falke TH, et al. Abnormalities of the uterus and cervix after diethylstilbestrol exposure: correlation of findings on MR and hysterosalpingography. *AJR Am J Roentgenol* 1989;153:1235–1238.

15 **Answer B.** Though it is a rare complication, intrauterine device placement is a risk factor for tubal *Actinomyces israelii* infection. Like *Actinomyces* infection elsewhere, tubal *Actinomyces* is characterized by a locally aggressive infection that destroys tissue planes. Abscesses, fistulae, and sinus tracts are common, and it can resemble tuberculosis and malignancy. Due to its rarity, routine antibiotic prophylaxis for patients with intrauterine devices is not recommended.

References: American College of Obstetricians and Gynecologists. ACOG Practice Bulletin No. 121: Long-acting reversible contraception: implants and intrauterine devices. *Obstet Gynecol* 2011;118:184–196.
Marret H, Wagner N, Ouldamer L, et al. Pelvic actinomycosis: just think of it. *Gynecol Obstet Fertil* 2010;38:307–312.
Rezvani M, Shaaban AM. Fallopian tube disease in the nonpregnant patient. *Radiographics* 2011;31:527–548.

16 **Answer A.** The fallopian tube microinserts are in a normal position, and there is bilateral fallopian tube occlusion. It is common for normally positioned inserts to assume the tortuous course of the fallopian tubes. Therefore, the device may be foreshortened or superimposed during fluoroscopy (e.g., the right-sided insert in this case).

Fallopian tube microinserts are a minimally invasive method of permanent sterilization placed through a hysteroscopic approach. Hysterosalpingography (HSG) is typically performed 3 months after microinsert placement to (1) determine whether the devices remain appropriately positioned and (2) to evaluate tubal patency. An estimated 5% to 15% of women who receive these devices will still have patent tubes (i.e., incomplete sterilization) at 3 months. In these cases, other means of contraception are continued until tubal occlusion can be verified on a follow-up HSG.

The most common fallopian tube microinsert is composed of an inner coil and an outer coil (Essure device [Conceptus, Mountain View, CA]). The inner coil is within and lateral to the outer coil. Correct device placement is verified by meeting the following criteria: (1) intratubal positioning of the lateral tip of the inner coil with <50% of the length of the inner coil in the uterine cavity or (2) <30 mm of distance between the medial tip of the inner coil and the uterine cornua. Indicators that a device is malpositioned include the following: (1) ≥50% of the inner coil is in the uterine cavity, (2) ≥30 mm of distance between the medial tip of the inner coil and the uterine cornua, or (3) migration outside the fallopian tube.

The inner and outer coil and their marker tips for the left tubal microinsert are shown below:

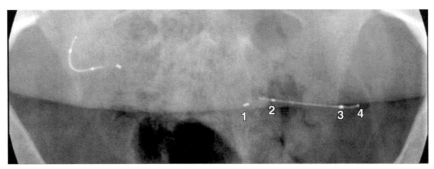

1. *Outer coil, medial tip*
2. *Inner coil, medial tip*
3. *Outer coil, lateral tip*
4. *Inner coil, lateral tip*

Persistent tubal patency (i.e., incomplete sterilization) is defined as retrograde contrast material entering the peritoneal cavity, or retrograde contrast material entering the fallopian tube past the lateral tip of the outer coil. If one or both tubes remain patent by these criteria, other means of contraception should be used and a repeat HSG should be performed in 3 months.

References: Guelfguat M, Gruenberg TR, Dipoce J, et al. Imaging of mechanical tubal occlusion devices and potential complications. *Radiographics* 2012;32:1659–1673.
Rodriguez AM, Kilic GS, Vu TP, et al. Analysis of tubal patency after essure placement. *J Minim Invasive Gynecol* 2013;20:468–472.
Wittmer MH, Famuyide AO, Creedon DJ, et al. Hysterosalpingography for assessing efficacy of Essure microinsert permanent birth control device. *AJR Am J Roentgenol* 2006;187:955–958.

17 **Answer C.** In the United States, vesicovaginal fistulae are most often iatrogenic (e.g., following hysterectomy or pelvic radiotherapy). In third world countries, many vesicovaginal fistulae are due to obstetrical trauma from prolonged labor (Answer C). Repair of a simple vesicovaginal fistula is most often performed using a transvaginal approach, and there is a high technical success rate. In the setting of a complex fistula and/or a recurrent fistula related to prior radiotherapy, a tissue interposition graft may be necessary to promote fistula closure.

Human papillomavirus infection (Answer A) is associated with cervical cancer, genital warts, and vaginal cancer. Although vaginal cancer is a possible cause of vesicovaginal fistula formation, no mass was seen on physical examination, and the patient has not had any pelvic radiation therapy.

Clonorchis sinensis (i.e., liver fluke, Answer B) infects the biliary tree and gallbladder and can lead to the development of cholangiocarcinoma. It does not typically infect the urogenital tract.

There is no known dietary predisposition to vesicovaginal fistula formation (Answer D). However, in the United States, colovesical fistulae are most commonly caused by prior diverticulitis, which does have an association with a low-fiber, high-carbohydrate diet.

References: Elkins TE. Surgery for the obstetric vesicovaginal fistula: a review of 100 operations in 82 patients. *Am J Obstet Gynecol* 1994;170:1108–1120.
Lee D, Dillon BE, Lemack GE, et al. Long-term functional outcomes following nonradiated vesicovaginal repair. *J Urol* 2014;191:120–124.
Pshak T, Nikolavsky D, Terlecki R, et al. Is tissue interposition always necessary in transvaginal repair of benign, recurrent vesicovaginal fistulae? *Urology* 2013;82:707–712.

18 **Answer B.**   Vaginal cancer is a rare malignancy. In the United States, the most common cell type is squamous cell carcinoma (~85%) and the most common risk factor is human papillomavirus infection. In fact, the majority of patients diagnosed with squamous cell carcinoma of the vagina have human papillomavirus DNA detectable within their tumor specimens. Prior radiation therapy (Answer A) is a risk factor for squamous cell carcinoma, but this is a less common association than human papillomavirus infection. The risk factors for cervical and vaginal cancer are similar. Interestingly, vaginal cancers that involve the cervix are classified as cervical cancers.

Adenocarcinoma of the vagina is the commonest form of vaginal cancer in patients under the age of 20, but overall, it is less common than squamous cell carcinoma, which becomes more common as patients age. Adenocarcinoma of the vagina is associated with in utero diethylstilbestrol exposure (Answer C). *Chlamydia trachomatis* infection is not a known risk factor for vaginal adenocarcinoma (Answer D).

References: Creasman WT, Phillips JL, Menck HR. The National Cancer Data Base report on cancer of the vagina. *Cancer* 1998;83:1033–1040.

Daling JR, Madeleine MM, Schwartz SM, et al. A population-based study of squamous cell vaginal cancer: HPV and cofactors. *Gynecol Oncol* 2002;84:263–270.

19 **Answer B.**   The images demonstrate a circumscribed T2-hypointense hypovascular solid ovarian mass. In the context of developing pleural effusions and ascites, this is compatible with an ovarian fibroma producing Meigs syndrome. CA-125 levels are often elevated in this condition. The secondary findings of Meigs syndrome (e.g., ascites, pleural fluid) typically resolve completely following removal of the responsible ovarian mass. Patients with Meigs syndrome who undergo ipsilateral oophorectomy have a similar survival to patients who do not have Meigs syndrome. The prognosis of Meigs syndrome differs dramatically from that of metastatic ovarian cancer: the prognosis of Meigs syndrome is excellent, and the prognosis of metastatic ovarian cancer is dismal.

The differential diagnosis of a T2-hypointense adnexal mass includes leiomyoma (pedunculated or broad ligament fibroid), fibroma, fibrothecoma, cystadenofibroma, Brenner tumor, endometriosis, and scar tissue. This differential diagnosis can be narrowed by determining whether the mass arises from the ovary (thereby excluding a typical leiomyoma) and whether the mass enhances (solid vs. cystic).

References: Dockerty MB, Masson JC. Ovarian fibromas: a clinical and pathologic study of two hundred and eighty-three cases. *Am J Obstet Gynecol* 1944;47:741–752.

Jeong YY, Outwater EK, Kang HK. Imaging evaluation of ovarian masses. *Radiographics* 2000;20:1445–1470.

Siegelman ES, Outwater EK. Tissue characterization in the female pelvis by means of MR imaging. *Radiology* 1999;212:5–18.

20 **Answer A.**   Neither CA-125 nor pelvic ultrasound has been shown to be effective in screening for ovarian cancer in average-risk women (either alone or in combination). This is because ovarian cancer is rare in average-risk women, resulting in a low positive predictive value for identified abnormalities. Remember that unlike sensitivity and specificity, positive predictive value and negative predictive value are dependent on the prevalence of disease in the studied population. Therefore, the harms and costs of screening may outweigh the benefits in this setting. Trials studying various methods of ovarian cancer screening in selected at-risk populations are underway in an effort to improve identification of early-stage ovarian cancer.

References: Finkler NJ, Benacerraf B, Lavin PT, et al. Comparison of serum CA-125, clinical impression, and ultrasound in the preoperative evaluation of ovarian masses. *Obstet Gynecol* 1988;72:659–664.

Jacobs I. Screening for early ovarian cancer. *Lancet* 1988;2:171–172.

Jacobs I, Stabile I, Bridges J, et al. Multimodal approach to screening for ovarian cancer. *Lancet* 1988;1:268–271.

United States Preventive Task Force (USPSTF). Screening for ovarian cancer. 2012. http://www.uspreventiveservicestaskforce.org/uspstf/uspsovar.htm. Accessed 3/2014.

21 **Answer D.** The investigator should instead contrast the growth rate of ovarian carcinomatosis in the setting of standard-of-care systemic therapy against that of an IND- and IRB-approved novel therapeutic agent. It is unethical to deny patients standard-of-care therapy to determine the natural history of a disease or to use placebo therapy when there is an established effective treatment.

There is a modern-age parallel to this ethical question with the Tuskegee syphilis experiment. In this unethical experiment, conducted by the U.S. Public Health Service, African American sharecroppers with syphilis were denied treatment with curative penicillin so that the natural history of the disease could be studied. This unethical behavior led to the death of over 100 study participants and caused a revolution in the methods of protection for human subjects. In particular, the Belmont Report on the Ethical Principles and Guidelines for the Protection of Human Subjects of Research was published, the Office for Human Research Protections was created, and Institutional Review Boards were formalized.

References: Lerner BH. Sins of omission—cancer research without informed consent. *N Engl J Med* 2004;351:628–630.

The Belmont Report. Ethical Principles and guidelines for the protection of human subjects of research. The National Commission for the Protection of Human Subjects of Biomedical and Behavioral Research. Office of the Secretary 1979.

22 **Answer B.** The images demonstrate a cyst within the anterolateral vaginal wall compatible with a Gartner duct cyst. Gartner duct cysts are benign congenital abnormalities of the mesonephric (Wolffian) duct that arise within the vaginal wall superior to the inferior margin of the pubic symphysis. Gartner duct cysts are most commonly incidental findings of no clinical significance. In some cases, they can exert mass effect upon the urethra (causing urinary symptoms), can become infected, or can arise in association with other congenital urogenital tract abnormalities.

Bartholin gland cysts (Answer A) usually arise inferior to the inferior margin of the pubic symphysis within the posterolateral inferior vaginal wall near the labia. Like Gartner duct cysts, Bartholin gland cysts are often incidental findings that may become infected. Urethral diverticula (Answer C) arise anterior to the vagina in the periurethral tissues above the level of the inferior margin of the pubic symphysis. Urethral diverticula can be complicated by infection, stone formation, and urothelial carcinoma development. Urethral diverticula are hypothesized to develop from rupture of infected periurethral glands. Skene gland cysts (Answer D) are inferiorly located paired periurethral cysts that arise lateral to the external urethral meatus. Like Gartner duct cysts and Bartholin gland cysts, Skene gland cysts can become infected.

References: Hahn WY, Israel GM, Lee VS. MRI of female urethral and periurethral disorders. *AJR Am J Roentgenol* 2004;182:677–682.

Siegelman ES, Outwater EK, Banner MP, et al. High-resolution MR imaging of the vagina. *Radiographics* 1997;17:1183–1203.

23 **Answer A.** The apparent lack of flow within the normal-sized and otherwise normal-appearing left ovary is likely technical. Ovarian torsion is very unlikely given that the ovaries are normal and similar in size. Ovarian enlargement is an early and consistent finding in patients with ovarian torsion. In several published series, the volume of the torsed ovary was 12 to 28 times the volume of the unaffected ovary. Unlike for the evaluation of testicular torsion, the presence or absence of flow on Doppler ultrasound is unreliable for the evaluation of ovarian torsion. This is for two key reasons: (1) the ovaries have a dual blood supply and (2) the depth of the ovaries from the transducer is generally much greater than it is for the testicles.

References: Albayram F, Hamper UM. Ovarian and adnexal torsion: spectrum of sonographic findings with pathologic correlation. *J Ultrasound Med* 2001;20:1083–1089.

Chang HC, Bhatt S, Dogra VS. Pearls and pitfalls in diagnosis of ovarian torsion. *Radiographics* 2008;28:1355–1368.

Lubner MG, Simard ML, Peterson CM, et al. Emergent and nonemergent nonbowel torsion: spectrum of imaging and clinical findings. *Radiographics* 2013;33:155–173.

Servaes S, Zurakowski D, Laufer MR, et al. Sonographic findings of ovarian torsion in children. *Pediatr Radiol* 2007;37:446–451.

24 **Answer B.** Risk factors for tubal ectopic pregnancy include (1) pelvic inflammatory disease (*Neisseria gonorrhoeae* infection, *Chlamydia trachomatis* infection), (2) prior ectopic pregnancy, (3) intrauterine device placement, and (4) infertility treatment (e.g., in vitro fertilization). Human papillomavirus infection (Answer A) and previous normal deliveries (Answers C and D) are not risk factors for ectopic pregnancy.

References: Breen JL. A 21 year survey of 654 ectopic pregnancies. *Am J Obstet Gynecol* 1970;106:1004–1019.

Levine D. Ectopic pregnancy. *Radiology* 2007;245:385–397.

25 **Answer A = 2, B = 3, C = 1.** The Belmont Report (1979) outlines the ethical principles and guidelines for the protection of human subjects of research. It was produced in response to the egregious and unethical Tuskegee syphilis study, in which African American citizens were denied treatment for active syphilis infection so that the natural history of the disease could be studied.

There are three basic ethical principles outlined in the Belmont Report that have direct application to the practice of human subjects research:

Ethical Principle	Application(s)
Respect for persons	Respect for persons leads to informed consent, in which the details of the study are provided to the study subjects in a method they can comprehend, permitting them the opportunity to provide voluntary assent to participate.
Beneficence	Beneficence leads to a balancing of study risks and study benefits, in which the risks to the subjects are minimized and the benefits to the subjects are maximized. Study subjects should only be exposed to risks when necessary. The benefits and risks must be "balanced," and that balance must in general favor the study subjects.
Justice	Justice leads to the appropriate selection of study subjects, in which there is a fair and equitable selection process for the inclusion of study subjects. Vulnerable populations (e.g., prisoners, the chronically ill) must be protected against oversampling by research teams who might exploit their captive state for sake of convenience.

Reference: The Belmont Report. Ethical Principles and guidelines for the protection of human subjects of research. The National Commission for the Protection of Human Subjects of Biomedical and Behavioral Research. Office of the Secretary 1979.

26 **Answer B.** The most common location (60% to 80%) for an ectopic pregnancy to develop is within the ampullary segment of the fallopian tube. Therefore, the paratubal regions should be scrutinized in at-risk women in an effort to identify an extrauterine gestational sac or a complex adnexal mass. However, a substantial minority of women with ectopic pregnancy will have a "normal" pelvic ultrasound. Therefore, lack of visualization of an adnexal mass is an insensitive sign for ectopic pregnancy.

Uterine ectopic pregnancies (Answer A) are rare, and there are two main types: scar ectopic pregnancy and interstitial ectopic pregnancy. Scar ectopic pregnancies develop at the site of cesarean section scars. They can be diagnosed by localizing the gestational sac to the cesarean section scar in the anterior lower uterine segment without evidence of myometrium between the sac and the bladder wall. Interstitial pregnancy is an ectopic pregnancy that develops in the interstitial segment of the fallopian tube. It should be considered when the gestational sac is located in the high lateral endometrial canal near the cornua, and the thickness of the overlying myometrium is ≤4 mm.

Ovarian ectopic pregnancy is very rare (Answer C). In fact, if a complex cystic adnexal mass is identified in the setting of suspected ectopic pregnancy, the most important thing to determine is whether the mass arises from the ovary. If it does arise from the ovary, it is unlikely to represent an ectopic pregnancy (e.g., corpus luteum). If it does not arise from the ovary, it is highly likely to represent an ectopic pregnancy (95% of the time). Intra-abdominal ectopic pregnancies (Answer D) and cervical ectopic pregnancies (Answer E) are rare.

References: Breen JL. A 21 year survey of 654 ectopic pregnancies. *Am J Obstet Gynecol* 1970;106:1004–1019.

Levine D. Ectopic pregnancy. *Radiology* 2007;245:385–397.

27 Answer A.   The images demonstrate a cyst within the lateral inferior vaginal wall near the labia compatible with a Bartholin gland cyst. Although usually asymptomatic incidental findings, Bartholin gland cysts can become infected. Infected Bartholin gland cysts are exquisitely painful, and management of an infected Bartholin gland cyst usually consists of antibiotic therapy and drainage.

References: Bhide A, Nama V, Patel S, et al. Microbiology of cysts/abscesses of Bartholin's gland: review of empirical antibiotic therapy against microbial culture. *J Obstet Gynaecol* 2010;30:701–703.

Hahn WY, Israel GM, Lee VS. MRI of female urethral and periurethral disorders. *AJR Am J Roentgenol* 2004;182:677–682.

Siegelman ES, Outwater EK, Banner MP, et al. High-resolution MR imaging of the vagina. *Radiographics* 1997;17:1183–1203.

28 Answer B.   The imaging demonstrates multiple tiny saclike contrast material–filled collections along the isthmic segment of the fallopian tube consistent with salpingitis isthmica nodosa. This condition is believed to result from scarring related to prior pelvic inflammatory disease (*Neisseria gonorrhoeae* infection, *Chlamydia trachomatis* infection) or in some cases endometriosis. It is a strong risk factor for infertility and tubal ectopic pregnancy.

References: Creasy JL, Clark RL, Cuttino JT, et al. Salpingitis isthmica nodosa: radiologic and clinical correlates. *Radiology* 1985;154:597–600.

Krysiewicz S. Infertility in women: diagnostic evaluation with hysterosalpingography and other imaging techniques. *AJR Am J Roentgenol* 1992;159:253–261.

Majmudar B, Henderson PH, Semple E. Salpingitis isthmica nodosa: a high-risk factor for tubal pregnancy. *Obstet Gynecol* 1983;62:73–78.

Simpson WL Jr, Beitia LG, Mester J. Hysterosalpingography: a reemerging study. *Radiographics* 2006;26:419–431.

29 Answer C.   The imaging is compatible with a hydrosalpinx. Note the "incomplete septation" projecting within the lumen of the fluid-filled structure representing infolding of the wall of the tube. Common causes of hydrosalpinx include (1) pelvic inflammatory disease, (2) tubal ligation, (3) endometriosis, and (4) hysterectomy. A hydrosalpinx can be complicated by pus (i.e., pyosalpinx) or hemorrhage (i.e., hemosalpinx).

A hydrosalpinx can be differentiated from cystic ovarian masses (Answers A, B, and D) by its extraovarian location and longitudinal shape. It is common for a hydrosalpinx to fold on itself, giving the impression of a multilocular cystic mass. A key to the diagnosis is realizing that the "septations" within a hydrosalpinx are folds that incompletely span the lumen and not true septations. When a hydrosalpinx is imaged in cross section, thickened longitudinal folds may project into the lumen of the fallopian tube and give the appearance of mural nodules (i.e., so-called "cogwheel" sign). The true linear nature of these longitudinal folds is best appreciated on long-axis or 3D imaging.

References: Benjaminov O, Atri M. Sonography of the abnormal fallopian tube. *AJR Am J Roentgenol* 2004;183:737–742.

Kim MY, Rha SE, Oh SN, et al. MR imaging findings of hydrosalpinx: a comprehensive review. *Radiographics* 2009;29:495–507.

Rezvani M, Shaaban AM. Fallopian tube disease in the nonpregnant patient. *Radiographics* 2011;31:527–548.

30   **Answer A = 3, B = 1, C = 4, D = 2.**   The fallopian tube has four main segments.

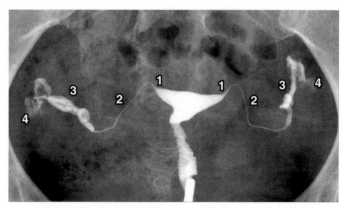

1 = interstitial, 2 = isthmic, 3 = ampullary, 4 = infundibular

From medial to lateral, they include the interstitial segment (the segment that tunnels through the myometrium), the isthmic segment (the thinnest and longest segment where salpingitis isthmica nodosa develops), the ampullary segment (the lateral dilated segment where ectopic pregnancy is most common), and the infundibulum (the lateral-most funnel-shaped segment that receives the ovum and contains fimbriae).

References: Rezvani M, Shaaban AM. Fallopian tube disease in the nonpregnant patient. *Radiographics* 2011;31:527–548.

Simpson WL Jr, Beitia LG, Mester J. Hysterosalpingography: a reemerging study. *Radiographics* 2006;26:419–431.

Retroperitoneum

QUESTIONS

1   A 22-year-old male with right lower quadrant pain undergoes a CT of the abdomen and pelvis. The only abnormality is shown below. What is the best next step?

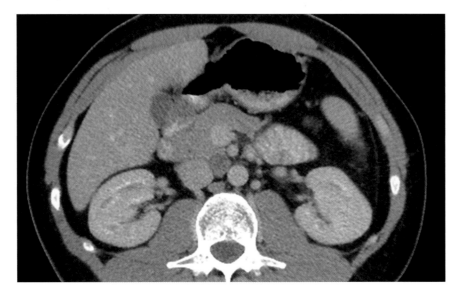

   A. Percutaneous biopsy
   B. Whole-body PET-CT
   C. Scrotal ultrasound
   D. Metaiodobenzylguanidine (MIBG) study

2   A 62-year-old male presents with right groin pain. A hernia is suspected, and a CT of the abdomen and pelvis is performed. An incidental 5.1-cm fusiform infrarenal aortic aneurysm is identified. There are no comparison images. At what aneurysm sac size is repair indicated for an asymptomatic abdominal aortic aneurysm in an "average-risk" patient?

   A. 4.0 cm
   B. 4.5 cm
   C. 5.0 cm
   D. 5.5 cm

3 A 50-year-old male presents with an enlarged left external iliac lymph node. Percutaneous biopsy is planned. Which of the following approaches is least likely to result in a complication?

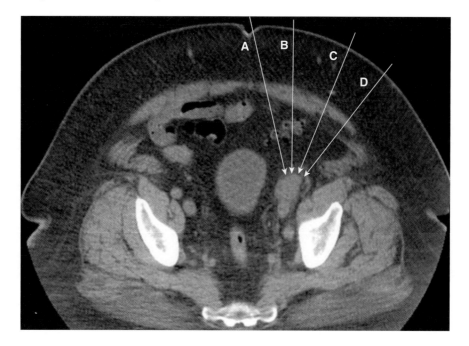

A. A
B. B
C. C
D. D

4 A 42-year-old male with pancreatitis and complicated peripancreatic fluid collections presents for catheter drainage. In which space is the fluid collection posterior to the left kidney located?

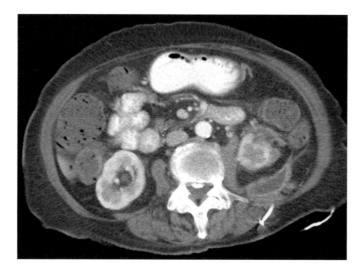

A. Anterior pararenal space
B. Posterior pararenal space
C. Perirenal space
D. Interfascial plane
E. Left paracolic gutter

5 A 60-year-old female with fatigue and no comorbidities undergoes a CT of the abdomen and pelvis demonstrating multiple enlarged retroperitoneal lymph nodes. A percutaneous core needle biopsy is performed under conscious sedation with a 15-cm-long 18-gauge end-firing biopsy device with a 2-cm throw. Six specimens are obtained, and the patient is taken to recovery.

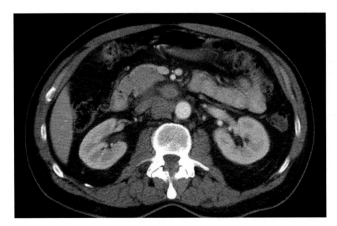 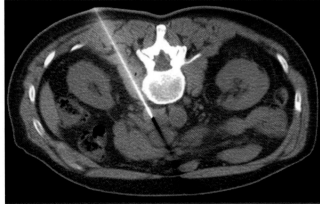

One hour later, the patient stands up for the first time since the biopsy, becomes queasy, and nearly loses consciousness. She is returned to her bed, and vital signs are obtained. (1) heart rate 40 bpm, (2) blood pressure 80/40 mm Hg, and (3) SpO$_2$ 100% on room air. She has no abdominal pain or ecchymosis. Two minutes later, she is asymptomatic, and her vital signs are (1) heart rate 72 bpm, (2) blood pressure 115/65 mm Hg, and (3) SpO$_2$ 100% on room air. What is the best next step?

A. Observation
B. Unenhanced CT
C. CT angiogram
D. Embolization

6 A 22-year-old male with metastatic testicular cancer undergoes a contrast-enhanced CT of the abdomen and pelvis. There is a single-comparison contrast-enhanced CT of the abdomen and pelvis performed 6 months ago. In addition to development of a new lesion, what defines "progressive disease" according to RECIST 1.1?

A. A ≥20% increase in the sum of diameters of the target lesions, with an absolute increase of at least 5 mm
B. A ≥30% increase in the sum of diameters of the target lesions, with an absolute increase of at least 5 mm
C. A ≥20% increase in the diameter of any single target lesion, with an absolute increase of at least 5 mm
D. A ≥30% increase in the diameter of any single target lesion, with an absolute increase of at least 5 mm

7 Which of the following structures is located in the anterior pararenal space?
A. Kidney
B. Duodenum
C. Transverse colon
D. Stomach

8   A 30-year-old female with right lower quadrant pain undergoes an abdominal MRI. Axial and sagittal T1-weighted contrast-enhanced GRE with fat saturation and axial and sagittal T2-weighted FSE sequences are presented below. What is the most likely diagnosis?

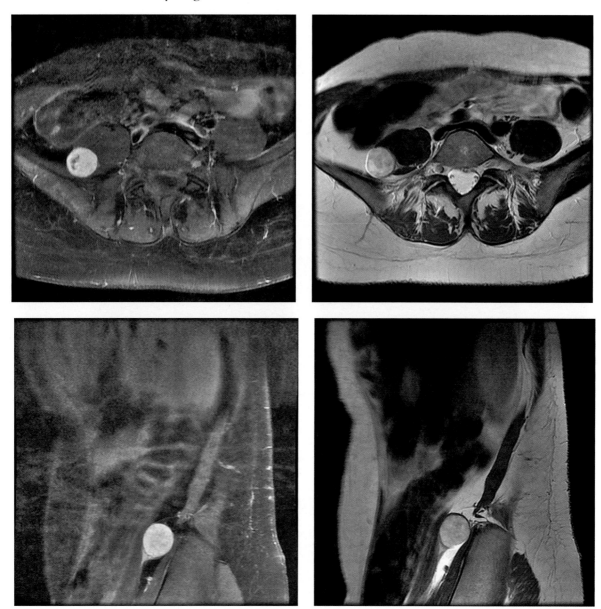

A. Paraganglioma
B. Nerve sheath tumor
C. Aneurysm
D. Metastasis

9   A 54-year-old male with stage V chronic kidney disease undergoes an unenhanced MR angiogram of his abdominal aorta. What best explains the "dark" appearance of fast-flowing blood on spin echo imaging?

A. Fast-flowing blood has a long T1.
B. Fast-flowing blood has a short T2.
C. Fast-flowing blood is only exposed to either a 90-degree or a 180-degree RF pulse.
D. Fast-flowing blood is always exposed to both a 90-degree and a 180-degree RF pulse.

10 A 25-year-old female stabbing victim undergoes a CT of the chest, abdomen, and pelvis. A 13-cm hemorrhage is identified in the right perirenal space related to a 3-cm renal laceration. Her hemoglobin is 7.1 g/dL. What best predicts this patient's need for operative management?

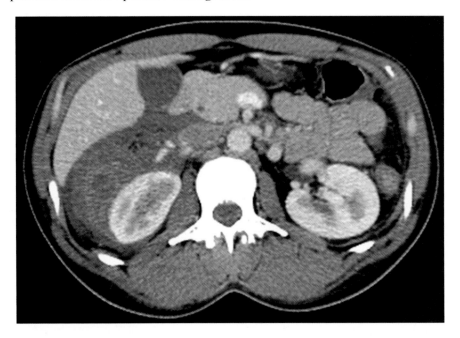

A. Mechanism of injury
B. AAST injury grade
C. Hemoglobin level
D. Size of the hematoma
E. Width of the laceration

11 A 51-year-old female with a 2.0-cm solid inferior pole right renal mass undergoes percutaneous radiofrequency ablation with two thermal ablation probes. An image from the ablation is shown below. What poses the greatest risk to this patient?

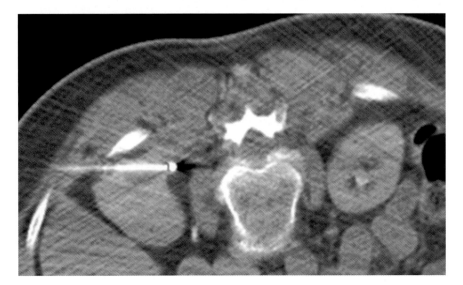

A. Nerve injury
B. Collecting system injury
C. Vascular injury
D. Incomplete treatment

12 A 65-year-old male with a remote history of colon cancer undergoes abdominal
    MRI after an incidental renal mass is discovered on surveillance CT imaging.
    Two unenhanced 2D axial gradient-recalled echo (GRE) images obtained from
    different imaging volumes are shown below. What is the most likely explanation
    for the appearance of the veins (left image) and arteries (right image)?

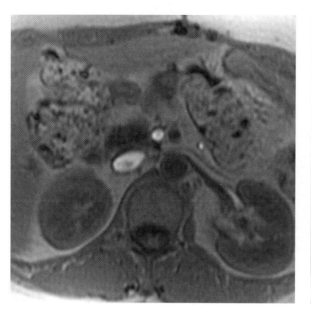
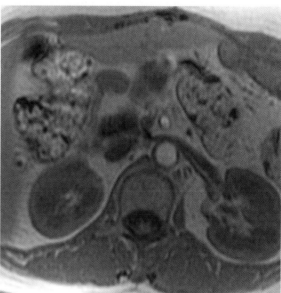

A. Unsaturated residual longitudinal magnetization entering the image volume
B. Unsaturated residual transverse magnetization entering the image volume
C. Saturated residual longitudinal magnetization entering the image volume
D. Saturated residual transverse magnetization entering the image volume

13 A 56-year-old asymptomatic male with microscopic hematuria undergoes a CT
    urogram that shows anterior displacement of the kidneys and duodenum. What
    is the best next step?

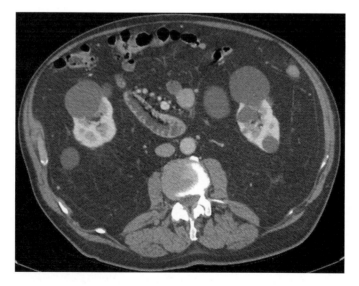

A. Clinical management (benign finding)
B. Percutaneous biopsy
C. Prophylactic ureteric stents
D. Operative debulking

14   A 70-year-old male with dyspnea and long-standing pulmonary fibrosis undergoes a contrast-enhanced CT, and a lobular solid mass is identified. Representative images in the axial (left) and coronal (right) plane are shown below. What is the most likely diagnosis?

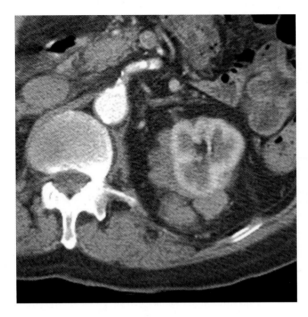 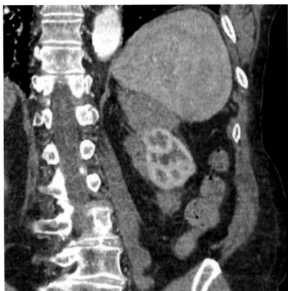

A. Renal cell carcinoma
B. B-cell lymphoma
C. Splenic angiosarcoma
D. Adrenocortical carcinoma

15   A 70-year-old male with a 40-pack-year smoking history and L2-L3 spondylodiscitis presents with acute flank pain, and a contrast-enhanced CT of the abdomen and pelvis is performed. The maximum infrarenal aortic caliber is 3.5 cm. What is the best next step?

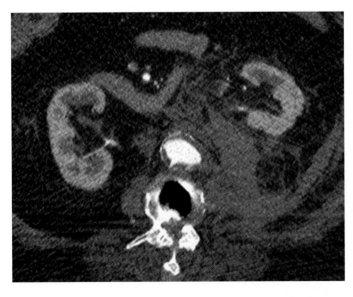 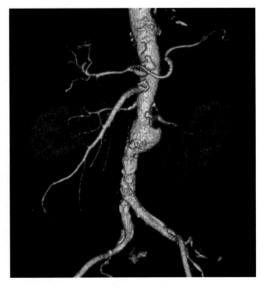

A. Volume replacement and observation
B. Volume replacement and intravenous antibiotics
C. Volume replacement and emergent aortic endograft placement
D. Volume replacement and emergent operative repair

16 What are the typical findings of retroperitoneal Erdheim-Chester disease?

    A. Diffusely enlarged sausage-shaped pancreas with a rind of peripancreatic fibrosis

    B. Bilateral perirenal and pararenal soft tissue masses with associated ureteric obstruction

    C. Unilateral locally aggressive solid mass of the renal capsule with or without calcifications

    D. Bilateral renal and perirenal masses that displace but do not invade nearby structures

17 A 35-year-old female with fever and low back pain undergoes a contrast-enhanced CT of the abdomen and pelvis. The patient lives in the United States and has no relevant history. What is the most likely offending organism?

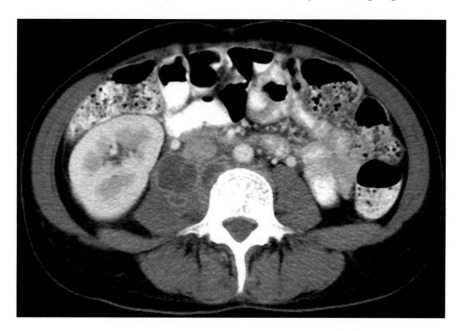

    A. *Staphylococcus aureus*

    B. *Mycobacterium tuberculosis*

    C. *Escherichia coli*

    D. *Bacteroides* species

18 A 70-year-old female with atrial fibrillation on warfarin therapy develops severe abdominal pain after a fall. What is the typical range of attenuation for clotted blood on an unenhanced CT of the abdomen?

    A. 0 to 20 HU

    B. 20 to 40 HU

    C. 40 to 70 HU

    D. 70 to 100 HU

19 A 60-year-old male with a 5.5-cm infrarenal aortic aneurysm undergoes percutaneous repair with an aortoiliac endograft. One year later, the sac size is 4.0 cm and a small type II endoleak is identified. What is the best next step?

    A. Annual observation

    B. Percutaneous embolization

    C. Surgical ligation

    D. Endograft excision

20 A 60-year-old male with vague low back pain undergoes a contrast-enhanced CT of the abdomen and pelvis. Which of the following diseases is associated with this imaging finding?

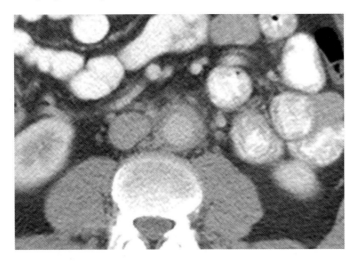

A. Renal cell carcinoma
B. Autoimmune pancreatitis
C. Autosomal dominant polycystic disease
D. *Schistosoma haematobium* infection

21 A 25-year-old female who is postoperative day 3 following an emergent cesarean section for fetal distress presents with sepsis and acute respiratory distress syndrome. An abdominal radiograph is performed. What is the most likely diagnosis?

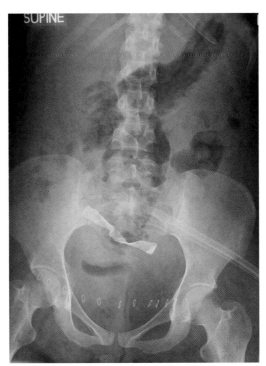

A. Necrotizing fasciitis
B. Large bowel obstruction
C. Retained foreign body
D. Malpositioned tube

22 A 54-year-old female who is postoperative day 9 following a partial right nephrectomy presents with persistent flank pain. Axial contrast-enhanced CT of the abdomen is performed (left), and coronal reconstructions are generated (right). What is the most likely diagnosis?

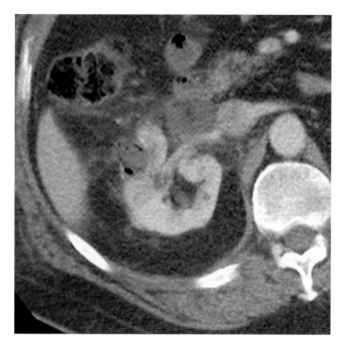 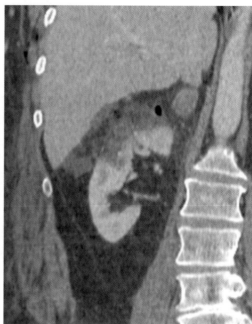

A. Normal postoperative appearance
B. Renal artery pseudoaneurysm
C. Collecting system injury
D. Renal abscess

23 Persistence of the right and left supracardinal veins can result in a "duplicated" or "double" IVC. When this variant manifests, into what structures do the right and left IVC usually drain?

A. Right IVC: right atrium; left IVC: azygous vein
B. Right IVC: azygous vein; left IVC: hemiazygous vein
C. Right IVC: right atrium; left IVC: left renal vein
D. Right IVC: right renal vein; left IVC: left renal vein

24 A 65-year-old male with stage V chronic kidney disease presents for an unenhanced MR angiogram. Conventional "black blood" spin echo sequences are planned. For a conventional spin echo–based sequence, when should the 180-degree refocusing pulse be applied?

A. Immediately before TE
B. Immediately after TE
C. TE/2
D. 2*TE

25 A 65-year-old male with Gleason 5 + 4 = 9 prostate cancer undergoes a contrast-enhanced CT of the abdomen and pelvis. What is the approximate sensitivity of morphologic CT imaging for the detection of nodal metastasis (on a node-by-node basis)?

A. 30%
B. 50%
C. 70%
D. 90%

26 A 68-year-old female undergoes a contrast-enhanced CT of the abdomen and pelvis that reveals a large retroperitoneal mass. What is the most likely cell type?

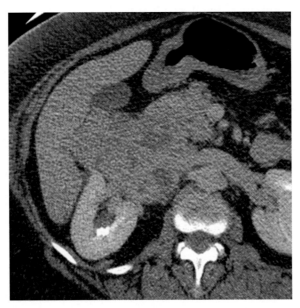

A. Liposarcoma
B. Leiomyosarcoma
C. Lymphoma
D. Leiomyoma
E. Lipoma

27 A 65-year-old male with lymphoma enrolls in a clinical trial and undergoes a contrast-enhanced CT reconstructed at 5-mm collimation. What criterion determines whether the lymph node depicted in the image would be considered a "target lesion" according to RECIST 1.1?

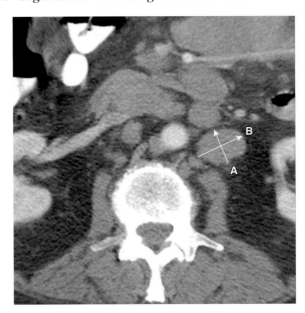

A. The node qualifies as a "target lesion" if line A is ≥10 mm.
B. The node qualifies as a "target lesion" if line A is ≥15 mm.
C. The node qualifies as a "target lesion" if line B is ≥10 mm.
D. The node qualifies as a "target lesion" if line B is ≥15 mm.

28 A 57-year-old female with adrenocortical carcinoma enrolls in a clinical trial and undergoes a contrast-enhanced CT reconstructed at 5-mm collimation. What criterion determines whether the mass depicted in the image would be considered a "target lesion" according to RECIST 1.1?

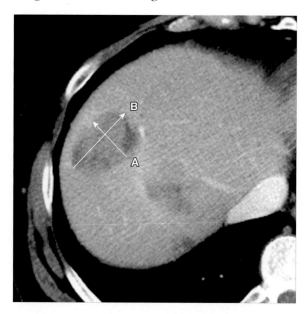

A. The mass qualifies as a "target lesion" if line A is ≥10 mm.
B. The mass qualifies as a "target lesion" if line A is ≥15 mm.
C. The mass qualifies as a "target lesion" if line B is ≥10 mm.
D. The mass qualifies as a "target lesion" if line B is ≥15 mm.

29 A 60-year-old male undergoes a CT angiogram. Isotropic images are acquired in the axial plane. Which of the following lines best represents how the aneurysm sac should be measured?

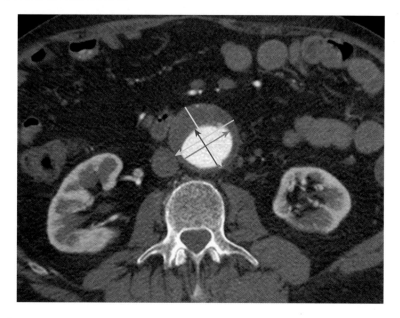

A. Blue
B. Yellow
C. Orange
D. Pink
E. The aneurysm sac should not be measured on this image.

30 A 60-year-old male with flank pain and hematuria undergoes a retroperitoneal ultrasound. A 4.5-cm solid renal mass is identified, and there is echogenic material in the renal vein and vena cava. Which of the following best distinguishes tumor thrombus from bland thrombus?

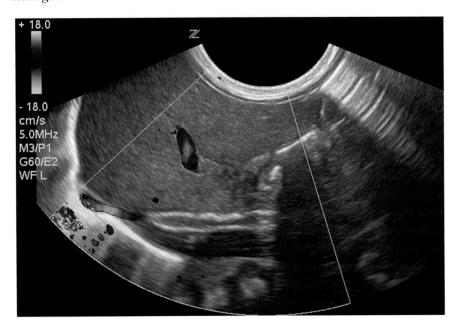

A. Tumor thrombus is echogenic and bland thrombus is hypoechoic.

B. Tumor thrombus has a systolic waveform and bland thrombus does not.

C. Tumor thrombus is central and bland thrombus is peripheral.

D. Tumor thrombus is mobile and bland thrombus is not.

ANSWERS AND EXPLANATIONS

1   **Answer C.**   The image demonstrates an enlarged low-attenuation interaortocaval lymph node near the insertion of the right gonadal vein. In a young male patient, isolated lymph node enlargement in this location is suggestive of metastatic testicular cancer. Of course, other etiologies are possible, and if the scrotal ultrasound is normal, the node would require further workup. Percutaneous biopsy (Answer A) is not the best first step because access to the node is challenging, and there are potentially noninvasive means of establishing the diagnosis (e.g., scrotal ultrasound). PET-CT (Answer B) is premature and probably unnecessary. An extra-adrenal paraganglioma, though possible, is less likely than a malignant lymph node, and therefore MIBG scan is not the best first step (Answer D).

Remember that in most patients, the right gonadal vein inserts upon the inferior vena cava just below the insertion of the right renal vein. The left gonadal vein inserts directly into the left renal vein. Nodal enlargement adjacent to either gonadal vein insertion site in an at-risk population is suggestive of testicular cancer, and scrotal ultrasound should be considered.

A generic differential diagnosis for an abnormal low-attenuation abdominal lymph node includes (1) germ cell tumor metastasis, (2) tuberculosis, (3) Whipple disease, (4) fungal infection, (5) necrotic metastasis, and (6) retroperitoneal lymphangioleiomyomatosis.

References: Pano B, Sebastia C, Bunesch L, et al. Pathways of lymphatic spread in male urogenital pelvic malignancies. *Radiographics* 2011;31:135–160.
Park JM, Charnsangavej C, Yoshimitsu K, et al. Pathways of nodal metastasis from pelvic tumors: CT demonstration. *Radiographics* 1994;14:1309–1321.

2   **Answer D.**   Current recommendations are that asymptomatic abdominal aortic aneurysms in average-risk patients should be repaired when ≥5.5 cm. This guideline represents a balancing of the risk of rupture and the risk of repair. The annual risk of rupture of an abdominal aortic aneurysm 5.0 to 5.9 cm is estimated to be between 3% and 15%. Other indications for repair include (1) symptomatic aneurysms, (2) aneurysm growth rate ≥0.5 cm within 6 months, and (3) ruptured aneurysms.

References: Brewster DC, Cronenwett JL, Hallett JW, et al. Guidelines for the treatment of abdominal aortic aneurysms. Report of a subcommittee of the Joint Council of the American Association for Vascular Surgery and Society for Vascular Surgery. *J Vasc Surg* 2003;37:1106–1117.
Hirsch AT, Haskal ZJ, Hertzer NR, et al. ACC/AHA 2005 Practice Guidelines for the management of patients with peripheral arterial disease (lower extremity, renal, mesenteric, and abdominal aortic): a collaborative report from the American Association for Vascular Surgery/Society for Vascular Surgery, Society for Cardiovascular Angiography and Interventions, Society for Vascular Medicine and Biology, Society of Interventional Radiology, and the ACC/AHA Task Force on Practice Guidelines. *Circulation* 2006;113:e463–e654.
Welch HG, Albertsen PC, Nease RF, et al. Estimating treatment benefits for the elderly: the effect of competing risks. *Ann Intern Med* 1996;124:577–584.

3   **Answer D.**   Approach D is least likely to result in a complication. Both approach A and approach B traverse the sigmoid colon, and approach C traverses the groove for the deep inferior epigastric vasculature. This groove can be identified by the characteristic fat-containing "notch" along the undersurface of the rectus musculature. In addition to avoiding structures along the needle path, it is also important to ensure that the needle throw does not exit the far wall of the lymph node and enter the external iliac vasculature behind it. Careful planning can allow proper selection of needle size, throw length, and approach vector.

References: Brant WE, Helms CA. *Fundamentals of diagnostic radiology*, 3rd ed. Philadelphia, PA: Lippincott Williams & Wilkins, 2006.
Funaki B, Lorenz JM, Van Ha TG. *Teaching atlas of vascular and non-vascular interventional radiology*, 1st ed. New York: Thieme, 2007.

4   **Answer D.**   The fluid collection has dissected into the interfascial plane bounding the perirenal space and posterior pararenal space. The crescent shape of the collection angling to an anterolateral point confirms the interfascial position. Note the fat posterior (posterior pararenal space) and anterior (perirenal space) to the collection distinguishing it from the other retroperitoneal spaces. In this case, there is also inflammatory debris in the posterior pararenal space manifesting as irregular and lobular soft tissue attenuation posterior to the collection.

The interfascial planes are potential spaces between the fasciae of the retroperitoneum that distend when infiltrated by a pathologic process; they are a common location for collections resulting from pancreatitis. Below is another example of pancreatitis with fluid in the anterior pararenal space (A) and posterior pararenal space (B). The perirenal space is indicated by (C).

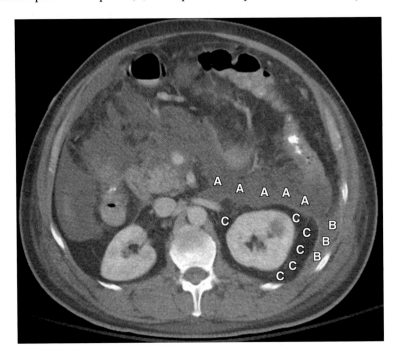

References: Ishikawa K, Idoguchi K, Tanaka H, et al. Classification of acute pancreatitis based on retroperitoneal extension: application of the concept of interfascial planes. *Eur J Radiol* 2006;60:445–452.
Molmenti EP, Balfe DM, Kanterman RY, et al. Anatomy of the retroperitoneum: observations of the distribution of pathologic fluid collections. *Radiology* 1996;200:95–103.

5   **Answer A.**   The clinical picture is most consistent with a vasovagal reaction, which is characterized by bradycardia and hypotension. Vasovagal reactions are uncommon, self-limited complications of minimally invasive procedures. They can be exacerbated by quick changes in position and are best managed by positional maneuvers, intravenous isotonic fluids, and observation.

The best next step for this now-asymptomatic patient is observation with serial vital sign monitoring. Review of the intraprocedural images demonstrates correct placement of the needle between the inferior vena cava and aorta. If the patient's symptoms were from bleeding, they would likely be accompanied by abdominal pain and tachycardia and would likely persist despite changes in position.

References: Kennedy DJ, Schneider B, Casey E, et al. Vasovagal rates in fluoroscopically guided interventional procedures: a study of over 8,000 injections. *Pain Med* 2013;14:1854–1859.

van Lieshout JJ, Wieling W, Karemaker JM, et al. The vasovagal response. *Clin Sci (Lond)* 1991;81:575–586.

6 **Answer A.**   According to RECIST 1.1, the "sum of diameters" is what is followed over time to monitor treatment response. "Progressive disease" is defined as (1) unequivocal development of a new lesion or (2) a ≥20% increase in the sum of diameters of all target lesions (minimum increase ≥5 mm) compared to the smallest sum of diameters measured at any point of time on the current study protocol.

Casual use of phrases like "disease progression" or "partial response" in radiology reports should be discouraged because these terms have specific definitions. The following table outlines definitions for the four major disease states that can be assigned on follow-up imaging according to RECIST 1.1:

RECIST 1.1 Response Assessment	Definition
Complete response (CR)	Resolution of all target lesions; lymph nodes may still be visible, but all pathologic lymph nodes (target and nontarget) must be <10 mm in short axis
Partial response (PR)	≥30% decrease in the sum of diameters compared to the baseline sum of diameters
Progressive disease (PD)	≥20% increase in the sum of diameters compared to the smallest sum of diameters ever measured on the current study protocol and an absolute increase in the sum of diameters ≥5 mm; any unequivocally new lesion is also considered progressive disease
Stable disease (SD)	Does not qualify for complete response, partial response, or progressive disease

References: Eisenhauer EA, Therasse P, Bogaerts J, et al. New response evaluation criteria in solid tumours: revised RECIST guideline (version 1.1). *Eur J Cancer* 2009;45(2):228–247.

Nishino M, Jagannathan JP, Ramaiya NH, et al. Revised RECIST guideline version 1.1: what oncologists want to know and what radiologists need to know. *AJR Am J Roentgenol* 2010;195:281–289.

7 **Answer B.**   The anterior pararenal space is bounded posteriorly by the anterior pararenal fascia (e.g., Gerota's fascia) and anteriorly by the peritoneum. It contains the retroperitoneal portions of the duodenum, the pancreas, the descending colon, and the ascending colon. Gas within the anterior pararenal space suggests duodenal perforation, infection, or iatrogenic manipulation.

References: Korobkin M, Silverman PM, Quint LE, et al. CT of the extraperitoneal space: normal anatomy and fluid collections. *AJR Am J Roentgenol* 1992;159:933–942.

Molmenti EP, Balfe DM, Kanterman RY, et al. Anatomy of the retroperitoneum: observations of the distribution of pathologic fluid collections. *Radiology* 1996;200:95–103.

8 **Answer B.**   The images demonstrate a hypervascular solid mass lateral to the psoas muscle along the course of the right femoral nerve consistent with a nerve sheath tumor (Answer B). The hyperintensity compared to skeletal muscle on T2-weighted images and the conical shape of the lower margin of the tumor as it blends with the femoral nerve fibers strongly support the diagnosis.

Although paragangliomas (Answer A) are hypervascular and can be found in the retroperitoneum along the sympathetic chain, they tend to be closer to midline and would not usually blend with a peripheral nerve as this mass is doing. In fact, of the listed options, only peripheral nerve sheath tumors tend to exhibit this morphology. An aneurysm (Answer C) would be expected to demonstrate absent signal on spin echo imaging (i.e., flow void) unless it was thrombosed (in which case, it would not be enhancing) or experiencing slow flow. An isolated hypervascular retroperitoneal metastasis (Answer D) would be unusual in a patient of this age without any other supportive clinical history.

References: Beaman FD, Kransdorf MJ, Menke DM. Schwannoma: radiologic-pathologic correlation. *Radiographics* 2004;24:1477–1481.

Lin J, Martel W. Cross-sectional imaging of peripheral nerve sheath tumors. *AJR Am J Roentgenol* 2001;176:75–82.

Rha SE, Byun JY, Jung SE, et al. Neurogenic tumors in the abdomen: tumor types and imaging characteristics. *Radiographics* 2003;23:29–43.

9 **Answer C.** Signal generation with spin echo MR imaging requires protons to be exposed to both a 90-degree excitation radiofrequency (RF) pulse followed by a 180-degree refocusing RF pulse. Protons that are not exposed to both RF pulses will not generate signal. Fast-flowing blood is a good example of this. Fast-flowing blood moving through the imaged section will only be exposed to a single RF pulse. This results in an intravascular signal void.

This principle is often exploited for so-called "black-blood" imaging in which the null signal within fast-flowing blood is used to produce image contrast. Slow-flowing blood will produce a signal because it remains in the slice long enough to be exposed to both pulses (90 and 180 degrees). Similarly, vessels moving within the slice plane, regardless of speed, will also experience both RF pulses. In some circumstances, the intravascular signal produced from slow-flowing blood might be mistaken for thrombus. To minimize this potential, saturation bands are sometimes applied at the edges of the imaging volume to saturate signal from inflowing blood.

References: Jung BA, Weigel M. Spin echo magnetic resonance imaging. *J Magn Reson Imaging* 2013;37:805–817.

McRobbie DW, Moore EA, Graves MJ, et al. *MRI: from picture to proton*, 2nd ed. New York: Cambridge University Press, 2007.

10 **Answer B.** The best predictor of nonobservational management is the AAST (American Association for the Surgery of Trauma) grade of injury, which stratifies risk based primarily on CT findings.

AAST Grade	Injury
1	Renal contusion or a nonexpanding subcapsular hematoma
2	Nonexpanding hematoma in perirenal space or a <1-cm renal laceration without collecting system injury
3	Renal laceration >1 cm without collecting system injury
4	Renal laceration involving collecting system, or main renal artery/vein injury with contained hemorrhage
5	Shattered kidney or avulsion of the renal hilum

Although the AAST injury scale has been shown to correlate with operative intervention and renal loss, it does not take into account active extravasation or pseudoaneurysm formation peripheral to the renal hilum, both of which are findings that may lead to catheter-directed management.

The majority of patients with renal trauma can be observed with no intervention.

References: Moore E, Shackford S, Packter H, et al. Organ injury scaling: spleen, liver, and kidney. *J Trauma* 1989;29:1664–1666.

Santucci RA, McAninch JW, Safir M, et al. Validation of the American Association for the Surgery of Trauma organ injury severity scale for the kidney. *J Trauma* 2001;50:195–200.

11 Answer A. The greatest risk to this patient is nerve damage. The ablation needle is immediately adjacent to the ipsilateral quadratus lumborum muscle without intervening tissue or fluid. If the ablation is performed without first displacing the muscle from the ablation zone, the ipsilateral ilioinguinal and iliohypogastric nerves that run along the anterior surface of the muscle will be threatened. Similarly, ablations performed adjacent to the lateral margin of the psoas muscle can threaten the ipsilateral genitofemoral nerve. These nerve-related complications can be minimized by using hydrodissection with inert fluid (e.g., 5% dextrose solution) or a "lever technique" to displace the kidney from the nearby muscle(s). Conductive electrolyte-containing solutions (e.g., normal saline) should be avoided during radiofrequency ablation.

Collecting system injury (Answer B) and vascular pedicle injury (Answer C) are unlikely due to the peripheral location of the mass. Incomplete treatment (Answer D) is unlikely given the small size (2.0 cm) of the tumor.

References: Boss A, Classen S, Kuczyk M, et al. Thermal damage of the genitofemoral nerve due to radiofrequency ablation of renal cell carcinoma: a potentially avoidable complication. *AJR Am J Roentgenol* 2005;185:1627–1631.

Kam AW, Littrup PJ, Walther MM, et al. Thermal protection during percutaneous thermal ablation of renal cell carcinoma. *J Vasc Interv Radiol* 2004;15:753–758.

Lee SJ, Choyke LT, Wood BJ. Use of hydrodissection to prevent nerve and muscular damage during radiofrequency ablation of kidney tumors. *J Vasc Interv Radiol* 2006;17:1967–1969.

12 Answer A. Hyperintense intravascular signal intensity at the margins of gradient-recalled echo image volumes occurs because of "flow-related enhancement," or so-called "time-of-flight effects." This is due to the influx of unsaturated spin isochromats into the image volume that are rich in preserved longitudinal magnetization conferred by the main magnetic field (B_o). The longitudinal magnetization is preserved and maximal because the inflowing spins have not yet been exposed to a 90-degree excitation pulse. Once they are exposed, their longitudinal magnetization will be converted to transverse magnetization. Over time, after multiple RF exposures and repetitive signal loss, the spins will be considered "saturated" and contribute little to the intravascular signal intensity. Saturation bands can be applied that presaturate inflowing blood.

References: McRobbie DW, Moore EA, Graves MJ, et al. *MRI: from picture to proton*, 2nd ed. New York: Cambridge University Press, 2007.

Wehrli FW. Time-of-flight effects in MR imaging of flow. *Magn Reson Med* 1990;14:187–193.

13 Answer A. Retroperitoneal lipomatosis is characterized by symmetric proliferation of the retroperitoneal fat, resulting in displacement of the kidneys and duodenum anteriorly and a narrowed, vertically oriented urinary bladder. Many patients identified to have this condition have coexisting urinary or bowel symptoms, but the management is clinical. The number of patients with asymptomatic retroperitoneal lipomatosis is likely underreported because abdominal imaging is generally performed in patients with abdominal symptoms. Prophylactic ureteric stenting (Answer C) and operative resection (Answer D) are not indicated.

Percutaneous biopsy (Answer B) is not required because the diagnosis is established by imaging. Benign (e.g., lipoma, myelolipoma, angiomyolipoma) and malignant (e.g., liposarcoma) fat-containing retroperitoneal tumors can be differentiated from retroperitoneal lipomatosis by their inherent asymmetry.

References: Craig WD, Fanburg JC, Henry LR, et al. Fat-containing lesions of the retroperitoneum: radiologic-pathologic correlation. *Radiographics* 2009;29:261–290.

Fogg LB, Smyth JW. Pelvic lipomatosis: a condition simulating pelvic neoplasm. *Radiology* 1968;90:558–564.

Heyns CF. Pelvic lipomatosis: a review of its diagnosis and management. *J Urol* 1991;146:267–273.

14 **Answer B.** The images demonstrate a lobular homogeneous perinephric soft tissue mass that abuts the left kidney and spleen without invasion. The most likely diagnosis is lymphoma. The mass does not appear to arise from the kidney or spleen, and therefore renal cell carcinoma (Answer A) and splenic angiosarcoma (Answer C) are unlikely. Adrenocortical carcinoma (Answer D) is not the best answer because these masses are typically large, heterogeneous, centrally necrotic, and centered on the adrenal gland.

The differential diagnosis for a primary perirenal mass includes lymphoma, sarcoma, and extraadrenal myelolipoma. The differential diagnosis for bilateral perirenal masses includes a variety of immune-related tumors and metastatic disease: (1) lymphoma, (2) mass-forming retroperitoneal fibrosis, (3) Erdheim-Chester disease, (4) extramedullary hematopoiesis, (5) Rosai-Dorfman disease, (6) Castleman disease, (7) Waldenström macroglobulinemia, and (8) metastatic disease.

References: Surabhi VR, Menias C, Prasad SR, et al. Neoplastic and non-neoplastic proliferative disorders of the perirenal space: cross-sectional imaging findings. *Radiographics* 2008;28:1005–1017.

Westphalen A, Yeh B, Qayyum A, et al. Differential diagnosis of perinephric masses on CT and MRI. *AJR Am J Roentgenol* 2004;183:1697–1702.

15 **Answer D.** The best next step for a ruptured aortic aneurysm in the setting of adjacent spondylodiscitis is volume replacement with emergent operative repair. Observation (Answer A) and antibiotic therapy (Answer B) will likely result in the death of the patient. Endovascular repair (Answer C), though feasible, is not optimal in the setting of an adjacent active infection due to the risk of infecting the graft.

In general, the likelihood of abdominal aortic aneurysm rupture is highly correlated with aneurysm sac size. Abdominal aortic aneurysms <4 cm rarely rupture, and most asymptomatic abdominal aortic aneurysms are not electively repaired until ≥5.5 cm. The small size of the ruptured aneurysm in this case suggests that the integrity of the aortic wall must be compromised. Given the adjacent spondylodiscitis, it is likely an infected (i.e., mycotic) aneurysm.

References: Fichelle JM, Tabet G, Cormier P, et al. Infected infrarenal aortic aneurysms: when is in situ reconstruction safe? *J Vasc Surg* 1993;17:635–645.

Huang YK, Ko PJ, Chen CL, et al. Therapeutic opinion on endovascular repair for mycotic aortic aneurysm. *Ann Vasc Surg* 2014;28(3):579–589.

Oderich GS, Panneton JM, Bower TC, et al. Infected aortic aneurysms: aggressive presentation, complicated early outcome, but durable results. *J Vasc Surg* 2001;34:900–908.

16 **Answer B.** Retroperitoneal Erdheim-Chester disease is characterized by perinephric soft tissue thickening, retroperitoneal soft tissue masses, ureteric obstruction, and histologic non-Langerhans histiocytosis. The disease is commonly associated with retro-orbital soft tissue masses, diabetes insipidus, and metaphyseal osteosclerosis.

A diffusely enlarged sausage-shaped pancreas with a rind of peripancreatic fibrosis (Answer A) is characteristic of autoimmune pancreatitis associated with IgG4 disease.

A unilateral locally aggressive solid mass of the renal capsule with or without calcifications (Answer C) is characteristic of sarcoma of the renal capsule.

A pattern of renal and bulky perirenal masses that displace but do not invade nearby structures (Answer D) is characteristic of retroperitoneal lymphoma.

References: Surabhi VR, Menias C, Prasad SR, et al. Neoplastic and non-neoplastic proliferative disorders of the perirenal space: cross-sectional imaging findings. *Radiographics* 2008;28:1005–1017.

Venkatanarasimha N, Garrido MC, Puckett M, et al. AJR teaching file: a rare multisystem disease with distinctive radiologic-pathologic findings. *AJR Am J Roentgenol* 2009;193:S49–S52.

Westphalen A, Yeh B, Qayyum A, et al. Differential diagnosis of perinephric masses on CT and MRI. *AJR Am J Roentgenol* 2004;183:1697–1702.

17   **Answer A.**   Psoas abscesses are rare in the United States and most commonly caused by *Staphylococcus aureus* infection resulting from hematogenous dissemination (80% to 90%). *Mycobacterium tuberculosis* infection (e.g., secondary dissemination from Pott disease of the spine) is a less common but important consideration because the antibiotic therapy differs, the organism is difficult to detect unless specifically sought, and patient isolation may be required in infected patients. Gut flora (e.g., *Escherichia coli, Bacteroides* species) can be seen in patients with a perforated viscus (e.g., diverticulitis, Crohn disease).

MR imaging of the spine should be considered in patients with a psoas abscess to evaluate for spondylodiscitis. Percutaneous drainage and prolonged antibiotic therapy are the mainstays of therapy. Operative debridement may be required if the spine is involved.

References: Dinc H, Onder C, Turhan AL, et al. Percutaneous drainage of tuberculous and nontuberculous psoas abscess. *Eur J Radiol* 1996;23:130–134.

Muckley T, Schultz T, Kirschner M, et al. Psoas abscess: the spine as a primary source of infection. *Spine* 2003;28:106–113.

Walsh TR, Reilly JR, Hanley E, et al. Changing etiology of iliopsoas abscess. *Am J Surg* 1992;163:413–416.

18   **Answer C.**   Clotted blood is typically 40 to 70 HU on unenhanced CT. This differs from the attenuation of free fluid (0 to 20 HU) and free-flowing extraluminal blood (20 to 40 HU). Free-flowing extraluminal blood is lower in attenuation than clotted blood because it has not yet formed a solid clot.

The iron in the hemoglobin of red blood cells contributes significantly to the attenuation of blood. Clots are higher in attenuation than intravascular and free-flowing extraluminal blood because as the clot forms, plasma is expressed, and the relative concentration of red blood cells is increased.

References: Hamilton JD, Kumaravel M, Censullo ML, et al. Multidetector CT evaluation of active extravasation in blunt abdominal and pelvic trauma patients. *Radiographics* 2008;28:1603–1616.

Katz DS, Lane MJ, Mindelzun RE. Unenhanced CT of abdominal and pelvic hemorrhage. *Semin Ultrasound CT MR* 1999;20:94–107.

Shanmuganathan K, Mirvis SE, Sover ER. Value of contrast-enhanced CT in detecting active hemorrhage in patients with blunt abdominal or pelvic trauma. *AJR Am J Roentgenol* 1993;161:65–69.

19   **Answer A.**   The sharp decrease in size of the aneurysm sac despite the presence of a small type II endoleak indicates that the sac is not under significant pressure, and therefore observation is the best choice. Many type II endoleaks will spontaneously thrombose and very few result in clinically significant sequelae. The stability of the aneurysm sac is the most important criterion guiding management. In general, persistent (>6 months) type II endoleaks associated with aneurysm sac growth (≥5 mm) should be treated, while asymptomatic type II endoleaks that spontaneously resolve or are associated with a stable or decreasing sac size can be observed.

References: Silverberg D, Baril DT, Ellozy SH, et al. An 8-year experience with type II endoleaks: natural history suggests selective intervention is a safe approach. *J Vasc Surg* 2006;44:453–459.

Steinmetz E, Rubin BG, Sanchez LA, et al. Type II endoleak after endovascular abdominal aortic aneurysm repair: a conservative approach with selective intervention is safe and cost-effective. *J Vasc Surg* 2004;306–313.

White SB, Stavropoulos SW. Management of endoleaks following endovascular aneurysm repair. *Semin Intervent Radiol* 2009;26:33–38.

20   Answer B.   IgG4-related sclerosing disease (as in this case) is characterized by a variety of findings, including (1) autoimmune pancreatitis, (2) retroperitoneal fibrosis, (3) sclerosing cholangitis, (4) renal masses, (5) thickening of the renal pelvis, (6) sclerosing mesenteritis, (7) lymph node enlargement, (8) salivary gland swelling, and (9) others.

Retroperitoneal fibrosis is characterized by desmoplastic periaortic soft tissue thickening that tethers and retracts nearby tissues. Ureteric obstruction is a feared complication that is managed with ureteric stenting or operative mobilization (ureterolysis, ureteric lateralization, and omental wrapping). Many cases of retroperitoneal fibrosis are idiopathic or medication induced. Several diseases can mimic idiopathic retroperitoneal fibrosis including (1) IgG4-related sclerosing disease, (2) inflammatory aortic aneurysm, (3) lymphoma, (4) metastatic disease, (5) Erdheim-Chester disease, (6) other autoimmune conditions, and (7) prior radiotherapy.

Differentiating benign retroperitoneal fibrosis from one of the malignant mimics (e.g., metastatic disease, lymphoma) is important. Although the risk of malignancy is small (<10%), the management is obviously different. Operative biopsy is the most reliable method of establishing the diagnosis due to the risk of sampling error with a percutaneous approach (i.e., metastatic disease presenting like retroperitoneal fibrosis will often have a mix of malignant cells and surrounding secondary reactive fibrosis). However, in patients who are not ideal operative candidates, percutaneous biopsy is often used and combined with imaging follow-up.

References: Koep L, Zuidema GD. The clinical significance of retroperitoneal fibrosis. *Surgery* 1977;81:250–257.

Scheel PJ Jr, Feeley N. Retroperitoneal fibrosis. *Rheum Dis Clin North Am* 2013;39:365–381.

Vlachou PA, Khalili K, Jang HJ, et al. IgG4-related sclerosing disease: autoimmune pancreatitis and extrapancreatic manifestations. *Radiographics* 2011;31:1379–1402.

21   Answer C.   The radiopaque tape in the center of the pelvis indicates a retained surgical sponge. Retained foreign bodies can be a source of sepsis, delayed healing, and litigation. Different manufacturers imbed different devices with different radiopaque strips; another example of a retained sponge is shown below. Unlike the index case, this sponge (just below the diaphragm in the right upper quadrant, surrounded by surgical clips) is embedded with a series of parallel metallic lines as opposed to a single metallic strip.

Although there is gas within the pelvic soft tissues of the index case (Answer A), this can be a normal finding postoperative day 3. There is no evidence of large bowel obstruction (Answer B) or tube malposition (Answer D).

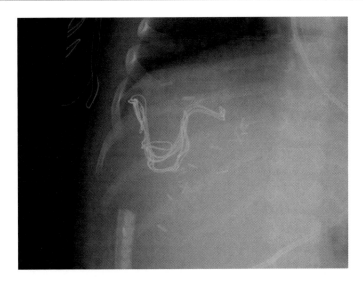

References: Hunter TB, Taljanovic MS. Foreign bodies. *Radiographics* 2003;23:731–757.
Manzella A, Filho PB, Albuquerque E, et al. Imaging of gossypibomas: pictorial review. *AJR Am J Roentgenol* 2009;193:S94–S101.

22 **Answer A.** The images demonstrate a fluid- and gas-containing lentiform structure within the partial nephrectomy bed consistent with a surgical bolster (Answer A). This is a commonly used intraoperative device intentionally left in situ for the promotion of hemostasis. On CT imaging, the bolster will often be fluid attenuation and contain foci of gas that can be misinterpreted as an abscess (Answer D). Clues that the finding is not an abscess include (1) time course (bolsters can be present for at least a month following the operation), (2) shape (the bolster "fits" into the partial nephrectomy bed), (3) tightly packed air bubbles (representing gas trapped within the interstices of the bolster), (4) lack of an enhancing wall, (5) and lack of an air–fluid level.

References: Pai D, Willatt JM, Korobkin M, et al. CT appearances following laparoscopic partial nephrectomy for renal cell carcinoma using a rolled cellulose bolster. *Cancer Imaging* 2010;10:161–168.
Sandrasegaran K, Lall C, Rajesh A, et al. Distinguishing gelatin bioabsorbable sponge and postoperative abdominal abscess on CT. *AJR Am J Roentgenol* 2005;184:475–480.

23 **Answer C.** Congenital variants of the IVC are varied and uncommon but are routinely seen on imaging studies of the abdomen and pelvis. "Duplicated" or "double" IVC results from persistence of the right and left supracardinal veins. In this condition, it is common for the right IVC to receive blood from the right common iliac vein and then drain into the right atrium, while the left IVC receives blood from the left common iliac vein and then drains into the left renal vein. This variant is clinically significant because failure to protect both sides of ingress in patients with DVT can lead to pulmonary embolism despite filter placement.

References: Kandpal H, Sharma R, Gamangatti S, et al. Imaging the inferior vena cava: a road less traveled. *Radiographics* 2008;28:669–689.
Restrepo CS, Eraso A, Ocazionez D, et al. The diaphragmatic crura and retrocrural space: normal imaging appearance, variants, and pathologic conditions. *Radiographics* 2008;28:1289–1305.

24 **Answer C.** Spin echo sequences are based on the principle of performing a 180-degree refocusing pulse TE/2 msec after the initial 90-degree excitation pulse. This is done to eliminate the static field inhomogeneities (e.g., inhomogeneity in the main magnetic field [B_0] and static local susceptibility effects) that contribute to T2* decay. The figure demonstrates the difference between T2 decay (blue line) and T2* decay (red line). The T2 time is the length of time it takes for the transverse magnetization (M_{xy}) to decay to 37% of its maximum signal due solely to spin–spin relaxation in the absence of static field inhomogeneities (e.g., after a spin echo sequence). The T2* time is the length of time it takes for the transverse magnetization to decay to 37% of its maximum signal without removal of static field inhomogeneities (e.g., after a gradient-recalled echo sequence). T2 decay is also referred to as spin–spin relaxation.

The 180-degree refocusing pulse occurs TE/2 msec after the 90-degree excitation pulse to allow symmetric and opposite dephasing to occur on either side of the 180-degree pulse. Fixed static field inhomogeneities cancel, and the spin echo is measured at TE.

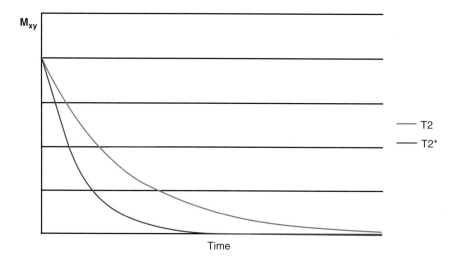

References: Jung BA, Weigel M. Spin echo magnetic resonance imaging. *J Magn Reson Imaging* 2013;37:805–817.

McRobbie DW, Moore EA, Graves MJ, et al. *MRI: from picture to proton*, 2nd ed. New York: Cambridge University Press, 2007.

25 **Answer A.** The approximate sensitivity of morphologic CT for the detection of prostate cancer nodal metastasis is 30%. This poor sensitivity is understandable because nodal metastatic disease is only detectable by CT when tumor expands the lymph node(s) beyond a certain size threshold (>1 cm in short axis is a commonly used threshold for most pelvic lymph node stations). In general, CT has a low sensitivity for nodal metastases, regardless of the primary tumor type.

References: Hricak H, Doms GC, Jeffrey RB, et al. Prostatic carcinoma: staging by clinical assessment, CT, and MR imaging. *Radiology* 1987;162:331–336.

Platt JF, Bree RI, Schwab RE. The accuracy of CT in the staging of carcinoma of the prostate. *AJR Am J Roentgenol* 1987;149:315–318.

Wolf JS Jr, Cher M, Dall'era M, et al. The use and accuracy of cross-sectional imaging and fine needle aspiration cytology for detection of pelvic lymph node metastases before radical prostatectomy. *J Urol* 1995;153:993–999.

26 **Answer B.** The most likely diagnosis for a large solid primary retroperitoneal mass that is centered around the IVC is leiomyosarcoma. It is the second most common primary malignancy of the retroperitoneum (liposarcoma is more common (Answer A), but the IVC involvement and lack of macroscopic fat in this case favor leiomyosarcoma). In general, large primary masses of the retroperitoneum are most often sarcoma (most common), lymphoma, or peripheral nerve sheath tumors. Lymphoma (Answer C) is usually thought of as a "soft" tumor that displaces but does not invade adjacent structures. Local invasion of adjacent structures would be uncommon for a benign mass (Answers D and E). Lipomas are composed entirely of macroscopic fat (Answer E).

Other masses that invade the IVC include (1) renal cell carcinoma, (2) adrenocortical carcinoma, and (3) hepatocellular carcinoma.

References: Hartman DS, Hayes WS, Choyke PL, et al. Leiomyosarcoma of the retroperitoneum and inferior vena cava: radiologic-pathologic correlation. *Radiographics* 1992;12:1203–1220.
Kandpal H, Sharma R, Gamangatti S, et al. Imaging the inferior vena cava: a road less traveled. *Radiographics* 2008;28:669–689.

27 **Answer B.**   RECIST 1.1 (**R**esponse **E**valuation **C**riteria **i**n **S**olid **T**umors v. 1.1) is a systematic imaging biomarker used to monitor disease response in patients with solid tumors. This system contains a series of rules that govern which masses and lymph nodes can be considered "target lesions" (i.e., lesions with a high likelihood of malignancy that can be followed and measured reliably over time). Lymph nodes qualify as "target lesions" in RECIST 1.1 if they are ≥15 mm in short axis. "Short axis" is defined as a maximum diameter measurement drawn perpendicular to the long axis measurement.

References: Eisenhauer EA, Therasse P, Bogaerts J, et al. New response evaluation criteria in solid tumours: revised RECIST guideline (version 1.1). *Eur J Cancer* 2009;45(2):228–247.
Nishino M, Jagannathan JP, Ramaiya NH, et al. Revised RECIST guideline version 1.1: what oncologists want to know and what radiologists need to know. *AJR Am J Roentgenol* 2010;195:281–289.

28 **Answer C.**   Unlike lymph nodes, which must be ≥15 mm in short axis, lesions within solid organs must be ≥10 mm in long axis to be considered "target lesions." This difference is because lymph nodes are normal structures, while lesions within organs are not.

Each patient can be assigned a maximum of five target lesions, of which no more than two can be within any given organ. Once all target lesions are assigned, the sum of their diameters is tabulated (long axis for lesions in organs, short axis for lymph nodes) to arrive at the "sum of diameters."

References: Eisenhauer EA, Therasse P, Bogaerts J, et al. New response evaluation criteria in solid tumours: revised RECIST guideline (version 1.1). *Eur J Cancer* 2009;45(2):228–247.
Nishino M, Jagannathan JP, Ramaiya NH, et al. Revised RECIST guideline version 1.1: what oncologists want to know and what radiologists need to know. *AJR Am J Roentgenol* 2010;195:281–289.

29 **Answer E.**   Aneurysm sacs should be measured along a plane perpendicular to the vascular center line (i.e., center line measurement). Convenience measurements made on directly acquired sections will under- or overrepresent the true aneurysm sac size and can have a deleterious effect on management. Specifically, size thresholds and growth rates are often key determinants guiding the decision to intervene upon an abdominal aortic aneurysm. If the measurements used for this decision making are erroneous, the decision making will be flawed.

The following is a typical aortic center line generated from a 3D workstation. Diameter measurements should be perpendicular to this center line extending from outer wall to outer wall at the maximum width. The diameter measurement performed in the upper left-hand image is at the superior margin of the aneurysm sac. A maximum caliber measurement of the abdominal aortic aneurysm would be made inferior to this where the aneurysm sac is largest.

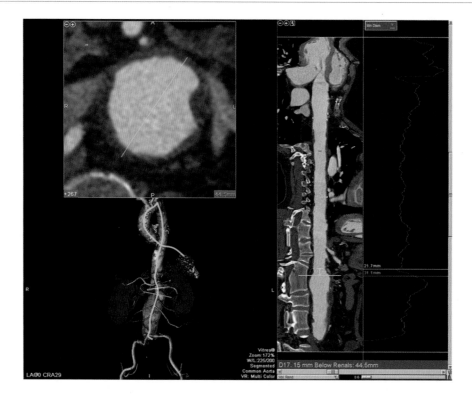

References. Cayne NS, Veith FJ, Lipsitz EC, et al. Variability of maximal aortic aneurysm diameter measurements on CT scan: significance and methods to minimize. *J Vasc Surg* 2004;39:811–815.

Hirsch AT, Haskal ZJ, Hertzer NR, et al. ACC/AHA 2005 Practice Guidelines for the management of patients with peripheral arterial disease (lower extremity, renal, mesenteric, and abdominal aortic): a collaborative report from the American Association for Vascular Surgery/Society for Vascular Surgery, Society for Cardiovascular Angiography and Interventions, Society for Vascular Medicine and Biology, Society of Interventional Radiology, and the ACC/AHA Task Force on Practice Guidelines. *Circulation* 2006;113:e463–e654.

30 **Answer B.**   The most specific feature for tumor thrombus is presence of vasculature within the thrombus. This can be identified on ultrasound as color flow or, more specifically, presence of an arterial spectral Doppler waveform within the vein. Barring artifacts, arterial spectral Doppler waveforms do not exist in veins unless there is neovascularity or an arteriovenous fistula. A venous spectral waveform is less specific because it could result from normal venous flow around the margins of the thrombus. On CT and MR, vasculature within the thrombus is confirmed with enhancement of the thrombus. Other features, including the size of the thrombus, its echogenicity or attenuation (Answer A), its location (Answer C), and its mobility (Answer D) are not reliable indicators. Tumor thrombus can expand the vein lumen to a greater degree than bland thrombus, but there is overlap in this presentation because acute bland thrombus is also expansile.

References: Hübsch P, Schurawitzki H, Susani M, et al. Color Doppler imaging of inferior vena cava: identification of tumor thrombus. *J Ultrasound Med* 1992;11:639–645.

Laissy JP, Menegazzo D, Debray MP, et al. Renal carcinoma: diagnosis of venous invasion with Gd-enhanced MR venography. *Eur Radiol* 2000;10:1138–1143.

10 Miscellaneous

QUESTIONS

1   A 32-year-old female trauma victim undergoes a contrast-enhanced CT of the abdomen and pelvis and an abnormality is detected in the right kidney. There is a small volume of ipsilateral perinephric fluid. The main right renal artery and main right renal vein are patent. What is the significance of the imaging findings in the right kidney?

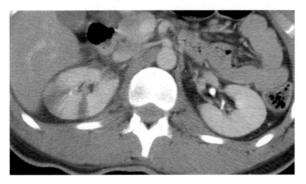 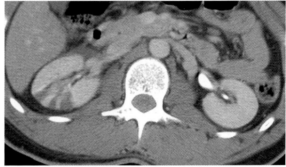

- A. Shattered kidney, operative management
- B. Renal contusions, conservative management
- C. Pyelonephritis, antibiotic therapy
- D. Renal infarcts, angiography and/or echocardiography

2   A retrospective cohort study evaluating the incidence of contrast-induced acute kidney injury (CI-AKI) compares acute kidney injury rates following CT in two groups: (1) patients who received contrast-enhanced CT as part of routine clinical care and (2) patients who received unenhanced CT as part of routine clinical care. Serum creatinine measurements drawn 48 hours after the CT are compared to serum creatinine measurements drawn prior to the CT. An increase at the 48-hour time point of ≥0.3 mg/dL is considered indicative of CI-AKI. All patients included in the study had all necessary serum creatinine measurements available. What source of bias is of greatest concern with this type of study design?

- A. Verification bias
- B. Selection bias
- C. Recall bias
- D. Lead-time bias

3   A 70-year-old male with a dilated left collecting system undergoes a retrograde pyelogram. What entity is classically associated with the imaging findings?

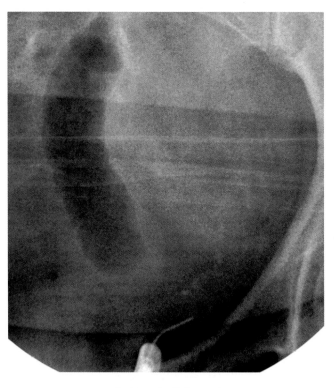 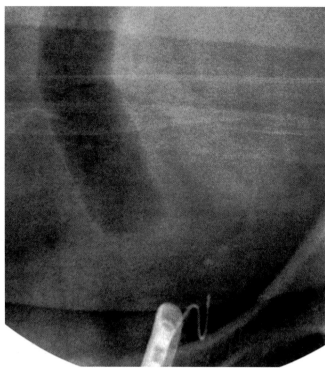

A. Urothelial carcinoma
B. Calculus disease
C. Blood clot
D. Fungal infection
E. *Schistosoma haematobium*

4   A 52-year-old female with chronic obstructive pulmonary disease on 2 L of home oxygen therapy undergoes a CT for right lower quadrant pain. A 1.5-cm cortically based left renal mass is identified. Biphasic renal mass protocol CT is performed demonstrating the following features: (1) unenhanced attenuation 50 HU, (2) nephrographic phase attenuation 100 HU, (3) no macroscopic fat, and (4) homogeneous enhancement. The unenhanced background renal parenchyma is 30 HU, the adjacent renal artery is 180 HU, and there are no comparison studies. What is the best next step?

A. Ignore (benign finding)
B. Percutaneous biopsy
C. Partial nephrectomy
D. Embolization

5   A new blood test is developed for prostate cancer screening. When the test is positive, a transrectal ultrasound (TRUS)-guided random prostate biopsy is performed. After decades of study, it is determined that patients diagnosed with prostate cancer through the screening program have improved survival. However, it is repeatedly noted that prostate cancers resulting from a screening-triggered biopsy are more likely to be variants with a slower growth rate. What type of screening bias results from the disproportionate identification of slowly progressive disease?

A. Reporting bias
B. Lead-time bias
C. Length bias
D. Overdiagnosis bias

6 Calculate the approximate voxel size of the 2D T2-weighted fast spin echo image shown below provided the following assumptions: (1) field of view = 16 cm × 16 cm, (2) phase-encoding matrix = 168, (3) frequency-encoding matrix = 228, (4) TE = 110 msec, (5) TR = 5,190 msec, (6) slice thickness = 3 mm, (7) interslice gap = 1 mm, (8) echo train length = 21.

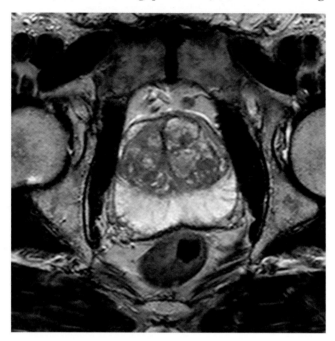

A. 0.95 mm × 0.70 mm × 3.00 mm
B. 0.95 mm × 0.70 mm × 4.00 mm
C. 1.43 mm × 1.05 mm × 3.00 mm
D. 1.43 mm × 1.05 mm × 4.00 mm
E. 0.14 mm × 0.11 mm × 3.00 mm
F. 0.10 mm × 0.07 mm × 4.00 mm
G. The voxel size cannot be calculated with the provided information.

7 A 59-year-old female with hematuria undergoes an intravenous pyelogram (IVP) demonstrating a mass in the left renal pelvis. What is the main reason that CT urography (CTU) has supplanted IVP for the detection of upper tract malignancy?

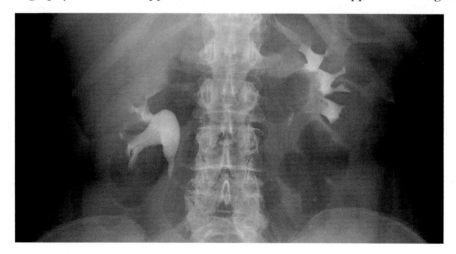

A. CTU requires less radiation than IVP.
B. CTU uses a lower dose of contrast material than IVP.
C. CTU detects less incidental findings than IVU.
D. CTU has a higher accuracy than IVU.

8 A 55-year-old female with no comorbidities undergoes percutaneous core biopsy of a 3.2-cm solid mass in the right perinephric space. The histology demonstrates epithelioid angiomyolipoma. What is the best next step?

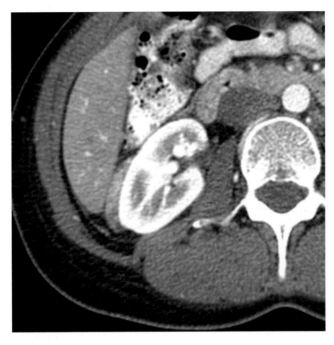

A. Observation (benign finding)
B. Repeat biopsy
C. Embolization
D. Operative resection

9 A 75-year-old male with elevated prostate specific antigen (PSA, 25 ng/mL) undergoes a 3.0-Tesla prostate MRI. What is the hyperintense elliptical structure identified along the midline?

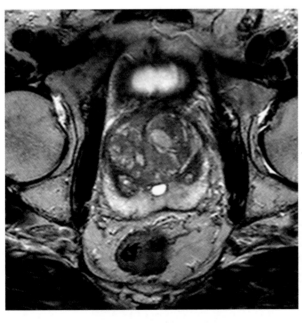 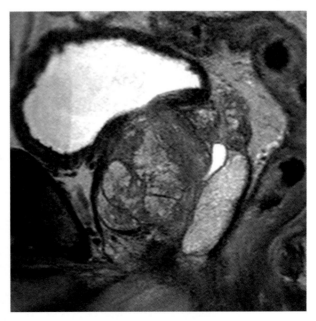

A. Glandular BPH nodule
B. Stromal BPH nodule
C. Utricle cyst
D. Prostate cancer

10 A 73-year-old male with Gleason 4 + 3 = 7 prostate cancer undergoes a 3.0-Tesla prostate MRI. What can be done to reduce the artifacts within the prostate gland?

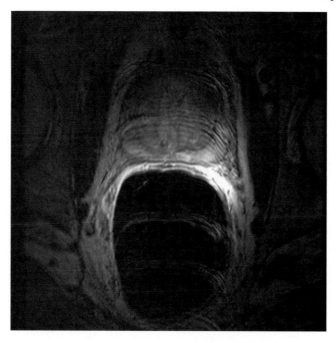

A. Change the frequency-encoding axis to: "left-to-right"
B. Change the phase-encoding axis to: "left-to-right"
C. Apply fat saturation using short tau inversion recovery (STIR)
D. Apply fat saturation using a spectrally selective radiofrequency pulse

11 A 50-year-old female with a left renal angiomyolipoma presents for treatment. At what size is embolization commonly considered for the treatment of an asymptomatic angiomyolipoma?

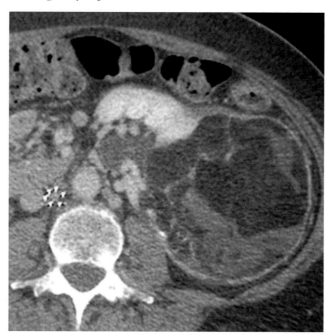

A. ≥2 cm
B. ≥4 cm
C. ≥6 cm
D. ≥8 cm

12 A 30-year-old male with acute left flank pain undergoes an unenhanced CT of the abdomen and pelvis. What is the most likely explanation for the abnormality in the left perinephric space?

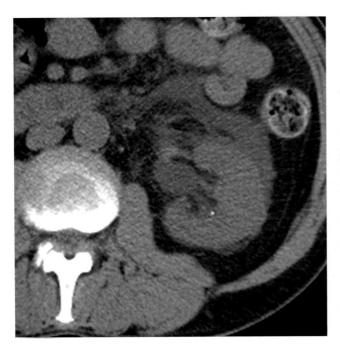 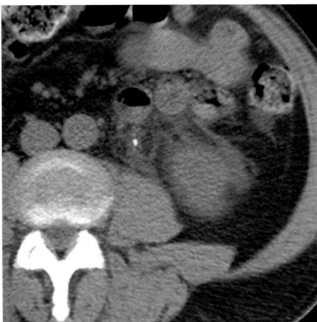

A. Urinoma

B. Abscess

C. Edema

D. Lymphoma

13 A 75-year-old female with stage IV chronic kidney disease (estimated glomerular filtration rate is 19 mL/min/1.73 m²), hypertension, peripheral vascular disease, and claudication symptoms presents for a CT angiogram of the abdomen and pelvis with runoff to the lower extremities. Which of the following prophylactic measures has the most supportive evidence as a technique to reduce this patient's risk of contrast-induced acute kidney injury?

A. Volume expansion with IV D5 0.45% NaCl

B. Volume expansion with IV 0.9% NaCl

C. Preprocedure administration of N-acetylcysteine

D. Preprocedure administration of sodium bicarbonate

14 A 70-year-old male presents for an ultrasound-guided percutaneous biopsy of an incidentally detected 2-cm homogeneously enhancing solid renal mass. What is the most common complication of this procedure?

A. Hemorrhage

B. Needle-track seeding

C. Renal abscess

D. Pneumothorax

E. Collecting system obstruction

F. Colonic injury

15 A 70-year-old female with a 2.0-cm heterogeneous solid renal mass presents for percutaneous renal mass biopsy. Which of the following approaches is most likely to yield a diagnostic result with the least risk of complication using an 18-gauge spring-loaded end-firing core biopsy device with a 1.0-cm or 2.0-cm throw length?

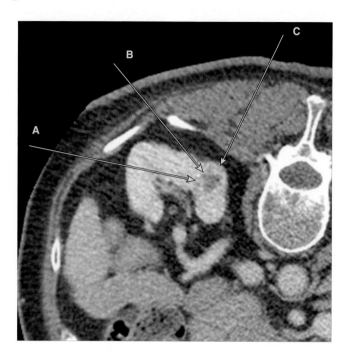

A. Angle A with a 1-cm throw length
B. Angle A with a 2-cm throw length
C. Angle B with a 1-cm throw length
D. Angle B with a 2-cm throw length
E. Angle C with a 1-cm throw length
F. Angle C with a 2-cm throw length

16 A 50-year-old female with back and flank pain undergoes an abdominal MRI. What is the most likely cause of the signal abnormality anterior to the common iliac arteries?

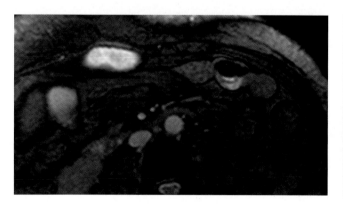
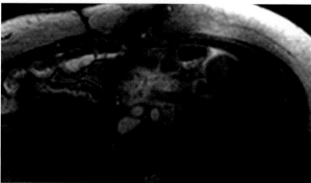

A. Magnetic field inhomogeneity
B. Inaccurate inversion time
C. Retroperitoneal fibrosis
D. Lymphoma

17 A 63-year-old male with metastatic prostate cancer undergoes a CT of the abdomen and pelvis. How should the current images be interpreted?

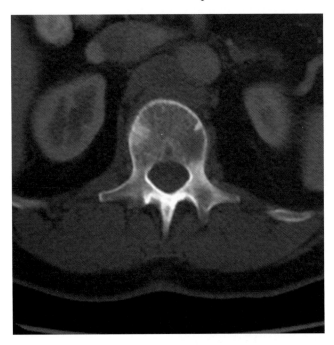 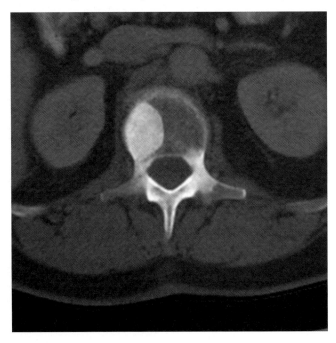

Nine months ago   *Current study*

A. Osseous metastatic disease; uncertain response
B. Osseous metastatic disease; progressive disease
C. Osseous metastatic disease; partial response
D. Osseous metastatic disease; stable disease

18 A 63-year-old male presents with scrotal discomfort and an ultrasound is performed. What is the most likely diagnosis?

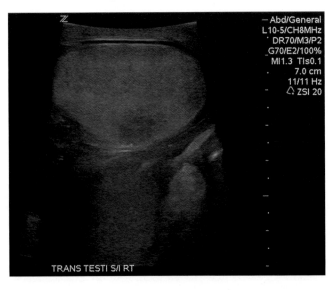 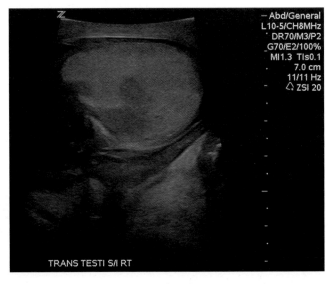

A. Seminomatous germ cell tumor
B. Nonseminomatous germ cell tumor
C. T-cell lymphoma
D. B-cell lymphoma

19 A 45-year-old female presents with an incidental finding. What is the most likely diagnosis?

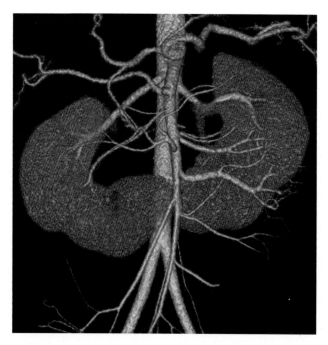

    A. Crossed-fused ectopia
    B. Horseshoe kidney
    C. Pelvic kidney
    D. Duplicated kidney

20 A 28-year-old female presents with lower abdominal pain and a CT is performed. What is the most likely antecedent history?

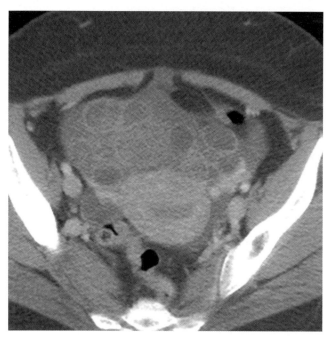 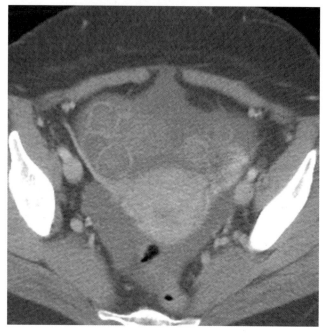

    A. Family history of ovarian cancer
    B. Hyperandrogenism and metabolic syndrome
    C. Recent normal menstruation
    D. Recent fertility treatment

21 A 40-year-old female with vague abdominal pain undergoes a CT of the abdomen and pelvis. What is the most likely diagnosis?

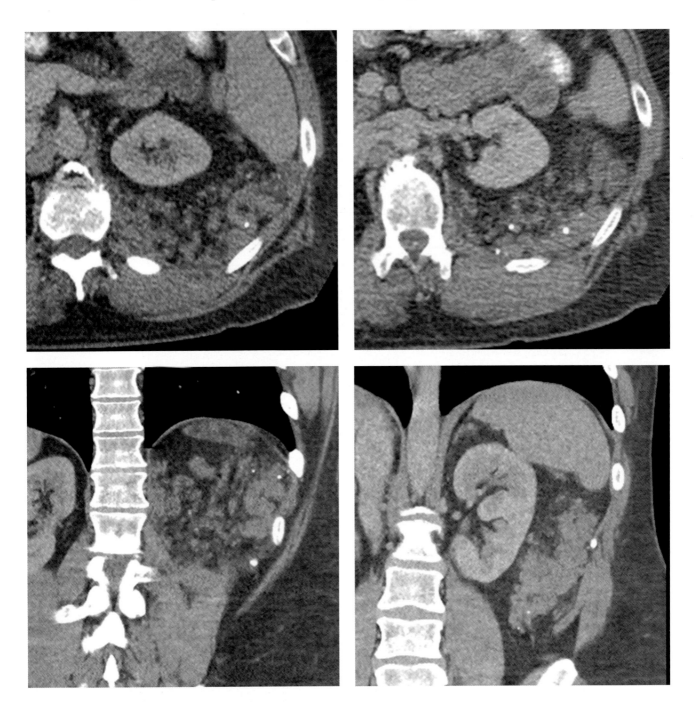

A. Lymphoma
B. Liposarcoma
C. Angiomyolipoma
D. Vascular malformation
E. Foreign body

22 A 33-year-old female with left lower quadrant pain undergoes a pelvic MRI. A nonenhancing abnormality is identified within the left ovary. What is the most likely cause of the T1 shortening within this abnormality?

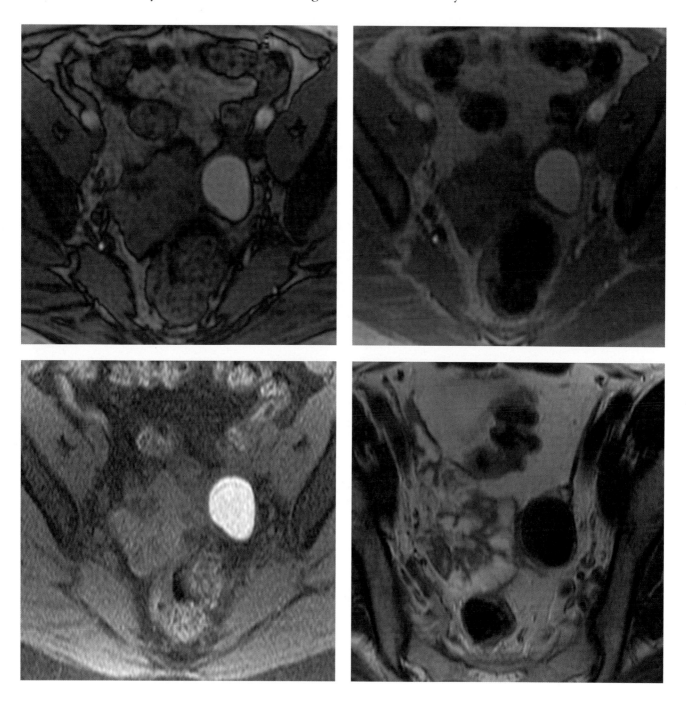

A. Fat
B. Protein
C. Hemorrhage
D. Melanin
E. Contrast material
F. Flow artifact
G. Calcium

23 A 50-year-old female with pelvic pain undergoes a pelvic MRI and a large necrotic mass is identified. What is the most likely diagnosis?

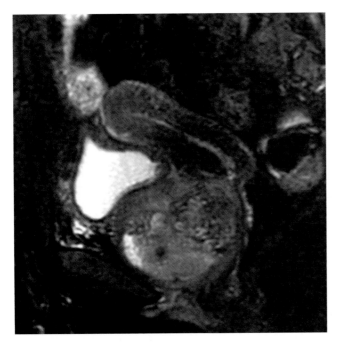 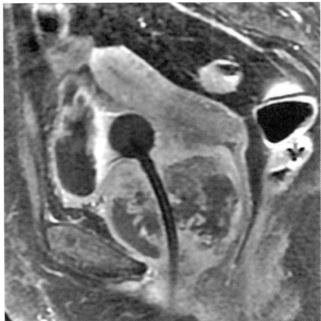

A. Cervical cancer

B. Vaginal cancer

C. Urethral cancer

D. Bladder cancer

E. Prostate cancer

24 A 70-year-old male with an incidentally detected 2-cm solid renal mass presents for a discussion regarding management. What is the commonly cited size threshold at which renal cell carcinoma is prone to metastasize?

A. 1 cm

B. 3 cm

C. 5 cm

D. 7 cm

25 Which of the following patients has the greatest risk of nephrogenic systemic fibrosis upon administration of gadolinium-based contrast material?

A. A 60-year-old male with acute kidney injury and eGFR 55 mL/min/1.73 m^2

B. A 40-year-old female with diabetes mellitus and eGFR 40 mL/min/1.73 m^2

C. A 50-year-old male with severe hypertension and eGFR 45 mL/min/1.73 m^2

D. A 70-year-old female with multiple myeloma and eGFR 60 mL/min/1.73 m^2

26 A radiology practice is interested in reducing radiation exposure to patients undergoing CT urography. Assuming that each of the following preserves the diagnostic accuracy of the examination, which will have the greatest effect on radiation dose reduction?

A. A 20% decrease in mA

B. A 20% decrease in kVp

C. A 20% decrease in pitch

D. A 20% decrease in z-axis coverage

27 A 70-year-old female with peripheral vascular disease and a suspected
paraneoplastic syndrome undergoes a CT of the chest, abdomen, and pelvis.
A 1.2-cm ovoid retrocrural mass is identified that measures 12 Hounsfield Units.
How should this finding be interpreted?

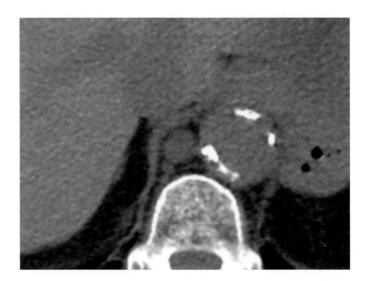

A. Normal variant, ignore
B. Enlarged lymph node, recommend biopsy
C. Enlarged lymph node, recommend upper endoscopy
D. Suspected paraganglioma, recommend MIBG
E. Suspected benign nerve sheath tumor, ignore

28 A 45-year-old average-size male with a psoas abscess is given conscious
sedation with midazolam IV and fentanyl IV for an ultrasound-guided drainage
catheter placement. During the procedure, the patient complains of ongoing
back pain, and so three additional doses of fentanyl IV are administered at
5, 10, and 15 minutes. At 20 minutes, the patient becomes hypoxic and his
respiratory rate is 6. Verbal and tactile stimulation has minimal effect. What is
the best next step?

A. Administer naloxone 0.2 mg IV q2–3 min until his respiratory rate is >10
B. Administer naloxone 2.0 mg IV q2–3 min until his respiratory rate is >10
C. Administer flumazenil 0.1 mg IV, may repeat q1 min, goal is respiratory
rate >10
D. Administer flumazenil 1.0 mg IV, may repeat q1 min, goal is respiratory
rate >10

29 A 55-year-old male with new-onset proteinuria is being scheduled for an
elective renal biopsy. He has a history of atrial fibrillation and is receiving
chronic warfarin therapy. According to the Society of Interventional Radiology
2012 consensus guidelines, what should be the target INR (International
Normalized Ratio) for this procedure?

A. INR < 1.9
B. INR < 1.7
C. INR < 1.5
D. INR < 1.3

30   A 20-year-old male with upper abdominal pain undergoes a contrast-enhanced
     CT of the abdomen and pelvis, and an abnormality is identified in his pelvis.
     Which of the following is strongly associated with this imaging finding?

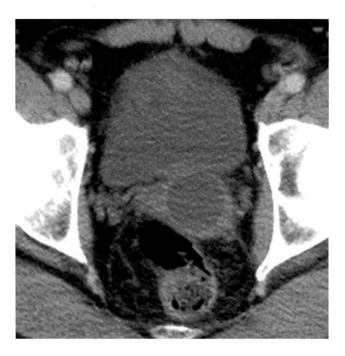

A. Chronic urinary retention
B. Ipsilateral renal agenesis
C. *Chlamydia trachomatis* infection
D. Prostate cancer

ANSWERS AND EXPLANATIONS

1   **Answer B.**   The images demonstrate a striated right nephrogram in the setting of trauma indicating multifocal contusion and/or laceration. This should be managed conservatively because the vessels are uninjured, the hilum and collecting system are intact, and there is only a small hematoma in the perinephric space. Follow-up imaging performed 2 years later (below) reveals cortical scarring at each site of injury but an otherwise intact, functioning kidney.

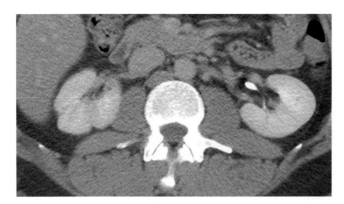 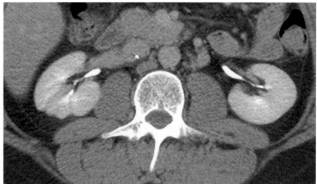

Other causes of a striated nephrogram include: (1) infarcts from a peripheral source (e.g., polyarteritis nodosa), (2) infarcts from a central source (e.g., endocarditis, renal artery injury), (3) renal vein thrombosis, (4) pyelonephritis, (5) glomerulonephritis, and (6) urinary tract obstruction.

A striated nephrogram is basically a multifocal incomplete delayed nephrogram in which some parts of the kidney are affected more than others. The differential diagnosis for a striated nephrogram is therefore similar to the differential diagnosis for a delayed nephrogram and follows a very simple rubric: (1) blood in, (2) blood out, (3) urine in, (4) urine out; when one or more of these four processes is disrupted, a delayed (or striated) nephrogram can result.

References: Kawashima A, Sandler CM, Corl FM, et al. Imaging of renal trauma: a comprehensive review. *Radiographics* 2001;21:557–574.
Santucci RA, McAninch JW, Safir M, et al. Validation of the American Association for the Surgery of Trauma organ injury severity scale for the kidney. *J Trauma* 2001;50:195–200.
Saunders HS, Dyer RB, Shifrin RY, et al. The CT nephrogram: implications for evaluation of urinary tract disease. *Radiographics* 1995;15:1069–1085.

2   **Answer B.**   Selection bias (Answer B) is the greatest threat to the described study design. Selection bias occurs when patients in one study group have fundamental differences that preclude direct comparison to another study group. With respect to the presented scenario, patients who receive unenhanced CT as part of routine clinical care are often shunted away from receiving intravascular contrast material for a particular reason and that reason in many cases directly relates to a concern for acute kidney injury. Therefore, we would expect that compared to patients receiving contrast-enhanced CT as part of routine clinical care, patients receiving unenhanced CT as part of routine clinical care would have a greater frequency of nephrotoxic risk factors, a higher incidence of chronic kidney disease, a lower mean glomerular filtration rate, and a higher incidence of acute kidney injury unrelated to contrast material.

Verification bias (Answer A) is a bias affecting studies of diagnostic tests. It occurs when the decision to perform the reference standard is partially or completely based on the results of the diagnostic test. Therefore, not all subjects receive the reference standard, over-estimating the sensitivity and under-estimating the specificity.

Recall bias (Answer C) is a bias affecting survey-based studies. It occurs when the subjects are asked to remember something about their past. Because memory is imperfect, the response(s) of the subjects are inaccurate, lending bias to the results.

Lead-time bias (Answer D) is a bias affecting studies of screening tests. It occurs when positive test results identify a disease earlier, but do nothing to affect the outcome. In other words, the time the patient dies is the same regardless of whether the screening study is performed, but the screening population appears to live longer because the disease is detected earlier.

References: Delgado-Rodriguez M, Llorca J. Bias. *J Epidemiol Community Health* 2004;58:635–641.

Gupta A, Roehrborn CG. Verification and incorporation biases in studies assessing screening tests: prostate-specific antigen as an example. *Urology* 2004;64:106–111.

3   **Answer A.**   The images demonstrate a "coiled catheter sign," which historically has been associated with urothelial carcinoma of the ureter. The soft tissue mass obstructs the ureter, preventing the wire or catheter from traversing it. Other mass-like causes of ureteric obstruction, such as calculi (Answer B), blood clots (Answer C), and fungal disease (Answer D), can usually be bypassed by a wire or catheter. *Schistosoma haematobium*–associated strictures (Answer E) are not usually mass-like and are rare in the United States.

References: Dyer RB, Chen MY, Zagoria RJ. Classic signs in uroradiology. *Radiographics* 2004;24:S247–S280.

Finby N, Begg CF. Carcinoma of the ureter: coiled catheter sign. *NY State J Med* 1963;15:63:2397–2399.

4   **Answer B.**   The question describes a small homogeneously enhancing solid renal mass in a patient with a significant comorbidity. The best option is percutaneous biopsy. A sizable minority of small solid renal masses <3 cm without macroscopic fat are benign (e.g., minimal fat angiomyolipoma, oncocytoma). When certain imaging or clinical features are present, biopsy should be considered before definitive therapy. In this case, the three features suggesting that this may represent a minimal fat AML include the following: (1) higher attenuation than background parenchyma on unenhanced CT (50 HU vs. 30 HU), (2) homogeneous enhancement, and (3) small size (1.5 cm). Although renal cell carcinoma is still the most likely diagnosis, the likelihood that this mass is benign is approximately 20%. Therefore, ignoring the finding (Answer A) and moving directly to definitive surgery (Answer C) are not the best choices. Embolization (Answer D) is used for the treatment of renal artery aneurysms, for prophylaxis against hemorrhage in the setting of an AML larger than 4 cm, and for preoperative risk reduction in patients with bulky renal cell carcinoma. The mass is unlikely to be an aneurysm because of the substantial difference in postcontrast attenuation (180 HU – 100 HU = 80 HU) between the mass and the adjacent renal artery.

References: Caoili EM, Davenport MS. Role of percutaneous needle biopsy for renal masses. *Semin Intervent Radiol* 2014;31:20–26.

Silverman SG, Gan YU, Mortele KJ, et al. Renal masses in the adult patient: the role of percutaneous biopsy. *Radiology* 2006;240:6–22.

Silverman SG, Israel GM, Herts BR, et al. Management of the incidental renal mass. *Radiology* 2008;249:16–31.

Silverman SG, Mortele KJ, Tuncali K, et al. Hyperattenuating renal masses: etiologies, pathogenesis, and imaging evaluation. *Radiographics* 2007;27:1131–1143.

5 **Answer C.** Length bias is a type of bias affecting screening studies in which slowly progressive disease is identified disproportionately more often by the screening test than rapidly progressive disease. Rapidly progressive disease results in death more quickly and therefore has less of an opportunity to be detected by screening. Length bias overinflates the survival benefits of screening by diagnosing a greater fraction of patients with clinically indolent disease.

Reporting bias (Answer A) is a type of bias affecting survey-based studies. It occurs when the study participants under- or over-report the truth. It occurs when the study participants have a reason to collude with the investigators or to hide the truth from them. For example, a survey-based study conducted by a Psychology professor investigating academic dishonesty among college students would likely result in an underreporting of negative behaviors.

Lead-time bias (Answer B) is a type of bias affecting screening studies. It occurs when positive test results identify a disease earlier, but do nothing to affect the outcome. In other words, the time the patient dies is the same regardless of whether the screening study is performed, but the screening population appears to live longer because the disease is detected earlier. Lead-time bias overinflates the survival benefits of screening.

Overdiagnosis bias (Answer D) is a type of bias affecting screening studies. It occurs when the screening test identifies a disease that would otherwise have no effect on patient outcome. This includes entities that are technically malignant but may be clinically irrelevant (e.g., low-volume Gleason sum 6 prostate cancer). Overdiagnosis bias overinflates the survival benefits of screening by detecting disease that would not have affected the survival of the patient.

References: Delgado-Rodriguez M, Llorca J. Bias. *J Epidemiol Community Health* 2004; 58:635–641.
Woolfe S, Harris R. The harms of screening. *JAMA* 2012;307:565–566.

6 **Answer A.** The voxel size for a 2D MR image is calculated with the following formula: (FOV/phase encoding steps) × (FOV/frequency encoding steps) × (slice thickness). For a 3D MR image, the final term is (FOV/phase encoding steps in the z-axis) instead of (slice thickness). The interslice gap is not included in the voxel size calculation because the interslice gap contributes no signal and is not part of the image. Working the calculation gives the following:

1. 160 mm/168 phase encoding steps = 0.95 mm
2. 160 mm/228 frequency encoding steps = 0.70 mm
3. 3 mm slice thickness
4. Voxel size = 0.95 mm × 0.70 mm × 3.00 mm

Notice that the in-plane resolution (0.95 mm × 0.70 mm) is generally superior to the through-plane resolution (3.00 mm).

Reference: McRobbie DW, Moore EA, Graves MJ, et al. *MRI: from picture to proton*, 2nd ed. New York: Cambridge University Press, 2007.

7 **Answer D.** The accuracy of CT urography (CTU) is substantially greater than the accuracy of intravenous pyelography (IVP) for the detection of upper tract malignancy. This is the principle explanation for the rapid shift in utilization away from IVP and toward CTU. However, CTU also has costs associated with its use. In particular, it is more expensive, the radiation dose tends to be higher (Answer A), and it detects more incidental findings unrelated to the urinary tract (Answer C). The contrast material dose used for both studies is relatively similar (Answer B). CTU is now considered a routine part of clinical care for the management of patients with hematuria, while IVP is now performed rarely in the United States.

References: Cowan NC, Turney BW, Taylor NJ, et al. Multidetector computed tomography urography for diagnosing upper urinary tract urothelial tumour. *BJU Int* 2007;99:1363–1370.
Gray Sears CL, Ward JF, Sears ST, et al. Prospective comparison of computerized tomography and excretory urography in the initial evaluation of asymptomatic microhematuria. *J Urol* 2002;168:2457–2460.
Jinzaki M, Matsumoto K, Kikuchi E, et al. Comparison of CT urography and excretory urography in the detection and localization of urothelial carcinoma of the upper urinary tract. *AJR Am J Roentgenol* 2011;196:1102–1109.
Silverman SG, Leyendecker JR, Amis ES. What is the current role of CT urography and MR urography in the evaluation of the urinary tract? *Radiology* 2009;250:309–323.

8 Answer D. Epithelioid angiomyolipoma is an aggressive variant of angiomyolipoma that can locally recur and metastasize to other sites. Therefore, in a young patient with no comorbidities, resection (Answer D) is the best next step.

Observation (Answer A) is not appropriate because epithelioid angiomyolipoma is an aggressive tumor. Repeat biopsy (Answer B) is not necessary because a definitive diagnosis has already been established. Embolization (Answer C) is not indicated because the mass is relatively small and resection is the definitive management.

Unfortunately, there are no imaging characteristics that allow a noninvasive diagnosis of epithelioid angiomyolipoma to be made. It can mimic renal cell carcinoma, minimal fat angiomyolipoma, and classic angiomyolipoma with macroscopic fat.

References: Froemming AT, Boland J, Cheville J, et al. Renal epithelioid angiomyolipoma: imaging characteristics in nine cases with radiologic-pathologic correlation and review of the literature. *AJR Am J Roentgenol* 2013;200:W178–W186.
Ryan MJ, Francis IR, Cohan RH, et al. Imaging appearance of renal epithelioid angiomyolipomas. *J Comput Assist Tomogr* 2013;37:957–961.
Varma S, Gupta S, Talwar J, et al. Renal epithelioid angiomyolipoma: a malignant disease. *J Nephrol* 2011;24:18–22.

9 Answer C. Utricle cysts represent benign fluid-filled distention of the prostatic utricle. The prostatic utricle is a Müllerian duct derivative that arises at the level of the verumontanum along the posterior margin of the prostatic urethra between the insertions of the ejaculatory ducts. Utricle cysts are therefore midline structures that do not enhance. Historically, prostatic utricle cysts have had an association with a variety of genitourinary malformations, but when detected by prostate MR in older men, they are generally of no clinical significance.

The structure is not a BPH (benign prostatic hyperplasia) nodule (Answers A and B) because it is posterior to the transition zone. It is not a prostate cancer (Answer D) because it has a classic imaging appearance for a prostatic utricle cyst, and it is markedly hyperintense to background parenchyma on T2-weighted images (i.e., prostate cancer is usually hypointense to background parenchyma on T2-weighted images).

References: Curran S, Akin O, Agildere AM, et al. Endorectal MRI of prostatic and periprostatic cystic lesions and their mimics. *AJR Am J Roentgenol* 2007;188:1373–1379.
Nghiem HT, Kellman GM, Sandberg SA, et al. Cystic lesions of the prostate. *Radiographics* 1990;10:635–650.

10 Answer B. The dominant artifacts propagating across the prostate gland in the image from the question are due to rectal peristalsis. The motion is visible only along the phase-encoding axis because the phase-encoding axis takes much more time to acquire than the frequency-encoding axis. By changing the phase-encoding axis to "left-to-right," motion-related artifacts will also change direction and their effect on the prostate gland will be minimized. An example is below:

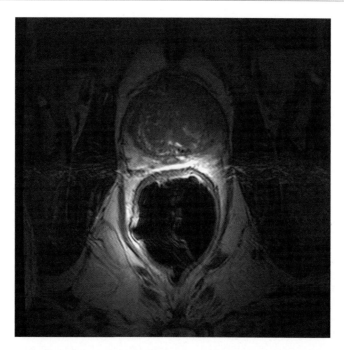

In general, the phase-encoding axis in abdominal and pelvic imaging is set to "anterior-to-posterior" because that is the shortest distance in a rectangular field of view. This enables the scan to be completed in the shortest amount of time (i.e., phase encoding takes time, frequency encoding takes so little time as to be negligible). In certain applications (e.g., prostate MRI), it is advantageous to change the phase-encoding direction to minimize motion-related artifact along the tissues of interest. Rectal peristalsis is exacerbated by rectal distention and use of an endorectal coil, and minimized by use of antiperistaltic agents (e.g., glucagon).

References: Hadgire SS, Eberhardt SC, Borczuk R, et al. Interpretation and reporting multiparametric prostate MRI: a primer for residents and novices. *Abdom Imaging* 2014. doi: 10/1007/s00261-014-0097-x

McRobbie DW, Moore EA, Graves MJ, et al. *MRI: from picture to proton*, 2nd ed. New York: Cambridge University Press, 2007.

11 **Answer B.** Renal angiomyolipoma (AML) is a benign renal mass that, when large, has a propensity toward spontaneous hemorrhage. Asymptomatic renal AMLs ≥4 cm and symptomatic AMLs regardless of size are considered for embolization.

The noninvasive diagnosis of a renal AML is based on the detection of macroscopic fat within a solid renal mass. Even small quantities of fat are diagnostic with rare exception (e.g., osseous metaplasia in a renal cell carcinoma [suspected when the fat-containing mass is also calcified or shows aggressive growth]). Some renal AMLs do not contain macroscopic fat and are termed "minimal fat AMLs." Like typical AMLs, "minimal fat AMLs" are also benign, but they cannot be easily distinguished from renal cell carcinoma on imaging. Therefore, they are most often diagnosed by biopsy or by resection for presumed renal cell carcinoma.

References: Davenport MS, Neville AM, Ellis JH, et al. Diagnosis of renal angiomyolipoma with Hounsfield unit thresholds: effect of size of region of interest and nephrographic phase imaging. *Radiology* 2011;260:158–165.

Rimon U, Duvdevani M, Garniek A, et al. Ethanol and polyvinyl alcohol mixture for transcatheter embolization of renal angiomyolipoma. *AJR Am J Roentgenol* 2006;187:762–768.

Soulen MC, Faykus MH, Shlansky-Goldberg RD, et al. Elective embolization for prevention of hemorrhage from renal angiomyolipomas. *J Vasc Interv Radiol* 1994;5:587–591.

12 **Answer A.**   The images demonstrate a moderate volume of simple-appearing fluid in the left perinephric space, mild left collecting system dilation, and a calculus in the left proximal ureter. This constellation of findings is compatible with a ruptured fornix and urinoma formation secondary to calculus-related urinary tract obstruction. Abscess (Answer B) and lymphoma (Answer D) are unlikely given the other imaging findings (i.e., obstructing stone). Additionally, the perinephric abnormality is fluid attenuation without other complicating features.

The fornix is the weakest point of the collecting system. Paired fornices of each calyx straddle the renal medulla. Pressurized states (e.g., obstruction) can lead to forniceal rupture and collecting system decompression, with leakage of urine into the perinephric space. Forniceal rupture can be distinguished from reactive perirenal edema (Answer C) by the volume of fluid in the perinephric space; reactive edema is typically small volume and urine from forniceal rupture is typically moderate or greater volume. Forniceal rupture is usually a self-limited abnormality that responds to conservative management if the obstruction can be relieved. If the obstruction is ongoing, ureteric stenting is performed to divert the urine away from the leak.

References: Doehn C, Fiola L, Peter M, et al. Outcome analysis of fornix ruptures in 162 consecutive patients. *J Endourol* 2010;24:1869–1873.
Dunnick NR, Sandler CM, Newhouse JH. *Textbook of Uroradiology*, 5th ed. Philadelphia: Lippincott Williams & Wilkins, 2012.
Kalafatis P, Zougkas K, Petas A. Primary ureteroscopic treatment for obstructive ureteral stone-causing fornix rupture. *Int J Urol* 2004;11:1058–1064.

13 **Answer B.**   The prophylactic measure that has the most consistent evidence supporting its use for the prevention of contrast-induced acute kidney injury ("CIN") is volume expansion with isotonic fluids (Answer B, 0.9% NaCl is "normal saline"). D5 0.45% NaCl (Answer A, "half-normal saline" with 5% dextrose) is a hypotonic solution that is less adept at volume expansion. Studies investigating N-acetylcysteine (Answer C) and sodium bicarbonate (Answer D) for the prevention of contrast-induced acute kidney injury have had mixed and inconclusive results.

References: American College of Radiology Committee on Drugs and Contrast Media. *Manual on Contrast Media*, 9th ed. Reston, VA: American College of Radiology, 2013.
McCullough PA. Contrast-induced acute kidney injury. *J Am Coll Cardiol* 2008;51:1419–1428.

14 **Answer A.**   The most common complication of percutaneous renal mass biopsy is hemorrhage. In fact, the majority of patients will experience some degree of hemorrhage, but this is typically self-limiting and of no clinical relevance. Persistent bleeding through the cannula often can be controlled percutaneously with stylet placement and/or use of a hemostatic slurry. Rarely, a pseudoaneurysm can develop that requires embolization.

Other complications of percutaneous renal mass biopsy are rare (e.g., needle track seeding [Answer B], infection [Answer C], pneumothorax [Answer D], collecting system obstruction [Answer E, usually from clot formation], damage to adjacent viscera [Answer F]).

References: Silverman SG, Gan YU, Mortele KJ, et al. Renal masses in the adult patient: the role of percutaneous biopsy. *Radiology* 2006;240:6–22.
Uppot RN, Harisinghani MG, Gervais DA. Imaging-guided percutaneous renal biopsy: rationale and approach. *AJR Am J Roentgenol* 2010;194:1443–1449.

15 **Answer E.**   The best approach is Angle C using a 1-cm throw length. Unlike the liver, in which it is often prudent to include normal parenchyma between the capsular entry site and the target, it is usually best with renal mass biopsies to enter the mass transgressing as little normal parenchyma as possible (or if possible, none at all). The bleeding risk of renal mass biopsy goes up with the length of normal parenchymal transgression and the depth of entry into the hilum. Using a throw length of the same size as the mass (2.0 cm) along Angle C (Answer F) would very likely breach the far wall of the mass and risk damage to the renal hilum.

References: Caoili EM, Davenport MS. Role of percutaneous needle biopsy for renal masses. *Semin Intervent Radiol* 2014;31:20–26.

Silverman SG, Gan YU, Mortele KJ, et al. Renal masses in the adult patient: the role of percutaneous biopsy. *Radiology* 2006;240:6–22.

16 **Answer A.** The signal abnormality in the retroperitoneum and mesentery most likely represents incomplete fat saturation. Fat saturation can be obtained using a variety of techniques, each with its own advantages and limitations. In this case, the fat saturation on the images is obviously heterogeneous. Compare the degree of fat saturation in the mesentery with that in the subcutaneous tissues. This suggests that the sequence was performed using a spectral fat suppression technique. With this technique, fat protons are selectively targeted based on their resonance frequency. This is feasible because fat and water protons precess at different frequencies. However, precession frequency is dependent on magnetic field strength (i.e., Larmor frequency). If the magnetic field is inhomogeneous, different regions of the body will experience different magnetic field strengths, causing the fat protons in those regions to precess at different frequencies than the magnet expects. When the spectral fat suppression pulse is applied, the fat in affected regions will not be precessing at the expected frequency and will not be suppressed.

Answer B (inappropriate inversion time) refers to another method of fat saturation that is based on the T1 time of fat. This method employs a 180-degree inversion RF pulse to null the signal from fat. As the fat protons recover from the 180-degree inversion RF pulse across the null point (i.e., zero signal), the excitation RF pulse is applied, resulting in zero signal contribution from fat. Such inversion recovery techniques (e.g., STIR) tend to provide more homogeneous fat saturation than spectral fat suppression techniques because they are not as affected by magnetic field inhomogeneity (T1 times are fixed properties of tissue and not dependent on the local magnetic field strength). However, unlike spectral fat saturation, which selectively targets the precession frequency of fat, inversion recovery techniques affect all tissues with a similar T1 time as fat. Therefore, inversion recovery techniques are not typically useful for contrast-enhanced sequences (due to the unpredictable T1-shortening effects of gadolinium-based contrast media).

Retroperitoneal fibrosis (Answer C) and lymphoma (Answer D) are not the best choices because the signal abnormality anterior to the iliac bifurcation does not distort the adjacent anatomy despite crossing tissue planes (both intraperitoneal and retroperitoneal fat are affected).

References: Delfaut EM, Beltran J, Johnson G, et al. Fat suppression in MR imaging: techniques and pitfalls. *Radiographics* 1999;19:373–382.

McRobbie DW, Moore EA, Graves MJ, et al. *MRI: from picture to proton*, 2nd ed. New York: Cambridge University Press, 2007.

17 **Answer A.** Increasing size of sclerotic bone metastases on CT imaging is nonspecific; it can represent disease progression (i.e., growing metastases) or response to therapy (i.e., so-called CT flare phenomenon). Therefore, Tc-99m MDP bone scintigraphy is used instead of CT to monitor treatment response in most patients with sclerotic osseous metastases. Notice that the Tc-99m MDP bone scintigraphy studies performed in the same patient show minimal change between the two study dates, in contradistinction to the CT findings.

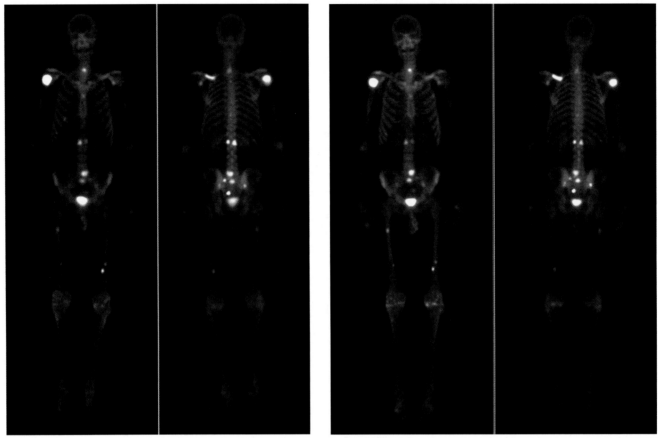

Nine months ago   *Index study*

In general, CT is insensitive for bone metastases and is ineffective at monitoring treatment response for sclerotic lesions. Lytic bone lesions can be more reliably measured and followed on CT because the lytic component often represents a soft tissue mass with visible margins. RECIST 1.1 criteria reflect this by allowing lytic bone lesions ≥10 mm to be considered target lesions and disallowing sclerotic bone lesions (regardless of size) from being considered target lesions.

References: Costelloe CM, Chuang HH, Madewell JE, et al. Cancer response criteria and bone metastases: RECIST 1.1, MDA, and PERCIST. *J Cancer* 2010;1:80–92.
Messiou C, Cook G, Reid AH, et al. The CT flare response of metastatic bone disease in prostate cancer. *Acta Radiol* 2011;52:557–561.

18 **Answer D.** In men over the age of 50, testicular lymphoma (Answer D) is more common than seminomatous (Answer A) and nonseminomatous (Answer B) germ cell malignancies. Testicular lymphoma is usually an aggressive diffuse large B-cell lymphoma (>75%) with a poor prognosis and a high rate of extranodal recurrence, particularly in the contralateral testicle and central nervous system. Treatment usually consists of ipsilateral orchiectomy, radiation to the contralateral testicle, and systemic therapy.

References: Fonseca R, Habermann TM, Colgan JP, et al. Testicular lymphoma is associated with a high incidence of extranodal recurrence. *Cancer* 2000;88:154–161.
Gundrum JD, Mathiason MA, Moore DB, et al. Primary testicular diffuse large B-cell lymphoma: a population-based study on the incidence, natural history, and survival comparison with primary nodal counterpart before and after the introduction of Rituximab. *J Clin Oncol* 2009;27:5227–5232.
Huyghe E, Matsuda T, Thonneau P. Increasing incidence of testicular cancer worldwide: a review. *J Urol* 2003;170:5–11.

19 **Answer B.** The 3D-rendered image demonstrates a horseshoe kidney, which is a congenital anomaly resulting from fusion of the lower poles of the kidneys. This condition predisposes affected patients to blunt injury of the horseshoe isthmus (i.e., the tissue connecting the lower poles), stone formation, urinary tract infection, and other congenital anomalies. Many patients with a horseshoe kidney have aberrant and accessory renal vasculature.

Crossed-fused ectopia (Answer A) is a congenital fusion anomaly in which the kidneys are on the same side of the retroperitoneum ("crossed"). Crossed-fused ectopia is associated with similar complications as horseshoe kidney. Pelvic kidney (Answer C) is a congenital anomaly in which there is an inferiorly located kidney that during embryologic development failed to ascend into the upper retroperitoneum. In patients with a pelvic kidney, there will usually be a vacant ipsilateral renal fossa. Congenital duplication (Answer D) is a congenital anomaly in which there are two collecting systems arising from a single kidney.

References: Dunnick NR, Sandler CM, Newhouse JH. *Textbook of uroradiology*, 5th ed. Philadelphia: Lippincott Williams & Wilkins, 2012.
Dyer RB, Chen MY, Zagoria RJ. Classic signs in uroradiology. *Radiographics* 2004;24:S247–S280.

20 **Answer D.** The images demonstrate enlarged multifollicular ovaries with ascites suggestive of ovarian hyperstimulation syndrome. Ovarian hyperstimulation syndrome is an iatrogenic complication of ovulation induction characterized by bilateral ovary enlargement (i.e., ovarian edema), numerous ovarian cysts, ascites, and pelvic pain. Although the majority of patients undergoing ovulation induction (65%) develop a mild form of this syndrome, 0.5% to 5% develops a severe and potentially life-threatening version that requires hospitalization. Third spacing and capillary leak result in peritoneal and pleural exudates, volume depletion, and hemoconcentration; thromboembolic complications can be deadly. Ovarian hyperstimulation syndrome also predisposes to ovarian torsion, which can be difficult to diagnose in this setting because the ovaries are already enlarged and edematous.

The imaging findings are not normal (Answer C) because normal ovaries are not this large and would have smaller follicles. Bilateral primary ovarian neoplasms (Answer A) would be unusual in a patient of this age. Polycystic ovary syndrome (PCOS, Answer B) can be associated with enlarged multicystic ovaries, but the degree of ovarian enlargement and the presence of ascites make PCOS much less likely.

References: Delvigne A, Rozenberg S. Epidemiology and prevention of ovarian hyperstimulation syndrome (OHSS): a review. *Hum Reprod Update* 2002;8:559–577.
Pedrosa I, Zeikus EA, Levine D, et al. MR imaging of acute right lower quadrant pain in pregnant and nonpregnant patients. *Radiographics* 2007;27:721–743.

21 **Answer D.** The images demonstrate a lobular nonaggressive mass in the left posterior pararenal space containing numerous tubular components and small calcifications that resemble phleboliths. The tissue planes are respected and the mass does not extend into adjacent compartments. The most likely diagnosis is a venolymphatic malformation (Answer D).

Although lymphoma (Answer A) and sarcoma (Answer B) are common causes of a large retroperitoneal mass, it would be unusual for these entities to have phleboliths or a tubular configuration. Angiomyolipoma (Answer C) is not the best answer because the mass lacks macroscopic fat, contains calcifications, and is separate from the kidney. Extra-renal angiomyolipoma is very rare, and angiomyolipomas do not usually contain calcifications. The fat within the mass is likely due to interdigitated normal retroperitoneal fat. A foreign body

(Answer E) likely would be surrounded by chronic inflammation, but the fat surrounding this mass is normal.

References: Burrows PE. Vascular malformations involving the female pelvis. *Semin Intervent Radiol* 2008;25:347–360.

Shanbhogue AK, Fasih N, Macdonald DB, et al. Uncommon primary pelvic retroperitoneal masses in adults: a pattern-based approach. *Radiographics* 2012;32:795–817.

22   Answer C.   The images demonstrate a T1-hyperintense mass within the left ovary on unenhanced images. It does not lose signal intensity on the fat-suppressed T1-weighted image, indicating that it is not composed of fat (i.e., it is not a dermoid). Therefore, the primary differential considerations are a hemorrhagic cyst or an endometrioma. Both are hyperintense to background tissue on T1-weighted images due to the presence of hemorrhage. In this case, endometrioma is the most likely diagnosis because of the hypointense appearance on the T2-weighted image ("T2-shading"). However, T2-shading is not specific for endometrioma; hemorrhagic cysts and hemorrhagic neoplasms can also have "T2 shading."

The other possible answers listed in the question also shorten T1 but are not likely explanations in this case. A short list of things that shorten T1 includes: (1) fat, (2) protein, (3) hemorrhage, (4) melanin, (5) gadolinium-containing contrast material, (6) time-of-flight flow artifact, and (7) calcium.

References: Corwin MT, Gerscovich EO, Lamba R, et al. Differentiation of ovarian endometriomas from hemorrhagic cysts at MR imaging: utility of the T2 dark spot sign. *Radiology* 2014;271:126–132.

Lee SI. Radiological reasoning: imaging characterization of bilateral adnexal masses. *AJR Am J Roentgenol* 2006;187:S460–S466.

23   Answer C.   The images demonstrate a large necrotic rounded mass centered about the female urethra (identified by the presence of a Foley catheter). It is sometimes difficult to localize the origin of a large mass, but in this case, of the likely candidates for a large pelvic mass, a urethral neoplasm is most likely.

A cervical cancer (Answer A) is unlikely because the nearby cervix is uninvolved (see the sagittal T2w image). The vagina is contacted by the mass (Answer B), but the epicenter of the mass is the urethra. Likewise, the mass contacts the bladder (Answer D), but the mass is largely below the level of the bladder neck. Prostate cancer (Answer E) is not a reasonable diagnostic consideration in this female patient.

References: Del Gaizo A, Silva AC, Lam-Himlin DM, et al. Magnetic resonance imaging of solid urethral and peri-urethral lesions. *Insights Imaging* 2013;4:461–469.

Fisher M, Hricak H, Reinhold C, et al. Female urethral carcinoma: MRI staging. *AJR Am J Roentgenol* 1985;144:603–604.

Grivas PD, Davenport M, Montie JE, et al. Urethral cancer. *Hematol Oncol Clin North Am* 2012;26:1291–1314.

24   Answer B.   It is rare for a renal cell carcinoma smaller than 3 cm to metastasize. In addition, most renal cell carcinomas are slow growing, with a mean growth rate of approximately 3 mm per year. These facts have contributed to a change in thinking regarding the management of small solid renal masses. Percutaneous biopsy and active surveillance are now receiving greater attention. Many elderly patients with a small solid renal mass will die of causes unrelated to their renal mass, even if that mass does prove to be malignant.

References: Chawla SN, Crispen PL, Hanlon AL, et al. The natural history of observed enhancing renal masses: meta-analysis and review of the world literature. *J Urol* 2006;175:425–431.

Thompson RH, Hill JR, Babeyev Y, et al. Metastatic renal cell carcinoma risk according to tumor size. *J Urol* 2009;182:41–45.

25 **Answer A.** Estimated glomerular filtration rate (eGFR) is unreliable in the setting of acute kidney injury; therefore, the listed eGFR for the patient in Answer A is not accurate. The two key risk factors for nephrogenic systemic fibrosis (NSF) are (1) eGFR <30 mL/min/1.73 m^2 and (2) acute kidney injury. Among patients with one or both of these conditions, gadolinium-based contrast media are relatively or absolutely contraindicated; those on dialysis and those receiving a "high-risk" agent are at greatest risk. "High-risk" agents as defined by the FDA and ACR include: (1) gadodiamide [Omniscan], (2) gadoversetamide [OptiMARK], and (3) gadopentetate dimeglumine [Magnevist].

Risk factors for chronic kidney disease (e.g., Answers B, C, D) in the absence of acute kidney injury or an eGFR <30 mL/min/1.73 m^2 have not been associated independently with NSF.

References: ACR Committee on Drugs and Contrast Media. *ACR Manual on Contrast Media* v.9. Reston, VA: American College of Radiology, 2013.
U.S. Food and Drug Administration. Information for healthcare professionals: Gadolinium-based contrast agents for magnetic resonance imaging. Accessed 4, 2014. http://www.fda.gov/drugs/drugsafety/postmarketdrugsafetyinformationforpatientsandproviders/ucm142884.htm

26 **Answer B.** Of the listed options, a 20% decrease in kVp will result in the greatest radiation dose reduction. This is because kVp has an exponential relationship with dose, while mA (Answer A), pitch (Answer C), and z-axis coverage (Answer D) have a linear relationship. Reducing the pitch (Answer C) will increase the dose to the patient, not decrease it.

References: Costello JE, Cecava ND, Tucker JE, et al. CT radiation dose: current controversies and dose reduction strategies. *AJR Am J Roentgenol* 2013;201:1283–1290.
Maldjian PD, Goldman AR. Reducing radiation dose in body CT: a primer on dose metrics and key CT technical parameters. *AJR Am J Roentgenol* 2013;200:741–747.
McCollough CH, Primak AN, Christner J. Strategies for reducing radiation dose in CT. *Radiol Clin N Am* 2009;47:27–40.

27 **Answer A.** A water-attenuation oval-shaped mass in the retrocrural space is consistent with a distended cisterna chyli, which is a normal variant. The cisterna chyli is a lymphatic reservoir that receives lymph from the lumbar region and intestines before ascending into the thorax as the thoracic duct. It is commonly visible on cross-sectional imaging. No further imaging or work-up is required. The importance of this finding is differentiating it from solid tissue, such as an enlarged retrocrural lymph node (Answers B and C) or a posterior mediastinal mass (Answers D and E). In both cases (an enlarged lymph node or a mediastinal mass), the attenuation of the abnormality typically would be >20 Hounsfield Units.

References: Pinto PS, Sirlin CB, Andrade-Barreto OA, et al. Cisterna chyli at routine abdominal imaging: a normal anatomic structure in the retrocrural space. *Radiographics* 2004;24:809–817.
Restrepo CS, Eraso A, Ocazionez D, et al. The diaphragmatic crura and retrocrural space: normal imaging appearance, variants, and pathologic conditions. *Radiographics* 2008;28:1289–1305.

28 **Answer A.** The patient is suffering from iatrogenic opioid-induced respiratory depression. The best next step is to administer 0.2 mg naloxone IV over 30 seconds, with redosing every 2 to 3 minutes until the patient's respiratory rate is >10.

Naloxone is the reversal agent for opioids (e.g., fentanyl), and flumazenil is the reversal agent for benzodiazepines (e.g., midazolam). The initial adult dose for the treatment of oversedation is 0.2 mg for naloxone (may repeat every

2 to 3 minutes) and 0.1 to 0.2 mg for flumazenil (may repeat every minute, maximum dose is 1 mg). The dose for both agents is lower for the treatment of oversedation compared to the treatment of a suspected overdose. Additionally, flumazenil is dosed more carefully because it can induce seizures in patients who are benzodiazepine dependent and/or who have a seizure history. Naloxone can be dosed more liberally, although patients who are opioid dependent can experience significant pain after its use.

References: ASA Task Force on Sedation and Analgesia by Non-Anesthesiologists. Practice guidelines for sedation and analgesia by non-anesthesiologists. *Anesthesiology* 2002;96:1004–1017.
Johnson S. Sedation and analgesia in the performance of interventional procedures. *Semin Intervent Radiol* 2010;27:368–373.
Martin ML, Lennox PH. Sedation and analgesia in the interventional radiology department. *J Vasc Interv Radiol* 2003;14:1119–1128.

29 **Answer C.** A renal biopsy is considered by the Society of International Radiology (SIR) to be a procedure with a "significant risk" of bleeding; therefore, the recommended INR target for an elective renal biopsy is <1.5.

The SIR released consensus guidelines in 2012 for the periprocedural management of coagulation status and hemostasis risk in patients subjected to percutaneous image-guided procedures. All image-guided percutaneous procedures were stratified into three general categories of risk: (1) low bleeding risk (e.g., thoracentesis, catheter exchange), (2) moderate bleeding risk (e.g., core liver biopsy, drain placement), and (3) significant bleeding risk (e.g., core renal biopsy, TIPS placement). General management recommendations were provided for each category, with the caveat that clinical factors may influence decision making (e.g., an emergent procedure, a patient with multiple comorbidities, use of hemostatic agents).

The SIR management recommendations for each category of risk are shown below:

Parameter	Low Risk	Moderate Risk	Significant Risk
INR	Correct to <2.0	Correct to <1.5	Correct to <1.5
aPTT	No consensus	No consensus	Stop/reverse heparin if >1.5× control
Platelets	Transfuse if <50,000	Transfuse if <50,000	Transfuse if <50,000
Clopidogrel	Hold 5 days prior	Hold 5 days prior	Hold 5 days prior
Aspirin	Do not hold	Do not hold	Hold 5 days prior
Fractionated heparin	Hold one dose prior	Hold one dose prior	Hold 24 hours or two doses prior

Reference: Patel IJ, Davidson JC, Nikolic B, et al. Consensus guidelines for periprocedural management of coagulation status and hemostasis risk in percutaneous image-guided interventions. *J Vasc Interv Radiol* 2012;23:727–736.

30 **Answer B.**   The image demonstrates a circumscribed cyst arising from the left seminal vesicle (note the "claw" sign along the medial and lateral margins) consistent with a seminal vesicle cyst. This is most commonly a congenital abnormality that is associated with ipsilateral renal agenesis or dysgenesis in 60% to 70% of cases. Other associations of seminal vesicle cysts include (1) vas deferens agenesis, (2) ectopic ureteral insertion, and (3) autosomal dominant polycystic kidney disease [ADPKD]. When present in ADPKD, the seminal vesicle cysts are commonly bilateral.

Chronic urinary retention (Answer A) is associated with bladder diverticula, which can resemble perivesical cystic lesions. In this case, the "claw" of soft tissue along the medial and lateral margins of the cyst joining it with the seminal vesicle is helpful for differentiation. Seminal vesicle cysts can be acquired after birth, but there is not a clear association with *Chlamydia trachomatis* infection (Answer C). Prostate cancer can invade the seminal vesicles (Answer D), but that usually presents as a solid mass, not a cystic structure, and prostate cancer would be rare in a 20-year-old patient.

References: Kim B, Kawashima A, Ryu JA, et al. Imaging of the seminal vesicle and vas deferens. *Radiographics* 2009;29:1105–1121.

Shebel HM, Farg HM, Kolokythas O, et al. Cysts of the lower male genitourinary tract: embryologic and anatomic considerations and differential diagnosis. *Radiographics* 2013;33:1125–1143.